INTERVENTIONAL CARDIOLOGY CLINICS

www.interventional.theclinics.com

Editor-in-Chief

MATTHEW J. PRICE

Controversies in the Management of STEMI

October 2016 • Volume 5 • Number 4

Editor

TIMOTHY D. HENRY

ELSEVIER

1600 John F. Kennedy Boulevard • Suite 1800 • Philadelphia, Pennsylvania, 19103-2899

http://www.theclinics.com

INTERVENTIONAL CARDIOLOGY CLINICS Volume 5, Number 4
October 2016 ISSN 2211-7458, ISBN-13: 978-0-323-46317-1

Editor: Lauren Boyle
Developmental Editor: Susan Showalter

Interventional Cardiology Clinics (ISSN 2211-7458) is published quarterly by Elsevier Inc., 360 Park Avenue South, New York, NY 10010-1710. Months of issue are January, April, July, and October. Subscription prices are USD 195 per year for US individuals, USD 436 for US institutions, USD 100 per year for US students, USD 195 per year for Canadian individuals, USD 520 for Canadian institutions, USD 150 per year for Canadian students, USD 295 per year for international individuals, USD 520 for international institutions, and USD 150 per year for international students. To receive student/resident rate, orders must be accompanied by name of affiliated institution, date of term, and the *signature* of program/residency coordinator on institution letterhead. Orders will be billed at individual rate until proof of status is received. Foreign air speed delivery is included in all *Clinics* subscription prices. All prices are subject to change without notice. **POSTMASTER:** Send address changes to *Interventional Cardiology Clinics*, Elsevier Health Sciences Division, Subscription Customer Service, 3251 Riverport Lane, Maryland Heights, MO 63043. **Customer Service: Telephone: 1-800-654-2452** (U.S. and Canada); **1-314-447-8871** (outside U.S. and Canada). **Fax: 1-314-447-8029. E-mail: journalscustomerservice-usa@elsevier.com (for print support); journalsonlinesupport-usa@elsevier.com (for online support).**

Reprints. For copies of 100 or more of articles in this publication, please contact the Commercial Reprints Department, Elsevier Inc., 360 Park Avenue South, New York, NY 10010-1710. Tel.: 212-633-3874; Fax: 212-633-3820; E-mail: reprints@elsevier.com.

CONTRIBUTORS

EDITOR-IN-CHIEF

MATTHEW J. PRICE, MD
Assistant Professor, Scripps Translational
Science Institute; Director of the Cardiac
Catheterization Laboratory, Scripps Green
Hospital, La Jolla, California

EDITOR

TIMOTHY D. HENRY, MD
Director, Division of Cardiology; Professor,
Department of Medicine, Cedars-Sinai
Medical Center, Los Angeles, California

AUTHORS

USMAN BABER, MD, MS
Assistant Professor of Medicine, Department
of Cardiology, The Mount Sinai Hospital,
New York, New York

**AMERJEET S. BANNING, BSc(Hons),
MB BS, MRCP**
Clinical Research Fellow, Leicester
Cardiovascular Biomedical Research Unit,
Department of Cardiovascular Sciences, The
National Institute of Health Research (NIHR),
University Hospitals of Leicester National
Health Service (NHS) Trust, Glenfield Hospital,
University of Leicester, Leicester, United
Kingdom

TAYLOR C. BAZEMORE, MD
Department of Internal Medicine, Duke
University Medical Center, Durham,
North Carolina

FREDY BOJANINI, MD
Lumen Foundation, Miami, Florida

ROBERTO BOTELHO, MD, PhD
Lumen Foundation, Miami, Florida

JAMIL CADE, MD
Lumen Foundation, Miami, Florida

WARREN J. CANTOR, MD
Associate Professor of Medicine, Division of
Cardiology, Southlake Regional Health
Center, Newmarket, Ontario, Canada;
Department of Medicine, University of
Toronto, Toronto, Ontario, Canada

MARCO CASTILLO, MD
Lumen Foundation, Miami, Florida

JUAN CORAL, MD
Lumen Foundation, Miami, Florida

DAVID COX, MD, FSCAI, FACC
Interventional Cardiologist, Associate Director
of Cardiac Catheterization Laboratory;
Director of Cardiovascular Research,
Department of Cardiology, Lehigh Valley
Heath Network, Allentown, Pennsylvania

XUMING DAI, MD, PhD
Division of Cardiology, University of North
Carolina at Chapel Hill, Chapel Hill, North
Carolina

STAVROS G. DRAKOS, MD, PhD
Director of Cardiac Mechanical Support;
Associate Professor of Medicine, Division of
Cardiovascular Medicine, University of Utah
School of Medicine, Salt Lake City, Utah

ALEXANDRA FERRÉ, MD
Lumen Foundation, Miami, Florida

CHRISTOPHER B. FORDYCE, MD, MHS, MSc
Duke Clinical Research Institute, Durham, North Carolina

ROSS F. GARBERICH, MS
Minneapolis Heart Institute Foundation, Abbott Northwestern Hospital, Minneapolis, Minnesota

J. LEE GARVEY, MD
Professor, Department of Emergency Medicine, Carolinas Medical Center, Charlotte, North Carolina

ANTHONY H. GERSHLICK, BSc, MB BS, FRCP
Professor of Interventional Cardiology, Leicester Cardiovascular Biomedical Research Unit, Department of Cardiovascular Sciences, The National Institute of Health Research (NIHR), University Hospitals of Leicester National Health Service (NHS) Trust, Glenfield Hospital, University of Leicester, Leicester, United Kingdom

CHRISTOPHER B. GRANGER, MD
Duke Clinical Research Institute, Durham, North Carolina

RAFAEL HARARI, MD
Cardiology Fellow, Department of Cardiology, The Mount Sinai Hospital, New York, New York

TIMOTHY D. HENRY, MD
Director, Division of Cardiology; Professor, Department of Medicine, Cedars-Sinai Medical Center, Los Angeles, California

BRIAN E. JASKI, MD
San Diego Cardiac Center, Sharp Healthcare, San Diego, California

BYUNG-SOO KO, MD
Interventional Cardiology Fellow, Division of Cardiovascular Medicine, University of Utah School of Medicine, Salt Lake City, Utah

DAVID C. LANGE, MD
Division of Cardiology, Cedars-Sinai Heart Institute, Los Angeles, California

ALEXANDRA J. LANSKY, MD
Professor of Medicine, Director, Heart and Vascular Clinical Research Program, Yale University School of Medicine, New Haven, Connecticut

DAVID M. LARSON, MD
Associate Clinical Professor, University of Minnesota Medical School, Minneapolis Heart Institute Foundation, Abbott Northwestern Hospital, Minneapolis, Minnesota; Division of Cardiology, Ridgeview Medical Center, Waconia, Minnesota

MICHEL R. LE MAY, MD
Division of Cardiology, University of Ottawa Heart Institute, Ottawa, Canada

MICHAEL C. McDANIEL, MD
Director, Cardiac Catheterization Laboratory, Assistant Professor of Medicine, Division of Cardiology, Grady Memorial Hospital, Emory University School of Medicine, Atlanta, Georgia

PETER McKAVANAGH, MD, PhD
Division of Cardiology, St Michael's Hospital, Toronto, Ontario, Canada

SAMEER MEHTA, MD
Lumen Foundation, Miami, Florida

VIVIAN G. NG, MD
Yale University School of Medicine, New Haven, Connecticut

DANIELA PARRA, MD
Lumen Foundation, Miami, Florida

MARCO PERIN, MD
Lumen Foundation, Miami, Florida

S. TANVEER RAB, MD
Associate Professor of Medicine, Division of Cardiology/Interventional Cardiology, Emory University Hospital, Emory University School of Medicine, Atlanta, Georgia

SUNIL V. RAO, MD
Division of Cardiology, Department of Internal Medicine, Duke University Medical Center; Department of Cardiology, Durham VA Medical Center, Durham, North Carolina

IVAN C. ROKOS, MD
Associate Clinical Professor, Department of
Emergency Medicine, University of California,
Los Angeles, Los Angeles, California

JUAN RUSSO, MD
Division of Cardiology, University of Ottawa
Heart Institute, Ottawa, Canada

NEERAJ SHAH, MD, MPH
Cardiology Fellow, Department of Cardiology,
Lehigh Valley Heath Network, Allentown,
Pennsylvania

RASHMEE U. SHAH, MD, MS
Assistant Professor, Division of Cardiovascular
Medicine, University of Utah School of
Medicine, Salt Lake City, Utah

RAHUL P. SHARMA, MD
Cedars-Sinai Heart Institute, Los Angeles,
California

SIDNEY C. SMITH Jr, MD
Division of Cardiology, University of North
Carolina at Chapel Hill, Chapel Hill,
North Carolina

DION STUB, MD, PhD
Alfred and Western Hospital, Monash
University, Baker IDI Heart and Diabetes
Institute, Melbourne, Victoria, Australia

FREDERICK G.P. WELT, MD, MS
Associate Chief of Cardiology; Professor of
Medicine, Division of Cardiovascular
Medicine, University of Utah School of
Medicine, Salt Lake City, Utah

PABLO YÉPEZ, MD
Lumen Foundation, Miami, Florida

CONTENTS

Current guidelines recommend that communities create and maintain a regional system of ST-segment elevation myocardial infarction (STEMI) care that includes assessment and continuous quality improvement of emergency medical services and hospital-based activities. Availability and timely access is a challenge in many areas of the United States. This article reviews clinical trial data supporting the use of primary percutaneous coronary intervention as the optimal reperfusion strategy, and fibrinolysis as an option when this is not possible. It then describes the outcomes and benefits of implementing regional systems of STEMI care, and discusses ongoing challenges for STEMI system implementation, including inadequate data collection and feedback, and hospital and physician competition.

In the modern ST-elevation myocardial infarction (STEMI) system, the use of electrocardiogram by emergency medical services (EMS) personnel and the option to bypass emergency departments on route to a PCI-capable hospital is of particular importance. Through training and a standardized referral process, EMS personnel can now accurately diagnose and refer STEMI patients directly to the catheterization laboratory of a percutaneous coronary intervention–capable hospital. Regional STEMI models have been implemented successfully across North America, resulting in palpable reductions in door-to-balloon time, morbidity, and mortality.

Primary percutaneous coronary intervention (PCI) is the preferred reperfusion strategy for ST elevation myocardial infarction (STEMI). However, only one-third of hospitals in the US have PCI availability 24/7. For non-PCI hospitals, transfer remains the optimal strategy. For expected delays of greater than 120 minutes, a pharmacoinvasive strategy is recommended. In patients with evidence of failed reperfusion or hemodynamic instability, immediate rescue PCI should be performed. All other patients should undergo routine cardiac catheterization and PCI within 24 hours after fibrinolysis. A pharmacoinvasive strategy is best implemented within an organized regional STEMI system with prospective standardized transfer protocols.

First-medical-contact-to-device (FMC2D) times have improved over the past decade, as have clinical outcomes for patients presenting with ST-elevation myocardial infarction (STEMI). However, with improvements in FMC2D times, false activation of the cardiac catheterization laboratory (CCL) has become a challenging problem. The authors define false activation as any patient who does not warrant emergent coronary angiography for STEMI. In addition to clinical outcome measures for these patients, STEMI systems should collect data regarding the total number of CCL activations, the total number of emergency coronary angiograms, and the number revascularization procedures performed.

Timely reperfusion therapy reduces complications and improves survival in ST elevation myocardial infarction (STEMI). An effective chain of survival has been established for STEMIs occur in the community (outpatient STEMI). Recent studies have identified a subgroup of patients who develop STEMI while hospitalized for primary conditions, often not directly related to coronary artery disease (in-hospital STEMI or inpatient STEMI). This article summarizes current understanding of patient demographics, clinical characteristics, care delivery system and outcomes of in-hospital STEMI, comparing with outpatient STEMI. We also identified opportunities for quality improvement and proposed strategies and future directions to improve care for these patients.

Cardiovascular disease is the leading cause of death worldwide. Case-fatality rates for myocardial infarction (MI) in the United States have decreased over the past decades, in large part due to advances in the treatment of acute MI and secondary preventive therapy after MI. Antiplatelet therapy remains the cornerstone of treatment of MI. This article reviews the current state of antiplatelet therapy in ST-segment elevation MI.

Anticoagulation is essential in patients with ST elevation myocardial infarction (STEMI) to prevent further thrombosis and to maintain patency of the infarct-related artery after reperfusion. The various anticoagulant medications available for use in patients with STEMI include unfractionated heparin (UFH), low-molecular-weight heparin, fondaparinux, and bivalirudin, a direct thrombin inhibitor. The authors review the current anticoagulation strategies for patients with STEMI undergoing primary percutaneous coronary intervention (PCI), fibrinolysis, or no reperfusion. The authors present the latest evidence and controversies on this topic, with a focus on bivalirudin versus UFH in the setting of primary PCI for STEMI.

This article discusses the controversies surrounding the use of transradial versus transfemoral approaches in the management of patients with ST-segment elevation myocardial infarction, beginning with a review of the benefits of transradial percutaneous coronary intervention (PCI) in this population. The unanswered questions about the mechanism underlying the mortality benefit of transradial PCI are discussed, concluding with recommendations for safe and effective strategies for adoption of the transradial approach to optimize outcomes in these high-risk patients.

Coronary artery disease is the leading cause of death in women. Women with ST-segment elevation myocardial infarctions continue to have worse outcomes compared with men despite advancements in therapies. Furthermore, these differences are particularly pronounced among young men and women with myocardial infarctions. Differences in the pathophysiology of coronary artery plaque development, disease presentation, and recognition likely contribute to these outcome disparities. Despite having worse outcomes compared with men, women clearly benefit from aggressive treatment and the latest therapies. This article reviews the treatment options for ST-segment elevation myocardial infarctions and the outcomes of women after treatment with reperfusion therapies.

Cardiogenic shock represents a state of low cardiac output and systemic hypoperfusion resulting in insufficient end-organ perfusion and consequent multiorgan failure. The main cause of this complication in the context of acute ST-elevation myocardial infarction is left ventricular dysfunction secondary to poor myocardial perfusion. In over 50% of cardiogenic shock cases, there is evidence of significant coronary stenosis within noninfarct-related arteries. Persistent ischemia in the noninfarct territory may contribute to ongoing hypotension. Currently, ESC and ACC/AHA/SCAI guidelines advocate complete revascularization in the context of multivessel coronary artery disease in the context of cardiogenic shock, although the evidence is weak.

The prognosis in ST-elevation myocardial infarction has improved with coronary care units, revascularization, and anticoagulant strategies; however, cardiogenic shock (CS) remains a highly fatal condition. Controversies remain about optimal pharmacologic therapies, revascularization strategies, the role of mechanical circulatory support (MCS), and evidence-based patient selection. The current informed consent paradigm for clinical trials creates challenges testing treatments in CS patients, who are too ill to consent and require immediate treatment. Several trials are underway comparing revascularization strategies and MCS options. Although the prognosis is grim, careful, new and existing treatments could change the course of this condition in the coming years.

Cardiac arrest is a major cause of morbidity and mortality and accounts for nearly 500,000 deaths annually in the United States. In patients suffering out-of-hospital cardiac arrest, survival is less than 15%, with considerable regional variation. Although most deaths occur during the initial resuscitation, an increasing proportion occur in patients hospitalized after initially successful resuscitation. In these patients, the significant subsequent morbidity and mortality is due to "post cardiac arrest syndrome." Until recently, most single interventions have yielded little improvement in rates of survival; however, there is growing recognition that optimal treatment strategies during the postresuscitation phase may improve outcomes.

Public reporting provides transparency and improved quality of care. However, methods in estimating risk adjusted mortality in ST-segment myocardial infarction, particularly in cardiogenic shock and cardiac arrest are contentious. There are concerns that this has resulted in risk-averse behavior in publicly reporting states, resulting in suboptimal care in these patients.

Major disparities exist between developed and developing countries in the management of acute myocardial infarction (AMI). These pronounced differences result in significantly increased morbidity and mortality from AMI in different regions of the world. Lack of infrastructure, insurance, facilities, and skilled personnel are the major constraints. Primary percutaneous coronary intervention has revolutionized the treatment of AMI; however, its global use is limited by the listed constraints. Telemedicine provides an efficient methodology that can hugely increase access and accuracy of AMI management.

CONTROVERSIES IN THE MANAGEMENT OF STEMI

THE CLINICS ARE NOW AVAILABLE ONLINE!

Access your subscription at:
www.theclinics.com

PREFACE

Despite Dramatic Progress, Significant Controversy and Critical Challenges for Patients with ST-Segment Elevation MI

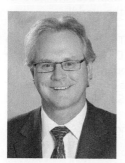

Timothy D. Henry, MD
Editor

Over the last two decades we have made remarkable progress in the treatment of ST-Segment Elevation Myocardial Infarction (STEMI). Although progress has been made in procedural aspects such as adjunctive pharmacology and stent technology, the major improvement has been the dramatic increase in the availability of the timely access to primary percutaneous coronary intervention (PCI). Still, we can and need to do better! The remaining controversies and challenges for patients with STEMI are the focus of this issue of *Interventional Cardiology Clinics*.

Perhaps the most significant advance has been the development of regional STEMI systems not only in the United States but also throughout the world. Fordyce and colleagues focus on not only the development of these STEMI systems but also the barriers to successful implementation. Russo and Le May review success and challenges in time-to-treatment, in particular for patients transferred from non-PCI centers. This is an important opportunity, as 50% to 75% of patients transferred from non-PCI centers are not treated within the guideline-recommended total door-to-balloon time of 120 minutes. Larson and colleagues then review the options available for patients with an expected delay and describe the growing body of evidence that supports a pharmacoinvasive approach.

The next two articles address two recent problems identified in contemporary STEMI care. With the increased focus on time-to-treatment, false activation of the cardiac cath lab has become a major issue in many regions of the country. Lange and colleagues review the reasons and potential solutions for this challenging issue. The worst place in America to have a STEMI is actually in the hospital! Dai and colleagues provide an excellent review of the literature and provide suggestions to improve the recognition and treatment of in-hospital STEMI.

Ongoing controversies that involve the primary PCI procedure are the focus of the next three articles. The availability of P2Y12 inhibitors has been a major advance, but there is still considerable disagreement regarding the optimal antiplatelet regimen. Drs Harari and Baber provide a wonderful review of the current literature. Then, Shah and Cox address the potentially even more controversial area of the optimal antithrombin. Finally, Drs Bazemore and Rao provide an excellent review of the relative merits of radial versus femoral access.

The next few articles provide insight into perhaps the most significant challenges we face if we are to make further progress over the next decade. More than half of STEMI patients have multivessel coronary disease, yet our knowledge on whether and when to treat nonculprit vessels remains woefully inadequate. Drs Banning and Gershlick provide an excellent review of the

Intervent Cardiol Clin 5 (2016) xiii–xiv
http://dx.doi.org/10.1016/j.iccl.2016.07.001
2211-7458/16/© 2016 Published by Elsevier Inc.

current data on multivessel disease in the setting of cardiogenic shock and discuss future directions. The two most common reasons STEMI patients still die in 2016 are related to complications from out-of-hospital cardiac arrest and advanced cardiogenic shock. Any further improvement in mortality will require a dramatic improvement in the care of these complex and high-risk patients. Sharma and Stub provide an overview of controversies in cardiac arrest, and Shah and colleagues provide a comprehensive view of the approach to patients with cardiogenic shock.

The final three articles provide important context to the field. Drs Ng and Lanksy discuss the well-known gender differences in STEMI, and Drs McDaniel and Rab review the complex issues involved in public reporting. Despite the improvements in outcomes and decreasing prevalence of STEMI in Europe and the United States, the global prevalence of STEMI continues to increase and the availability and timing of reperfusion therapy varies tremendously around the world. This major global challenge is the focus of our final article with a special emphasis on the potential of telemedicine.

My hope is that this wonderful collection of articles challenges us all to improve the care of STEMI patients throughout the world!

Timothy D. Henry, MD
Division of Cardiology
Department of Medicine
Cedars-Sinai Medical Center
127 South San Vicente Boulevard
Suite A3100
Los Angeles, CA 90048, USA
E-mail address:
henryt@cshs.org

Implementation of Regional ST-Segment Elevation Myocardial Infarction Systems of Care

Successes and Challenges

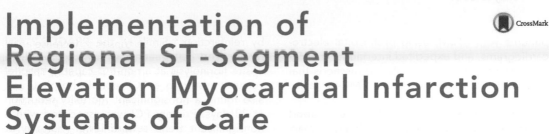

Christopher B. Fordyce, MD, MHS, MSc[a],*,
Timothy D. Henry, MD[b], Christopher B. Granger, MD[a]

KEYWORDS

- ST-segment elevation myocardial infarction • Reperfusion • Systems
- Primary percutaneous coronary intervention • Emergency medical services

---

KEY POINTS

- Timely reperfusion for acute myocardial infarction with ST-segment elevation is the most important treatment to improve early survival.
- Primary percutaneous coronary intervention is the ideal method of reperfusion but availability is a challenge in many areas of the United States.
- Providing patients with the earliest reperfusion calls for organized regional systems of care that include emergency medical services, non-PCI-capable hospitals, and PCI-capable hospitals working with regional protocols and continuously measuring and improving performance.
- Barriers to successful implementation of ST-segment elevation myocardial infarction (STEMI) systems include hospital and physician competition, system funding, EMS transport and finances, and inadequate data collection and feedback.
- Expanding STEMI systems throughout the world remains an important goal as well as expansion to other cardiovascular emergencies, such as out-of-hospital cardiac arrest, stroke, aortic dissection, and pulmonary embolism.

INTRODUCTION

Rapid coronary artery reperfusion is the foundation of treatment to improve survival for acute ST-segment elevation myocardial infarction (STEMI). Current guidelines strongly recommend that each community create and maintain a regional system of STEMI care that includes assessment and continuous quality improvement of emergency medical services (EMS) and hospital-based activities.[1] In this setting, primary percutaneous coronary intervention (PCI) is the preferred method of revascularization for acute STEMI, provided that it is performed promptly by skilled personnel.[1] Among patients undergoing PCI, clinical practice guidelines recommend first medical contact to device (FMC)-to-device time of less than 90 minutes for patients presenting to PCI-capable hospitals, and FMC-to-device time of less than 120 minutes for patients presenting to PCI-noncapable hospitals.[1] Standardization of regional STEMI reperfusion algorithms, consistent rapid identification of

---

[a] Duke Clinical Research Institute, 2400 Pratt Street, Durham, NC 27705, USA; [b] Cedars-Sinai Heart Institute, 127 South San Vicente Boulevard, Suite A3100, Los Angeles, CA 90048, USA
* Corresponding author.
E-mail address: christopher.fordyce@duke.edu

Intervent Cardiol Clin 5 (2016) 415–425
http://dx.doi.org/10.1016/j.iccl.2016.06.001
2211-7458/16/$ – see front matter © 2016 Elsevier Inc. All rights reserved.

patients with STEMI using prehospital electro-cardiograms, and expedited interfacility transfer using standardized protocols are methods that have all been shown to reduce FMC-to-device times.[2–4]

How have guidelines evolved to support STEMI regionalization, including timely primary PCI for an increasing proportion of patients with STEMI, and how successful has implementation of STEMI systems of care been? This article reviews clinical trial data supporting the use of primary PCI as the optimal reperfusion strategy, and fibrinolysis (ideally as part of a pharmacoinvasive strategy) as an option when this is not possible; describes the outcomes of regional systems of STEMI care, particularly in the United States; and discusses ongoing challenges for STEMI system implementation.

SUCCESSFUL ST-SEGMENT ELEVATION MYOCARDIAL INFARCTION REGIONALIZATION

Clinical Trial Evidence Supporting Primary Percutaneous Coronary Intervention as the Optimal Reperfusion Strategy

In the 1990s, trials comparing fibrinolytic therapy with primary PCI showed that primary PCI, if performed in a timely manner in high-volume centers, results in better survival than fibrinolysis.[5] At the same time, a meta-analysis demonstrated the superiority of transferring patients with STEMI who presented to non-PCI-capable centers for primary PCI, compared with on-site fibrinolysis.[6] The Danish Multicenter Randomized Study on Thrombolytic Therapy versus Acute Coronary Angioplasty in Acute Myocardial Infarction (DANAMI-2) trial, a well-designed, multicenter, randomized trial with 1572 patients including 24 referral hospitals and five PCI centers in Denmark, was stopped early when it demonstrated a significant reduction in the primary outcome of death, reinfarction, and stroke at 30 days (8% for primary PCI vs 13.7% for fibrinolysis; P<.001).[7] For those patients who were transferred for primary PCI from a non-PCI-capable site, the median time between randomization and arrival in the catheterization laboratory was 67 minutes, with 96% arriving within 120 minutes and the median time from first door to primary PCI was about 114 minutes (providing the basis for the current guideline recommendations). Importantly, the mortality benefit was most evident in the subgroup of high-risk patients (TIMI risk score ≥5 at presentation),[8] but the difference in the primary outcome favoring PCI remained significant at up to 7.8 years (11.7% vs 18.5%), driven mostly

by reinfarction.[9] Similarly, the PRAGUE-2 trial randomized 850 patients with acute STEMI to onsite fibrinolysis at a non-PCI-capable hospital versus transfer to a PCI-capable hospital, and also found a nonsignificant mortality reduction at 30 days. Primary PCI was associated with a nonsignificant trend toward lower mortality at 30 days (6.8% vs 10.0% with fibrinolysis) and benefits persisted at 5 years.[10,11]

Clinical Trial Evidence Supporting Fibrinolysis as a Viable Reperfusion Option

Ischemic time (time from symptom onset to reperfusion) drives the relative benefit of primary PCI compared with fibrinolysis. As ischemic time increases, outcomes are worse irrespective of reperfusion strategy. However, the benefits from reperfusion are lost more quickly with fibrinolytic therapy.[12]

Indeed, fibrinolytic therapy is most effective in less than or equal to 3 hours of symptom onset.[12,13] Evidence for which patients derive comparable benefits from fibrinolytic therapy to primary PCI comes from the STREAM study, which included 1892 patients with STEMI who presented within 3 hours after symptom onset and who were unable to undergo primary PCI within 1 hour.[14] These patients were randomized to undergo either primary PCI or fibrinolytic therapy with bolus tenecteplase (amended to half dose in patients ≥75 years of age), clopidogrel, and enoxaparin before transport to a PCI-capable hospital. There was no difference in the primary composite end point (death, shock, congestive heart failure, or reinfarction up to 30 days) between the fibrinolytic and PCI groups (12.4% vs 14.3%, respectively; relative risk, 0.86; 95% confidence interval, 0.68–1.09), and no difference in all-cause mortality at 1-year of follow-up.[15] Although the efficacy outcomes seemed similar to primary PCI, there was an increased rate of intracranial hemorrhage (1.0% vs 0.2%) for patients greater than or equal to 75 years old, resulting in a protocol amendment that called for a lower dose of fibrinolytics in this group. There is also reasonably strong evidence for benefit of routine transfer to receive urgent angiography ± PCI (a form of pharmacoinvasive therapy) within 3 to 24 hours.[16,17]

Implementation of Regional ST-Segment Elevation Myocardial Infarction Systems in the United States

Despite the promising results of DANAMI-2 and PRAGUE-2, many believed it would be challenging to replicate these results in North America with fragmented EMS systems and longer transportation times.[18] However, in 2002 the Minneapolis STEMI system was successfully implemented modeled after level 1 trauma systems in the United States (**Fig. 1**).[19] Rapid transfer of patients with STEMI from community hospitals up to 210 miles from a PCI center was safe and feasible using a standardized protocol with an integrated transfer system. The system was also successful in improving reperfusion times for patients presenting at PCI-noncapable hospitals with long transfer times using a pharmacoinvasive strategy.[20] In a consecutive unselected STEMI population, 30-day mortality was low, at 5.5%. Importantly, outcomes were similar with the pharmacoinvasive strategy, using half-dose fibrinolytic therapy, as with primary PCI despite more than an hour longer reperfusion time caused by the

long distance transfer. In 2007, a state-wide regional STEMI system was implemented in North Carolina with 65 hospitals and five regions: the Regional Approach to Cardiovascular Emergencies program. In Regional Approach to Cardiovascular Emergencies, there was successful shortening of reperfusion times for patients presenting directly to or transferred to a PCI-capable hospital.[21] The program expanded to then include all hospitals in North Carolina (21 PCI-capable, and 98 PCI noncapable), thus demonstrating the feasibility of regionalizing STEMI care to an entire state (**Fig. 2**).[22] Early adopters in predominately urban US STEMI systems of care include Los Angeles and Dallas.[23,24] **Table 1** compares the Minneapolis, North Carolina, Los Angeles, and Dallas systems, and the 16-region American Heart Association (AHA)

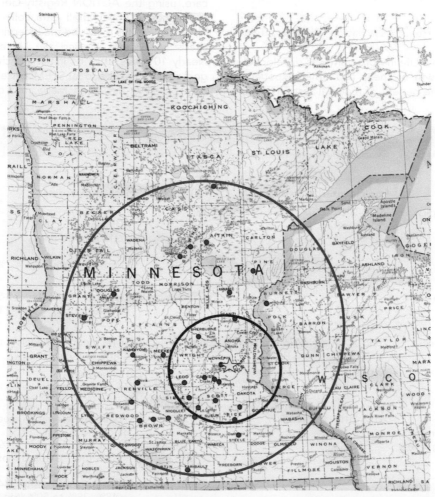

Fig. 1. Map of Minnesota with the PCI center (Abbott Northwestern Hospital) in Minneapolis (*yellow star*), zone 1 hospitals (<60 miles from PCI hospital; *blue circles*), and zone 2 hospitals (60–210 miles from PCI hospital; *red circles*). (*Adapted from* Henry TD, Sharkey SW, Burke MN, et al. A regional system to provide timely access to percutaneous coronary intervention for ST-elevation myocardial infarction. Circulation 2007;116(7):722; with permission.)

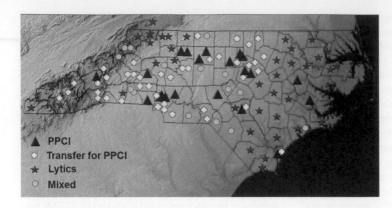

Fig. 2. North Carolina hospitals according to reperfusion strategy. PPCI, primary percutaneous coronary intervention. (*Adapted from* Jollis JG, Al-Khalidi HR, Monk L, et al. Regional Approach to Cardiovascular Emergencies (RACE) investigators. Expansion of a regional ST-segment-elevation myocardial infarction system to an entire state. Circulation 2012;126(2):190; with permission.)

▲ PPCI
○ Transfer for PPCI
★ Lytics
○ Mixed

Accelerator Program, which aimed to rapidly implement systems of care across multiple STEMI networks (discussed in more detail later).[25,26]

American Heart Association Mission: Lifeline Program

The Mission: Lifeline program was developed as an outgrowth of these and other experiences showing the benefit of regional systems of care

for STEMI.[27] A comprehensive review of best practices provided the basis for recommendations on how to establish regional systems of care, using the ACTION Registry-Get With the Guidelines as the overall data collection tool. The program has provided the blueprint for hundreds of systems around the United States. Nearly 10 years after its initial launch with the goal of creating the ideal STEMI system, significant progress has been made, but challenges

Table 1
Comparison of regional STEMI systems of care

System	Year(s) Implemented	Patients	Hospitals (PCI/Non-PCI)	Selected Outcomes[a]
Minneapolis	2003–2006	1345	1/30	DBT (median) PCI center: 65 min <60 miles: 95 min 60–210 miles: 120 min In-hospital mortality: 4.2%
North Carolina	2008–2009	6841	21/98	DBT (median) Direct to PCI center: 64–59 min Transfer to PCI center: 117–103 min
Los Angeles	2006–2007	476 (primary PCI)	30/44	DBT (% meeting guideline time) <50% to 90%
Dallas	2010–2012	3853; 928 undergoing primary PCI	15 PCI	DBT (median) 74–64 min
AHA Accelerator (16 regions)	2012–2013	23,809	171/313	FMC-to-device time (% meeting guideline times) Direct to PCI center: 50% to 55%; 45% to 57% (top 5 most improved regions) Transfer to PCI center: 44% to 48%; 38% to 50% (top 5 most improved regions)

Abbreviations: AHA, American Heart Association; DBT, door-to-balloon time.
[a] Preimplementation to postimplementation of STEMI system, where applicable.

remain.[28] **Fig. 3** is adapted from the original 2007 document, now modified to provide a contemporary view of the successes and ongoing challenges.

Facilitated by MISSION: Lifeline and development of transportation and transfer systems, PCI rates, and hospitals providing STEMI-related PCI have increased in the United States.[29] Furthermore, the expansion of STEMI networks continues internationally. Implementation of STEMI systems in several Western countries has been associated with reduced reperfusion times in Canada,[3,30–32] Australia,[33] Austria,[34] France,[35] and Italy,[36] with momentum for regionalization in such countries as Romania, China, South Africa, and Mexico.[37,38] Efforts in South America and Asia, with telemedicine as part of the Lumen Foundation (http://lumenglobal.org/), have also made important progress with a focus on low- and middle-income countries.[39]

Rapid Regionalization of Multiple ST-Segment Elevation Myocardial Infarction Networks: the American Heart Association Mission: Lifeline ST-Segment Elevation Myocardial Infarction Accelerator Program Demonstration Project

Despite the success of some regional systems in the United States, two decades of evidence, and the availability of the Mission: Lifeline resources, the reality is that 30% to 50% of patients still fail to meet guideline-recommended reperfusion times.[40–43] This is not the result of inadequate access to primary PCI, because the number of PCI-capable hospitals has increased by almost 50% over this time period and 90% of Americans live within 60 minutes of a PCI-capable facility (**Fig. 4**).[29,44–46] Rather, this is a result of the highly fragmented US health system comprising approximately 4750 acute care hospitals and more than

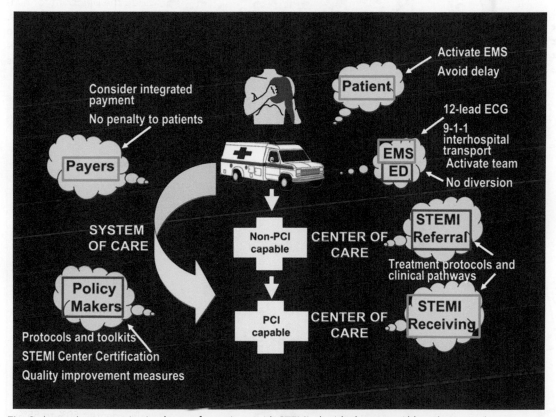

Fig. 3. Improving access to timely care for patients with STEMI: the ideal system. Although tremendous improvement has occurred in STEMI care since the publication of the initial Mission: Lifeline guidelines (*green boxes*), there are still many opportunities for improvement (*red boxes*). This includes ensuring emergency department bypass for patients with preactivation, more rapid door-in-door-out times for patients presenting to non-PCI-capable hospitals who then require transfer for primary PCI, and ongoing policy that supports transparent public reporting and encourages regional cooperation among key stakeholders. ECG, electrocardiogram. (*Adapted from* Jacobs AK, Antman EM, Faxon DP, et al. Development of systems of care for ST-elevation myocardial infarction patients: executive summary. Circulation 2007;116(2):226; with permission.)

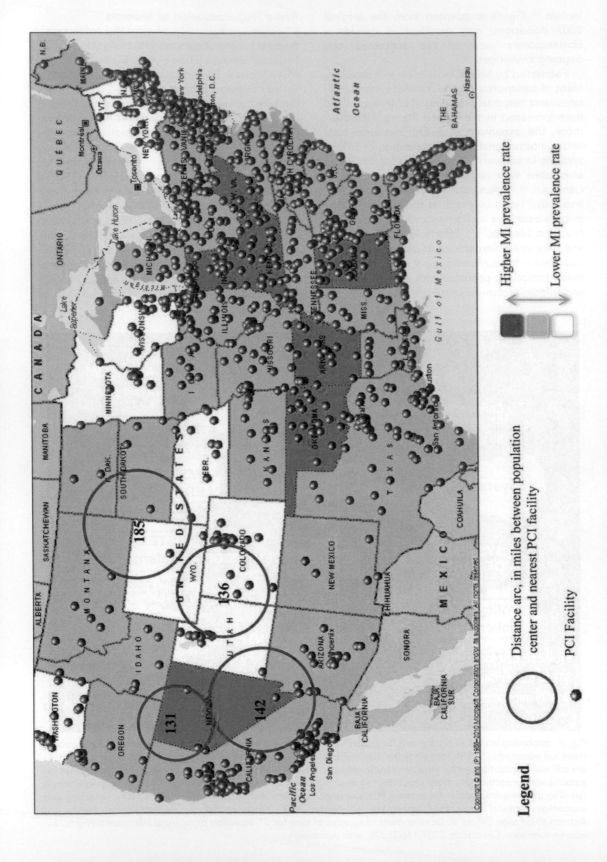

Legend

Distance arc, in miles between population center and nearest PCI facility

PCI Facility

Higher MI prevalence rate ← → Lower MI prevalence rate

15,000 EMS agencies. Therefore, building on successful efforts in organizing STEMI reperfusion systems on a regional basis, the Mission: Lifeline STEMI Accelerator Program Demonstration Project was developed to more completely implement Mission: Lifeline leveraging regional leadership, data collection, common protocols, and ongoing data review with timely feedback to increase the percentage of patients receiving primary PCI within guideline goals.[25]

The STEMI Systems Accelerator project intervention was organized and executed between March 2012 and July 2014 and involved 16 regions across the United States and included 23,809 patients with STEMI (18,267 patients who presented directly to a PCI-capable hospital and 5542 who were transferred from hospitals without PCI capability).[25,26] This work represented the largest effort ever attempted in the United States to organize STEMI care across multiple regions. There was a significant increase in the proportion of patients meeting guideline goals of FMC-to-device time, including those directly presenting via EMS (50% to 55%; $P<.001$) and transferred patients (44% to 48%; $P = .002$). Despite regional variability, the greatest gains occurred among patients in the five most-improved regions, increasing from 45% to 57% (direct EMS; $P<.001$)[26] and 38% to 50% (transfers; $P<.001$). A subsequent analysis found that there were significant differences in median FMC-to-device times among groups implementing prehospital activation (88 minutes for implementers, vs 89 minutes for pre-existing, vs 98 minutes for nonimplementers; $P<.001$ for comparisons).[47] Similarly, patients treated at hospitals implementing single-call transfer protocols had shorter median FMC-to-device times (112 vs 128 vs 152 minutes; $P<.001$). Emergency department bypass was also associated with shorter median FMC-to-device times for EMS direct presenters (84 vs 88 vs 94 minutes; $P<.001$) and transfers (123 vs 127 vs 167 minutes; $P<.001$). Taken together, the results of the Accelerator demonstration project show that a standardized approach of implementing regional

systems by bringing together stakeholders, establishing and implementing protocols, and reviewing data for continuous improvement can (and should) be done in nearly all regions of the United States.[26,47]

CHALLENGES TO ST-SEGMENT ELEVATION MYOCARDIAL INFARCTION REGIONALIZATION

Although STEMI reperfusion guidelines are nearly a decade old, up to 50% of patients in the United States fail to meet current reperfusion standards. Because 90% of Americans live within 60 minutes of a PCI-capable facility, this is not the results of inadequate access. Therefore, addressing current challenges is paramount to improving the quality of STEMI care in the United States.

Data Collection, Reporting, and Reimbursement

A major challenge to improving the care of patients with STEMI in the United States has been the lack of accurate and comprehensive data, the cornerstone of any quality improvement initiative. Data submitted to the Joint Commission and to registries, such as the National Registry for Myocardial Infarction, have been highly selective and have not included all patients with STEMI.[48] Likewise, ACTION-GWTG and CathPCI are both volunteer registries that exclude many complex and high-risk patients from the quality reports, and thus these may not be generalizable to the overall STEMI population. A recent report from three well-known large Massachusetts hospitals highlights this issue. More than a quarter of patients who underwent primary PCI were excluded from hospital quality reports collected by Centers for Medicare & Medicaid Services (CMS), and this percentage has grown substantially over time.[49] Of prime concern from a STEMI systems standpoint is that although 95% of CMS-reported cases met door-to-balloon time goals in 2011, this was true of only 61% of CMS-excluded cases. In fact, multiple studies have

Fig. 4. Geographic distance to nearest PCI-capable hospital (overlaid on state AMI prevalence rates). The distance arcs are overlaid on the MI prevalence rates delineated in the Centers for Disease Control and Prevention National Cardiovascular Disease Surveillance database. The four distance arcs on the map represent the greatest potential access difficulties in terms of transport times and would seem to most benefit from a regionalized transfer system involving air ambulances. The distances with the highest priority are those mapped over darker states. AMI, acute myocardial infarction. (*Adapted from* Langabeer JR, Henry TD, Kereiakes DJ, et al. Growth in percutaneous coronary intervention capacity relative to population and disease prevalence. J Am Heart Assoc 2013;2(6):e000370; with permission.)

reported that the odds of receiving primary PCI for STEMI are lower in areas that require public reporting of mortality after PCI.[50] Therefore, standardized data collection including the entire denominator of cases (complete case capture) is important to truly understand patient outcomes and identify knowledge gaps.

Economic and Political Barriers

There has been long-standing recognition that economics and politics weigh heavily when considering STEMI regionalization.[51] In the United States, these policies have contributed to the rapid adoption of cardiac catheterization laboratories but not necessarily the important next step of regionalizing care.[45,46] This has resulted in the creation of low-volume PCI centers, which are associated with worse in-hospital mortality compared with higher volume centers.[52]

At a local level, and also related to reimbursement, hospitals and cardiology group competition remain major barriers to regionalization. The best evidence supporting this comes from a report from the AHA Mission: Lifeline, which surveyed nearly 400 unique STEMI systems from 2008 to 2010.[28] The most common barriers were hospital competition (37%), EMS transport

and finances (26%), and competition between cardiology groups (21%). Other major reasons included lack of data collection and feedback (18%), lack of infrastructure support and funding (16%), and lack of bed availability (16%). Therefore, recognizing and then targeting these barriers by encouraging cooperation between key stakeholders at a regional level, through such programs as the AHA Accelerator program, remain essential to delivering optimal STEMI care.

SUMMARY

Based on a sound rational and on a wealth of experience, and supported as a class I recommendation in international practice guidelines, all communities should develop and maintain regional systems of care for treatment of STEMI. We have reviewed the history of STEMI systems and identified resources that can be used to develop such systems. The core elements are health care provider leadership and engagement; identifying funding (including from PCI center clinical services); establishing a data collection, sharing, and feedback mechanism; and establishing a plan for each hospital and EMS system in the region, with common protocols wherever

---

Box 1
Benefits of developing regional STEMI systems of care

- Faster FMC-to-device for patients presenting by EMS directly to primary PCI centers, including preactivating of the catheterization laboratory before hospital arrival
- Increasing the proportion of patients taken by EMS directly to primary PCI centers through bypassing non-PCI-capable hospitals with prehospital electrocardiogram diagnosis
- Faster first door to device times for patients with STEMI transferred from non-PCI-capable to PCI-capable hospitals
- Increased proportion of eligible patients who receive some reperfusion therapy because of reduced delays and better transportation protocols
- Improved use of guideline-based adjunctive pharmacology using standardized protocols
- Improved treatment of cardiac arrest, including primary PCI for appropriate patients
- Improved treatment of cardiogenic shock, including earlier transportation to centers capable of advanced shock management
- Improved treatment of aortic dissection and related emergencies, which also depend on rapid treatment to prevent mortality
- Platform for developing plans and protocols for optimizing regional care for other vascular emergencies, including stroke
- Improved quality improvement, communication, and feedback (immediate and periodic) across a region
- Opportunity for advancing coordinated and integrated care programs with emergency medical services, including training and motivating paramedics to provide state-of-art care
- Publicizing programs to increase public awareness of importance of recognizing symptoms and calling 9-1-1 and engaging in activities to improve community response to cardiovascular emergencies

possible. Sources for specific and detailed advice are found at http://www.heart.org/HEARTORG/HealthcareProfessional/Mission-Lifeline-Home-Page_UCM_305495_SubHomePage.jsp.

Although challenges remain, it is clear that regional STEMI systems provide more rapid and effective reperfusion to more patients with STEMI, with the knowledge that such treatment saves lives. There are numerous other important benefits listed in **Box 1**, including providing a platform for collaboration of hospitals with EMS for all cardiovascular emergencies[53] and for collecting data that allow one to address other opportunities to improve care.

REFERENCES

1. O'Gara PT, Kushner FG, Ascheim DD, et al. 2013 ACCF/AHA guideline for the management of ST-elevation myocardial infarction: a report of the American College of Cardiology Foundation/American Heart Association Task Force on Practice Guidelines. Circulation 2013;127(4):e362–425.
2. Curtis JP, Portnay EL, Wang Y, et al. The pre-hospital electrocardiogram and time to reperfusion in patients with acute myocardial infarction, 2000-2002: findings from the National Registry of Myocardial Infarction-4. J Am Coll Cardiol 2006; 47(8):1544–52.
3. Le May MR, So DY, Dionne R, et al. A citywide protocol for primary PCI in ST-segment elevation myocardial infarction. N Engl J Med 2008;358(3): 231–40.
4. Diercks DB, Kontos MC, Chen AY, et al. Utilization and impact of pre-hospital electrocardiograms for patients with acute ST-segment elevation myocardial infarction: data from the NCDR (National Cardiovascular Data Registry) ACTION (Acute Coronary Treatment and Intervention Outcomes Network) Registry. J Am Coll Cardiol 2009;53(2): 161–6.
5. Keeley EC, Boura JA, Grines CL. Primary angioplasty versus intravenous thrombolytic therapy for acute myocardial infarction: a quantitative review of 23 randomised trials. Lancet 2003;361(9351): 13–20.
6. Dalby M, Bouzamondo A, Lechat P, et al. Transfer for primary angioplasty versus immediate thrombolysis in acute myocardial infarction: a meta-analysis. Circulation 2003;108(15):1809–14.
7. Andersen HR, Nielsen TT, Rasmussen K, et al. A comparison of coronary angioplasty with fibrinolytic therapy in acute myocardial infarction. N Engl J Med 2003;349(8):733–42.
8. Thune JJ, Hoefsten DE, Lindholm MG, et al. Danish Multicenter Randomized Study on fibrinolytic

therapy versus acute coronary angioplasty in acute myocardial infarction (DANAMI)-2 investigators. Simple risk stratification at admission to identify patients with reduced mortality from primary angioplasty. Circulation 2005;112(13):2017–21.
9. Nielsen PH, Maeng M, Busk M, et al. Primary angioplasty versus fibrinolysis in acute myocardial infarction: long-term follow-up in the Danish acute myocardial infarction 2 trial. Circulation 2010; 121(13):1484–91.
10. Widimský P, Budesínský T, Vorác D, et al. Long distance transport for primary angioplasty vs immediate thrombolysis in acute myocardial infarction. Final results of the randomized national multicentre trial–PRAGUE-2. Eur Heart J 2003;24(1):94–104.
11. Widimský P, Bilkova D, Penicka M, et al. Long-term outcomes of patients with acute myocardial infarction presenting to hospitals without catheterization laboratory and randomized to immediate thrombolysis or interhospital transport for primary percutaneous coronary intervention. Five years' follow-up of the PRAGUE-2 Trial. Eur Heart J 2007;28(6):679–84.
12. Gersh BJ, Stone GW, White HD, et al. Pharmacological facilitation of primary percutaneous coronary intervention for acute myocardial infarction: is the slope of the curve the shape of the future? JAMA 2005;293(8):979–86.
13. Boersma E, Maas AC, Deckers JW, et al. Early thrombolytic treatment in acute myocardial infarction: reappraisal of the golden hour. Lancet 1996; 348(9030):771–5.
14. Armstrong PW, Gershlick AH, Goldstein P, et al. Fibrinolysis or primary PCI in ST-segment elevation myocardial infarction. N Engl J Med 2013;368(15): 1379–87.
15. Sinnaeve PR, Armstrong PW, Gershlick AH, et al. ST-segment-elevation myocardial infarction patients randomized to a pharmaco-invasive strategy or primary percutaneous coronary intervention: strategic reperfusion early after myocardial infarction (STREAM) 1-year mortality follow-up. Circulation 2014;130(14):1139–45.
16. Borgia F, Goodman SG, Halvorsen S, et al. Early routine percutaneous coronary intervention after fibrinolysis vs. standard therapy in ST-segment elevation myocardial infarction: a meta-analysis. Eur Heart J 2010;31(17):2156–69.
17. D'Souza SP, Mamas MA, Fraser DG, et al. Routine early coronary angioplasty versus ischaemia-guided angioplasty after thrombolysis in acute ST-elevation myocardial infarction: a meta-analysis. Eur Heart J 2011;32(8):972–82.
18. Henry TD. From concept to reality: a decade of progress in regional ST-elevation myocardial infarction systems. Circulation 2012;126(2):166–8.
19. Henry TD, Sharkey SW, Burke MN, et al. A regional system to provide timely access to percutaneous

coronary intervention for ST-elevation myocardial infarction. Circulation 2007;116(7):721–8.

20. Larson DM, Duval S, Sharkey SW, et al. Safety and efficacy of a pharmaco-invasive reperfusion strategy in rural ST-elevation myocardial infarction patients with expected delays due to long-distance transfers. Eur Heart J 2012;33(10):1232–40.

21. Jollis JG, Roettig ML, Aluko AO, et al. Implementation of a statewide system for coronary reperfusion for ST-segment elevation myocardial infarction. JAMA 2007;298(20):2371–80.

22. Jollis JG, Al-Khalidi HR, Monk L, et al. Regional Approach to Cardiovascular Emergencies (RACE) investigators. Expansion of a regional ST-segment-elevation myocardial infarction system to an entire state. Circulation 2012;126(2):189–95.

23. Rokos IC, French WJ, Koenig WJ, et al. Integration of pre-hospital electrocardiograms and ST-elevation myocardial infarction receiving center (SRC) networks: impact on door-to-balloon times across 10 independent regions. JACC Cardiovasc Interv 2009;2(4):339–46.

24. DelliFraine J, Langabeer J 2nd, Segrest W, et al. Developing an ST-elevation myocardial infarction system of care in Dallas County. Am Heart J 2013;165(6):926–31.

25. Bagai A, Al-Khalidi HR, Sherwood M. Regional systems of care demonstration project: mission: lifeline STEMI systems accelerator: design and methodology. Am Heart J 2014;167(1):15–21.e3.

26. Jollis JG, Al-Khalidi HR, Roettig ML, et al. Regional systems of care demonstration project: American Heart Association Mission: lifeline™ STEMI systems accelerator. Circulation 2016.

27. Jacobs AK, Antman EM, Faxon DP, et al. Development of systems of care for ST-elevation myocardial infarction patients: executive summary. Circulation 2007;116(2):217–30.

28. Jollis JG, Granger CB, Henry TD, et al. Systems of care for ST-segment-elevation myocardial infarction: a report from the American Heart Association's Mission: lifeline. Circ Cardiovasc Qual Outcomes 2012;5(4):423–8.

29. Shah RU, Henry TD, Rutten-Ramos S, et al. Increasing percutaneous coronary interventions for ST-segment elevation myocardial infarction in the United States: progress and opportunity. JACC Cardiovasc Interv 2015;8(1 Pt B):139–46.

30. Chan AW, Kornder J, Elliott H, et al. Improved survival associated with pre-hospital triage strategy in a large regional ST-segment elevation myocardial infarction program. JACC Cardiovasc Interv 2012;5(12):1239–46.

31. Mercuri M, Welsford M, Schwalm JD, et al. Providing optimal regional care for ST-segment elevation myocardial infarction: a prospective cohort study of patients in the Hamilton Niagara Haldimand Brant Local Health Integration Network. CMAJ Open 2015;3(1):E1–7.

32. Fordyce CB, Cairns JA, Singer J, et al. Evolution and impact of a regional reperfusion system for ST-elevation myocardial infarction. Can J Cardiol 2015. [Epub ahead of print].

33. Hutchison AW, Malaiapan Y, Jarvie I, et al. Prehospital 12-lead ECG to triage ST-elevation myocardial infarction and emergency department activation of the infarct team significantly improves door-to-balloon times: ambulance Victoria and MonashHEART Acute Myocardial Infarction (MonAMI) 12-lead ECG project. Circ Cardiovasc Interv 2009;2(6):528–34.

34. Kalla K, Christ G, Karnik R, et al. Implementation of guidelines improves the standard of care: the Viennese registry on reperfusion strategies in ST-elevation myocardial infarction (Vienna STEMI registry). Circulation 2006;113(20):2398–405.

35. Danchin N, Coste P, Ferrières J, et al. Comparison of thrombolysis followed by broad use of percutaneous coronary intervention with primary percutaneous coronary intervention for ST-segment-elevation acute myocardial infarction: data from the French registry on acute ST-elevation myocardial infarction (FAST-MI). Circulation 2008;118(3):268–76.

36. Ortolani P, Marzocchi A, Marrozzini C, et al. Clinical impact of direct referral to primary percutaneous coronary intervention following pre-hospital diagnosis of ST-elevation myocardial infarction. Eur Heart J 2006;27(13):1550–7.

37. Benedek I, Gyongyosi M, Benedek T. A prospective regional registry of ST-elevation myocardial infarction in Central Romania: impact of the stent for life initiative recommendations on patient outcomes. Am Heart J 2013;166(3):457–65.

38. Kaifoszova Z, Kala P, Alexander T, et al. Stent for life initiative: leading example in building STEMI systems of care in emerging countries. EuroIntervention 2014;10(Suppl T):T87–95.

39. Mehta S, Botelho R, Rodriguez D, et al. A tale of two cities: STEMI interventions in developed and developing countries and the potential of telemedicine to reduce disparities in care. J Interv Cardiol 2014;27(2):155–66.

40. Bagai A, Jollis JG, Dauerman HL, et al. Emergency department bypass for ST-Segment-elevation myocardial infarction patients identified with a pre-hospital electrocardiogram: a report from the American Heart Association Mission: lifeline program. Circulation 2013;128(4):352–9.

41. Dauerman HL, Bates ER, Kontos MC, et al. Nationwide analysis of patients with ST-segment-elevation myocardial infarction transferred for primary

percutaneous intervention: findings from the American Heart Association Mission: lifeline program. Circ Cardiovasc Interv 2015;8(5). pii:e002450.

42. Bagal A, Al-Khalidi HR, Munoz D, et al. Bypassing the emergency department and time to reperfusion in patients with prehospital ST-segment elevation: findings from the reperfusion in acute myocardial infarction in Carolina Emergency Departments Project. Circ Cardiovasc Interv 2013; 6(4):399–406.

43. Fosbol EL, Granger CB, Jollis JG, et al. The impact of a statewide pre-hospital STEMI strategy to bypass hospitals without percutaneous coronary intervention capability on treatment times. Circulation 2013;127(5):604–12.

44. Nallamothu BK, Bates ER, Wang Y, et al. Driving times and distances to hospitals with percutaneous coronary intervention in the United States: implications for prehospital triage of patients with ST-elevation myocardial infarction. Circulation 2006; 113(9):1189–95.

45. Concannon TW, Nelson J, Kent DM, et al. Evidence of systematic duplication by new percutaneous coronary intervention programs. Circ Cardiovasc Qual Outcomes 2013;6(4):400–8.

46. Langabeer JR, Henry TD, Kereiakes DJ, et al. Growth in percutaneous coronary intervention capacity relative to population and disease prevalence. J Am Heart Assoc 2013;2(6):e000370.

47. Fordyce CB, Al-Khalidi HR, Jollis JG, et al. Association of rapid care process implementation on reperfusion times across multiple STEMI networks: insights from the American Heart Association Mission: Lifeline STEMI Accelerator Program.

Orlando (FL): American Heart Association Scientific Sessions, 2015.

48. Campbell AR, Satran D, Larson DM, et al. ST-elevation myocardial infarction: which patients do quality assurance programs include? Circ Cardiovasc Qual Outcomes 2009;2(6):648–55.

49. Resnic FS, Normand SL, Piemonte TC, et al. Improvement in mortality risk prediction after percutaneous coronary intervention through the addition of a "compassionate use" variable to the National Cardiovascular Data Registry CathPCI dataset: a study from the Massachusetts Angioplasty Registry. J Am Coll Cardiol 2011;57(8):904–11.

50. Joynt KE, Blumenthal DM, Orav EJ, et al. Association of public reporting for percutaneous coronary intervention with utilization and outcomes among Medicare beneficiaries with acute myocardial infarction. JAMA 2012;308(14):1460–8.

51. Henry TD, Atkins JM, Cunningham MS, et al. ST-segment elevation myocardial infarction: recommendations on triage of patients to heart attack centers: is it time for a national policy for the treatment of ST-segment elevation myocardial infarction? J Am Coll Cardiol 2006;47:1339–45.

52. Kontos MC, Wang Y, Chaudhry SI, et al. Lower hospital volume is associated with higher in-hospital mortality in patients undergoing primary percutaneous coronary intervention for ST-segment-elevation myocardial infarction: a report from the NCDR. Circ Cardiovasc Qual Outcomes 2013;6(6):659–67.

53. Graham KJ, Strauss CE, Boland LL, et al. Has the time come for a national cardiovascular emergency care system? Circulation 2012;125(16):2035–44.

Time to Treatment
Focus on Transfer in ST-Elevation Myocardial Infarction

Juan Russo, MD, Michel R. Le May, MD*

KEYWORD
• Time to treatment • Door-to-balloon time • ST-elevation myocardial infarction

KEY POINTS
• In the modern ST-elevation myocardial infarction (STEMI) system, the use of electrocardiogram by emergency medical services (EMS) personnel and the option to bypass emergency departments on route to a PCI-capable hospital is of particular importance.
• Through training and a standardized referral process, EMS personnel can now accurately diagnose and refer STEMI patients directly to the catheterization laboratory of a percutaneous coronary intervention–capable hospital.
• Regional STEMI models have been implemented successfully across North America, and this has resulted in palpable reductions in door-to-balloon time, morbidity, and mortality.

Time to reperfusion is a key modulator of morbidity and mortality in patients with ST-elevation myocardial infarction (STEMI).[1–3] During STEMI, acute thrombotic occlusion of a coronary artery initiates an ischemic cascade, culminating in myocardial injury and necrosis. If reperfusion in the infarct-related artery (IRA) is not promptly re-established, ischemic myocardium at risk becomes irreversibly damaged, leading to poor patient outcomes, including death. Timely reperfusion in the IRA by pharmacologic and/or mechanical means can stop myocardial ischemia, reducing infarct size, morbidity, and mortality. Fibrinolytic therapy and primary percutaneous coronary intervention (PCI) are the 2 strategies currently available to achieve reperfusion.

PRIMARY PERCUTANEOUS CORONARY INTERVENTION VERSUS FIBRINOLYTIC THERAPY

The efficacy of primary PCI lies in its ability to provide rapid, complete, and sustained reperfusion of the IRA by mechanical means. A systematic review of 23 randomized controlled trials demonstrated that compared with fibrinolytic therapy, primary PCI was superior in reducing death, reinfarction, and stroke in patients with STEMI.[4] Primary PCI is also less costly than fibrinolytic therapy.[5]

TIME-DEPENDENT EFFICACY OF PRIMARY PERCUTANEOUS CORONARY INTERVENTION

Observations from early randomized trials demonstrated that the efficacy of primary PCI is highly time-dependent. In the Global Use of Strategies to Open Occluded arteries (GUSTO)-IIb substudy,[6] a strong inverse relationship between time to angioplasty and mortality was noted with 1.0% and 6.4% mortality rates when time to angioplasty was equal to or less than 60 minutes and equal to or greater than 90 minutes, respectively (Fig. 1). The association between timely reperfusion therapy and mortality led to the notion of the "golden hour" of

Division of Cardiology, University of Ottawa Heart Institute, 40 Ruskin Street, Ottawa K1Y 4W7, Canada
* Corresponding author.
E-mail address: mlemay@ottawaheart.ca

Intervent Cardiol Clin 5 (2016) 427–437
http://dx.doi.org/10.1016/j.iccl.2016.06.003

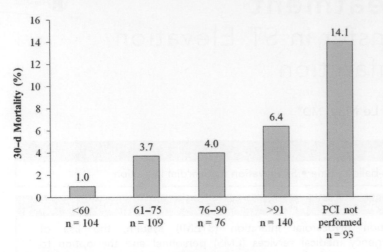

Fig. 1. Relationship between 30-day mortality and time from randomization to first balloon inflation in the GUSTO-IIb trial. Subjects assigned to PCI in whom PCI was not performed are also shown. (*Adapted from* Berger PB, Ellis SG, Holmes DR Jr, et al. Relationship between delay in performing direct coronary angioplasty and early clinical outcome in patients with acute myocardial infarction: results from the global use of strategies to open occluded arteries in Acute Coronary Syndromes (GUSTO-IIb) trial. Circulation 1999;100(1):17.)

primary PCI and an increased emphasis on its timely provision because "every minute of delay counts."[7] Thus, time to reperfusion emerged as a key indicator of the quality of care for STEMI patients managed with primary PCI. System delays, defined as the time from contact with the emergency medical services (EMS) to primary PCI and its components, prehospital delay, and door-to-balloon time (D2BT), all correlate with survival.[8] Accordingly, first medical contact has been recommended as a logical start time for measuring reperfusion therapy.[9–11] It has been defined as the time of EMS arrival on scene after the patient calls 9-1-1 or time of arrival at the emergency department when the patient arrives as a self-transport.[12] However, the time of arrival in the emergency department (door-time) has been generally adopted by most organizations as the standard start time for both scenarios because it is readily available in medical records

and it facilitates performance measurement.[13] Hence, D2BT has become the most widely used metric for primary PCI.

Data from the National Registry of Myocardial Infarction has corroborated the inverse relationship between D2BT and survival in patients referred for primary PCI.[2,3] Cannon and colleagues[2] evaluated 27,080 consecutive STEMI patients managed with primary PCI between 1994 and 1998, and found significantly higher in-hospital mortality when D2BT was greater than 2 hours. Shortly thereafter, McNamara and colleagues[3] reported on 29,222 patients treated with primary PCI within 6 hours of presentation between 1999 and 2002, and found a strong linear correlation between D2BT and in-hospital mortality (Fig. 2). In addition, D2BT correlated with mortality regardless of (1) time of symptom onset to hospital presentation and (2) baseline mortality risk. In a separate analysis,

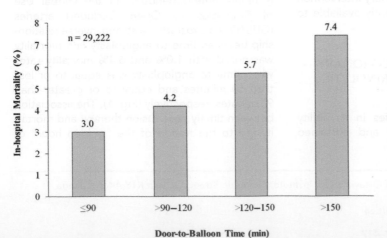

Fig. 2. In-hospital mortality and D2BT. In a cohort study of 29,222 STEMI subjects treated with PCI within 6 hours of presentation at 395 hospitals that participated in National Registry of Myocardial Infarction, longer D2BT was associated with increased in-hospital mortality. (*Data from* McNamara RL, Wang Y, Herrin J, et al. Effect of door-to-balloon time on mortality in patients with ST-segment elevation myocardial infarction. J Am Coll Cardiol 2006;47(11): 2180–6.)

Nallamothu and colleagues[14] reported that every 10-minute increase in D2BT increases the odds of death during the index admission by 9%. Recognizing the importance of timely reperfusion, the 2009 American College of Cardiology/American Heart Association (ACC/AHA) guidelines emphasized that D2BT be on an "as soon as possible" rather than a 90-minute benchmark.[15]

EVIDENCE TO SUPPORT TRANSFER FOR PRIMARY PERCUTANEOUS CORONARY INTERVENTION

Transfer of patients to PCI hospitals from non-PCI–capable hospitals can be associated with significant delays. However, 5 randomized trials reported that interhospital transfer for primary PCI was associated with superior clinical outcomes when compared with onsite fibrinolytic therapy at non-PCI–capable hospitals.[16–20] The favorable results from the largest of these trials, the Danish Trial in Acute Myocardial Infarction (DANAMI)-2, became the catalyst needed for regions to develop STEMI systems.[20] In DANAMI-2, the composite of death, reinfarction, and disabling stroke in subjects presenting at non-PCI hospitals was significantly lower in subjects transferred for primary PCI when compared with onsite fibrinolytic therapy, 8.5% and 14.2%, respectively. In subjects assigned to primary PCI, median time from admission to randomization was 22 minutes, and from randomization to first balloon inflation, 90 minutes. It was concluded that the transfer of patients to a PCI center for primary angioplasty is superior to onsite fibrinolytic therapy, provided that the transfer takes 2 hours or less.

EARLY IMPLEMENTATION OF PRIMARY PERCUTANEOUS CORONARY INTERVENTION: DOOR-TO-BALLOON TIMES ARE LONGER THAN EXPECTED

During the early implementation of primary PCI in health care systems, D2BTs were found to be significantly longer than those achieved in randomized controlled trials, particularly in patients requiring transfer from non-PCI hospitals and during off-hours.[21,22] Between January 1999 and December 2002, the D2BT for patients transferred for primary PCI in the United States was alarmingly high: the median D2BT was 180 minutes with only 4.2% and 15% of PCIs associated with a D2BT of less than 90 minutes and 120 minutes, respectively.[22] It was

recommended that improved systems were urgently needed to address these concerns.

GROWTH AND DEVELOPMENT OF ST-ELEVATION MYOCARDIAL INFARCTION SYSTEMS

DANAMI-2[20] provided awaited evidence to support a systematic application of primary PCI. This was further supported by Keeley and colleague's[4] quantitative review of randomized trials providing strong evidence of a survival benefit favoring primary PCI over fibrinolytic therapy. The timely publications of DANAMI-2 and Keeley and colleague's[4] analysis, in 2003, became the cornerstones for the growth and development of future STEMI systems.

Several factors needed to be considered in the United States and in Canada to develop a model to improve survival of STEMI patients with the use of systematic primary PCI. This would require a redesign of the traditional care of these patients, the development of new ambulance transport protocols, changes to physician referral patterns, and changes to emergency department protocols. Such a multisectoral project would require close collaboration of all stakeholders at the regional level while taking into consideration that the beneficial outcomes of primary PCI depend on the procedure being performed in high-volume centers by experienced interventional cardiologists.[23,24] Furthermore, the need for rapid transfer of STEMI patients to a PCI center would critically depend on the availability and training of the EMS personnel.[25–28]

In 2006, Bradley and colleagues,[29] and in 2007, Nallamothu and colleagues,[30] proposed strategies for reducing D2BT (Table 1). Key strategies included (1) prehospital electrocardiogram (ECG) and EMS early activation of the STEMI team, (2) emergency department bypass with direct transfer to the catheterization laboratory by EMS, (3) the emergency department activation of the catheterization laboratory without routine consultation with a cardiologist, and (4) single-call activation. The use of the prehospital ECG was strongly recommended because it significantly reduces the time to reperfusion. It gives the opportunity to make the diagnosis in the prehospital setting and alert the receiving hospital of an incoming STEMI patient.[25–28] Diagnostic quality 12-lead ECGs can be obtained in the majority of patients.[31] The EMS can then transmit the ECGs from a moving ambulance using cellular telephones.[32] Alternatively, the EMS can be trained at independently

Table 1
Strategies for reducing door-to balloon time

Hospital-Based Strategy	Description
Prehospital ECG and activation	Greater use of prehospital ECGs by EMS, with early activation of catheterization laboratory en route
Emergency department bypass	Direct transfer to the catheterization laboratory by EMS using prehospital ECGs
Process for triaging patients and rapidly obtaining ECG in the emergency department	Establishment of physical space and guidelines in the emergency department for obtaining ECGs during triage evaluations
Emergency department activation of the catheterization laboratory	Activation of the catheterization laboratory team by emergency medicine physicians without routine cardiology consultation
Single-call activation	Establishment of a single-call system for activating the entire catheterization laboratory team
Rapid arrival of PCI team at hospital	Establishment of the expectation that team members with be available to receive the patient 20–30 min after being paged
Process of performing PCI	Clearance of elective cases during routine work hours; preparation of angioplasty tables during off-hours; clear demarcation of roles for technical and nursing staff
Prompt data feedback	Routine data monitoring of performance with provision of prompt feedback
Senior management commitment	Organizational environment with strong support by senior management, as well as a culture that fosters and sustains organizational change directed at improving D2BT
Team-based approach	Emphasis on a team-based approach that provides seamless care from arrival of ambulance to balloon inflation before reperfusion: limit handoffs, 1 team, organizational support for continuous quality improvement

Abbreviation: ECG, electrocardiogram.

From Nallamothu BK, Bradley EH, Krumholz HM. Time to treatment in primary percutaneous coronary intervention. N Engl J Med 2007;357(16):1631–8; with permission. Copyright © 2007 Massachusetts Medical Society.

interpreting the ECG and then alerting the PCI center.[33]

In 2008, on implementing these strategies, the University of Ottawa Heart Institute published the results of a citywide protocol for primary PCI that showed that guideline D2BT were more often achieved when trained paramedics independently triaged and transported patients directly to a designated primary PCI center compared with cases in which patients were referred from non-PCI hospitals.[34] The data were collected in a real-world setting in which all STEMI patients were considered for primary PCI. As depicted in Fig. 3, D2BT of less than 90 minutes were achieved in 80% of patients transferred directly from the field, and in 12% of patients transferred from non-PCI hospitals. The design of such an STEMI system allowing EMS to transport patients directly to a primary PCI center has now been shown to be associated with a significant reduction in mortality.[35]

Other institutions have also reported on the feasibility of implementing strategies to improve time to reperfusion therapy. The Mayo Clinic adopted an STEMI protocol designed to coordinate systems of care for transfer of STEMI patients between hospitals. Median D2BT for interhospital STEMI transfers decreased from 117 minutes to 103 minutes, whereas median D2BT decreased from 64 to 59 minutes in patients presenting to the PCI center.[36] The Minneapolis Heart Institute developed a standardized regionalized PCI-based treatment system for STEMI patients for 30 hospitals up to 210 miles from a PCI center. In patients referred for primary PCI between 2003 and 2006, the median first D2BT for patients less than 60 miles (zone 1) and 60 to 210 miles (zone 2) from the PCI center was 95 minutes and 120 minutes, respectively.[37] The Reperfusion of Acute Myocardial Infarction in North Carolina Emergency Departments (RACE) study showed that the establishment of a coordinated statewide system could

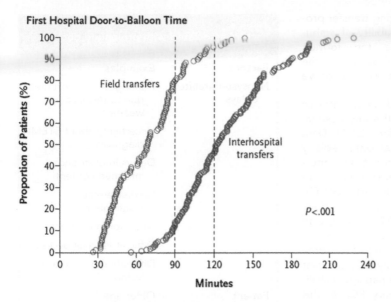

First Hospital Door-to-Balloon Time

Field transfers

Interhospital
transfers

$P<.001$

Proportion of Patients (%)

Minutes

Fig. 3. Cumulative door to balloon intervals in a citywide primary PCI program. Among patients who were transferred to a specialized center for primary PCI, D2BTs of less than 90 minutes were achieved in 80% of patients who were transferred directly from the field and in 12% of patients who were transferred from emergency departments. D2BTs of less than 120 minutes was achieved in 96% of patients transferred from the field and in 45% of patients transferred from emergency departments. (*From* Le May MR, So DY, Dionne R, et al. A citywide protocol for primary PCI in ST-segment elevation myocardial infarction. N Engl J Med 2008;358(3):236; with permission.)

significantly decrease delays in administering reperfusion therapy and improve the quality of care in STEMI patients. Median reperfusion times significantly improved: D2BT in patients presenting to PCI hospitals, 85 to 74 minutes, and in patients transferred to PCI hospital, 165 to 128 minutes. Door-to-needle times were also improved in patients treated with fibrinolytic therapy at non-PCI hospitals, 35 to 29 minutes.[38]

PERCUTANEOUS CORONARY INTERVENTION–RELATED DELAY: ROLE FOR FIBRINOLYTIC THERAPY

Primary PCI remains a resource intensive strategy requiring dedicated infrastructure, technical expertise, and organizational schemes to be implemented with the rapidity and reliability it requires.[39,40] In contrast, fibrinolytic therapy is readily available, portable, and administrable by a variety of health care practitioners. As a result, door-to-needle times are shorter and more predictable than D2BT in patients requiring transfer for primary PCI.[41] The concept of PCI-related delay (ie, D2BT minus door-to-needle time) has been suggested to clarify the impact of delaying reperfusion by choosing PCI over fibrinolytic therapy. In a pooled analysis of subjects enrolled in 25 randomized trials comparing primary PCI and fibrinolytic therapy, the risk of 30-day death was consistently reduced with primary PCI regardless of the PCI-related delay.[42] However, D2BT are

relatively short in randomized trials. When the impact of PCI-related delays on survival rates in real-world STEMI patients were assessed, the risk of death with PCI and fibrinolytic therapy were equal when the PCI-related delay was approximately 114 minutes.[41] Therefore, fibrinolytic therapy should be considered as a reperfusion strategy in settings where timely primary PCI is not consistently available (ie, when D2BT is anticipated to be greater than 120 minutes).[43]

SOURCES OF DOOR-TO-BALLOON TIME DELAYS

Longer than expected D2BT during early implementation of STEMI systems led to a strong interest in identifying sources of D2BT delays. The need for interhospital transfer for primary PCI has been consistently identified as a major contributor to PCI-related delays.[21] A critical component of the interhospital transfer process is the time spent in processing the STEMI patient in the emergency department of the sending hospital. A door-in-to-door-out (DIDO) time of 30 minutes or less is associated with lower in-hospital mortality[44] and has become a benchmark recommended by the 2013 ACC/AHA guidelines.[11] Thus, DIDO time has become a standard metric for measuring the efficiency of the sending hospital. The study by Miedema and colleagues[45] provides insights into causes of delay at sending hospitals. The most common causes of delay were (1) awaiting transport (26.4%) and (2) intrinsic emergency department delays (14.3%). Thus, standardizing transfer protocols and increasing the availability of ambulances would likely improve the former, whereas reassessing the clinical system in the emergency department would likely improve the latter.

In addition to system-related delays intrinsic to non-PCI–capable hospitals, the interhospital drive time can significantly prolong D2BT. Data from the National Cardiovascular Data Registry (NCDR) Acute Coronary Treatment and Intervention Outcomes Network Registry–Get With the Guidelines (ACTION Registry-GWTG) showed that the median interhospital drive time in the United States was 57 minutes, with less than 50% of subjects achieving D2BT of less than 120 minutes when the drive time exceeded 30 minutes.[46] Notably, a significant number of subjects in this study had a low likelihood of receiving timely primary PCI. In this cohort, the use of fibrinolytic therapy for timely reperfusion was infrequent and often delayed. These findings highlight the importance of considering fibrinolytic therapy as reperfusion therapy in settings where timely primary PCI is not reliably available.

Certain patient and index event characteristics can also be independent predictors of D2BT delays. Patients who are older, female, and free of chest pain on presentation consistently have longer D2BT.[21,22] The timing of presentation (off hours and weekends) or first-presentation hospital type (non-PCI–capable hospitals, low-volume PCI-capable hospitals, and academic centers) were also associated with significant increases in D2BT.[22] The mechanisms by which these factors affect D2BT are not entirely understood because they may reflect medical care in different settings and patient populations rather than a true deficiency of the STEMI system.

When examining the quality of STEMI systems, it is useful to examine the source and nature of D2BT delays. Nonsystem delays are prolongations in D2BT that do not reflect deficiencies in an STEMI system but rather represent necessary and often unavoidable time expenditures required for appropriate STEMI management (Table 2). Common nonsystem related delays include delays in obtaining informed consent, stabilization following cardiac arrest, the need for intubation, and difficult crossing target lesion during PCI.[47,48] Although nonsystem delays may not represent deficiencies in an STEMI system, they ultimately translate to a prolongation in D2BT with corollary increases in in-hospital mortality.[47]

| Table 2 | |
| Factors associated with prolonged door-to-balloon times | |
Factors	Examples
Nonsystem-related delays	Prolonged transport time due to distance or weather
	Uncertainty about STEMI diagnosis
	Delays in obtaining informed consent
	Cardiac arrest stabilization
	Need for intubation
	Difficult vascular access
	Difficulty crossing target lesion
Patient characteristics	Older age
	Female sex
	Not white race
	History of diabetes mellitus
	Prior coronary-artery bypass grafting
Index event characteristics	Absence of chest pain on presentation
	Anterior myocardial infarction
	Killip class >1
Hospital characteristics	Non-PCI–capable hospital
	Low-volume PCI-capable hospitals

Adapted from Brodie BR, Hansen C, Stuckey TD, et al. Door-to-balloon time with primary percutaneous coronary intervention for acute myocardial infarction impacts late cardiac mortality in high-risk patients and patients presenting early after the onset of symptoms. J Am Coll Cardiol 2006;47(2):290; and Nallamothu BK, Bates ER, Herrin J, et al. Times to treatment in transfer patients undergoing primary percutaneous coronary intervention in the United States: National Registry of Myocardial Infarction (NRMI)-3/4 analysis. Circulation 2005;111(6):764.

It has recently been reported that contemporary decreases in annual D2BT at a population level have not been associated with temporal improvements in mortality in the population of patients undergoing primary PCI.[49] This raised concerns around the true relationship between D2BT and survival. However on further evaluation of 150, 116 procedures in the NCDR CathPCI Registry, patient-specific D2BT was strongly and consistently associated with lower risk-adjusted in-hospital and 6-month mortality at the individual level.[40]

EVOLUTION OF GUIDELINES AND TIME TO REPERFUSION

Milestones relating to the evolution of STEMI ACC/AHA guidelines on time to reperfusion are listed in Table 3. Time-to-balloon inflation was first adopted as a performance standard in ACC/AHA STEMI guidelines in 1999.[50] Although previous guidelines suggested timely primary PCI as an alternative to fibrinolytic therapy, the 1999 update specified balloon inflation within 90 plus or minus 30 minutes of admission as a performance standard.[50]

In the 2004 ACC/AHA STEMI guidelines, the working definition of timely primary PCI was revised to first medical contact-to-balloon time within 90 minutes.[9] The 2004 guidelines also emphasized the importance of timely reperfusion therapy by strongly recommending fibrinolytic therapy in circumstances or settings where timely PCI is not available.

In 2008, the time from arrival to a non-PCI–capable hospital to discharge from non-PCI–capable hospital for primary PCI (ie, DIDO) was established as a formal ACC/AHA performance measure for quality of cardiovascular care.[51] In addition, D2BT as a performance measure for patients presenting to PCI-capable hospitals was expanded to include patients requiring transfer for primary PCI after presenting to a non-PCI–capable hospital.

STEMI pathways continued to evolve into regional STEMI systems, increasing the quality of care and efficiency through collaboration between neighboring hospital, EMS, and health care systems. In 2009, ACC/AHA guidelines recognized the importance of these systems by recommending the implementation of systems of care with basic tenets of the modern STEMI system: prehospital identification of STEMI and protocols for expedited transfer to PCI-capable hospitals.[15]

In the 2013 ACC/AHA STEMI guidelines, D2BT and DIDO times of 120 minutes and 30 minutes or less, respectively, were included as a benchmark for patients with STEMI presenting

Table 3
Evolution of guidelines or performance measurements regarding time to treatment of ST-elevation myocardial infarction patients

Year	Recommendations
1999[50]	Balloon inflation within 90 min of admission to hospital included as quality of care recommendation
2004[9]	Medical contact-to-balloon or D2BT of 90 min or less as benchmark (medical contact defined as arrival at the emergency department or contact with EMS). In settings where timely primary PCI is not available (ie, medical contact-to-balloon time within 90 min), fibrinolytic therapy should be performed (class I)
2006[10]	Median time from hospital arrival to PCI included in formal performance measures of cardiovascular care
2007[53]	First medical contact-to-balloon time within 90 min reinforced as a systems goal and quality of care measure in patients presenting to PCI-capable hospitals
2008[51]	Time from emergency department arrival at non-PCI–capable hospital to (1) emergency department discharge from referral facility for primary PCI and (2) primacy PCI at STEMI receiving facility added as performance measures No specific benchmark set due to controversy regarding what constitutes an unacceptable delay
2009[15]	Communities should develop an STEMI system of care that follows quality of care standards set forth by AHA that include transfer protocols, prehospital identification of STEMI, and multidisciplinary team assessment of clinical outcomes and performance measures
2013[11]	Addition of first medical contact-to-balloon time of 120 min or less as a system goal for patients undergoing transfer for primary PCI after presenting to non-PCI–capable hospital DIDO time of 30 min or less included at benchmark for non-PCI–capable hospitals transferring patients for primary PCI Reiteration of first medical contact-to-balloon time system goal of 90 min or less for patients presenting to PCI-capable hospitals In settings where timely primary PCI is not available (ie, medical contact-to-balloon time within 120 min), fibrinolytic therapy should be performed (class I)

to non-PCI–capable hospitals.[11] As with previous guidelines, the writing committee reiterated the importance of emphasizing timeliness and appropriateness, rather than simply choice, of reperfusion therapy, with fibrinolytic therapy indicated when anticipated first medical contact-to-balloon time exceeds 120 minutes. Fig. 4 depicts pathways and system goals for patients presenting with STEMI according to the guidelines.

THE MODERN ST-ELEVATION MYOCARDIAL INFARCTION SYSTEM: A WINDOW TO SHORTER DOOR-TO-BALLOON TIMES

The implementation of primary PCI for STEMI has significantly evolved over the last 2 decades into the modern STEMI system, which typically involves a collaborative effort by EMS systems, neighboring hospitals, and health care systems.[34] Fundamental components of the modern STEMI system include: the use of ECG by paramedics in the field; the option to bypass emergency departments on route to a PCI-capable hospital; the deployment of the PCI team by emergency department physicians without specialist consultation; and standardized protocols for medical assessment, treatment, and consent.[29,34,35,52] These basic tenets promote a rapid, standardized process for early STEMI diagnosis, management, and transfer, thereby increasing efficiency and collaboration at the departmental, hospital, and regional levels. Additionally, in many STEMI systems the efficacy of STEMI pathways has been further improved by the centralization of primary PCI (ie, a single PCI-capable hospital is responsible

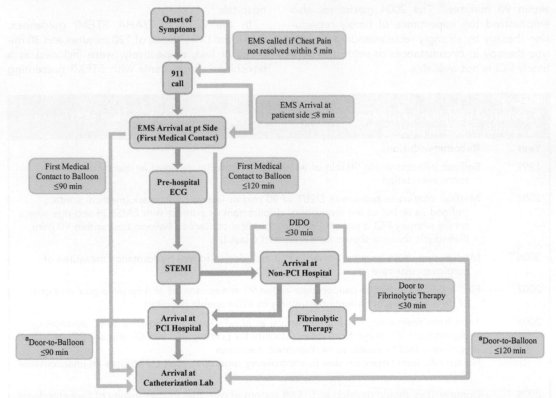

Fig. 4. Algorithm showing the steps associated with reperfusion therapy in STEMI patients and the recommended ACC/AHA guidelines to limit delays in reperfusion therapy. First medical contact-to-balloon time has become a formal quality of care measure and a major benchmark in the ACC/AHA STEMI guidelines. [a] In principle, first medical contact is the place where reperfusion can be initiated. In such cases, the 2004 guidelines indicated that the time of first medical contact for primary PCI (ie, start time) was arrival at the PCI hospital in situations in which EMS was not capable of administering prehospital fibrinolytic therapy. Because prehospital fibrinolytic therapy is seldom used in the United States, D2BT has been adopted as a quality of performance for measuring time to reperfusion. Pt, patient. (Data from Masoudi FA, Bonow RO, Brindis RG, et al. ACC/AHA 2008 statement on performance measurement and reperfusion therapy: a report of the ACC/AHA Task Force on Performance Measures (Work Group to address the challenges of Performance Measurement and Reperfusion Therapy). J Am Coll Cardiol 2008;52(24):2100–12.)

for the provision of primary PCI within a prespecified catchment area).[34] This process further standardizes and simplifies STEMI pathways for patients referred for primary PCI by paramedics or non-PCI–capable hospitals. It provides larger volumes to assigned PCI-capable hospitals, allowing the development and maintenance of primary PCI expertise, a known independent predictor of shorter D2BT and reduced mortality in STEMI.[14,39]

In the modern STEMI system, the use of ECG by EMS personnel and the option to bypass emergency departments on route to a PCI-capable hospital is of particular importance. Through training and a standardized referral process, EMS personnel can now accurately diagnose and refer STEMI patients directly to the catheterization laboratory of a PCI-capable hospital. Regional STEMI models have been implemented successfully across North America, and this has resulted in palpable reductions in D2BT, morbidity, and mortality.[34,35]

REFERENCES

1. Brodie BR, Hansen C, Stuckey TD, et al. Door-to-balloon time with primary percutaneous coronary intervention for acute myocardial infarction impacts late cardiac mortality in high-risk patients and patients presenting early after the onset of symptoms. J Am Coll Cardiol 2006;47(2):289–95.

2. Cannon CP, Gibson CM, Lambrew CT, et al. Relationship of symptom-onset-to-balloon time and door-to-balloon time with mortality in patients undergoing angioplasty for acute myocardial infarction. JAMA 2000;283(22):2941–7.

3. McNamara RL, Wang Y, Herrin J, et al. Effect of door-to-balloon time on mortality in patients with ST-segment elevation myocardial infarction. J Am Coll Cardiol 2006;47(11):2180–6.

4. Keeley EC, Boura JA, Grines CL. Primary angioplasty versus intravenous thrombolytic therapy for acute myocardial infarction: a quantitative review of 23 randomised trials. Lancet 2003; 361(9351):13–20.

5. Le May MR, Davies RF, Labinaz M, et al. Hospitalization costs of primary stenting versus thrombolysis in acute myocardial infarction: cost analysis of the Canadian STAT Study. Circulation 2003;108(21): 2624–30.

6. Berger PB, Ellis SG, Holmes DR Jr, et al. Relationship between delay in performing direct coronary angioplasty and early clinical outcome in patients with acute myocardial infarction: results from the global use of strategies to open occluded arteries in Acute Coronary Syndromes (GUSTO-IIb) trial. Circulation 1999;100(1):14–20.

7. De Luca G, Suryapranata H, Ottervanger JP, et al. Time delay to treatment and mortality in primary angioplasty for acute myocardial infarction: every minute of delay counts. Circulation 2004;109(10): 1223–5.

8. Terkelsen CJ, Sorensen JT, Maeng M, et al. System delay and mortality among patients with STEMI treated with primary percutaneous coronary intervention. JAMA 2010;304(7):763–71.

9. Antman EM, Anbe DT, Armstrong PW, et al. ACC/AHA guidelines for the management of patients with ST-elevation myocardial infarction; a report of the American College of Cardiology/American Heart Association Task Force on Practice Guidelines (Committee to Revise the 1999 Guidelines for the Management of patients with acute myocardial infarction). J Am Coll Cardiol 2004; 44(3):E1–211.

10. Krumholz HM, Anderson JL, Brooks NH, et al. ACC/AHA clinical performance measures for adults with ST-elevation and non-ST-elevation myocardial infarction: a report of the American College of Cardiology/American Heart Association Task Force on Performance Measures (Writing Committee to Develop Performance Measures on ST-Elevation and Non-ST-Elevation Myocardial Infarction). J Am Coll Cardiol 2006;47(1):236–65.

11. O'Gara PT, Kushner FG, Ascheim DD, et al. 2013 ACCF/AHA guideline for the management of ST-elevation myocardial infarction: a report of the American College of Cardiology Foundation/American Heart Association Task Force on Practice Guidelines. J Am Coll Cardiol 2013;61(4):e78–140.

12. Antman EM, Hand M, Armstrong PW, et al. 2007 focused update of the ACC/AHA 2004 guidelines for the management of patients with ST-elevation myocardial infarction: a report of the American College of Cardiology/American Heart Association Task Force on Practice Guidelines: developed in collaboration with the Canadian Cardiovascular Society endorsed by the American Academy of Family Physicians: 2007 Writing Group to review new evidence and update the ACC/AHA 2004 guidelines for the management of patients with ST-elevation myocardial infarction, writing on behalf of the 2004 Writing Committee. Circulation 2008;117(2): 296–329.

13. Masoudi FA, Bonow RO, Brindis RG, et al. ACC/AHA 2008 statement on performance measurement and reperfusion therapy: a report of the ACC/AHA Task Force on Performance Measures (Work Group to address the challenges of performance measurement and reperfusion therapy). J Am Coll Cardiol 2008;52(24):2100–12.

14. Nallamothu BK, Wang Y, Magid DJ, et al. Relation between hospital specialization with primary percutaneous coronary intervention and clinical outcomes

in ST-segment elevation myocardial infarction: National Registry of Myocardial Infarction-4 analysis. Circulation 2006;113(2):222–9.

15. Kushner FG, Hand M, Smith SC Jr, et al. 2009 focused updates: ACC/AHA guidelines for the management of patients with ST-elevation myocardial infarction (updating the 2004 guideline and 2007 focused update) and ACC/AHA/SCAI guidelines on percutaneous coronary intervention (updating the 2005 guideline and 2007 focused update) a report of the American College of Cardiology Foundation/American Heart Association Task Force on Practice Guidelines. J Am Coll Cardiol 2009;54(23):2205–41.

16. Widimsky P, Groch L, Zelizko M, et al. Multicentre randomized trial comparing transport to primary angioplasty vs immediate thrombolysis vs combined strategy for patients with acute myocardial infarction presenting to a community hospital without a catheterization laboratory. The PRAGUE study. Eur Heart J 2000;21(10):823–31.

17. Widimsky P, Budesinsky T, Vorac D, et al. Long distance transport for primary angioplasty vs immediate thrombolysis in acute myocardial infarction. Final results of the randomized national multicentre trial–PRAGUE-2. Eur Heart J 2003;24(1):94–104.

18. Vermeer F, Oude Ophuis AJ, vd Berg EJ, et al. Prospective randomised comparison between thrombolysis, rescue PTCA, and primary PTCA in patients with extensive myocardial infarction admitted to a hospital without PTCA facilities: a safety and feasibility study. Heart 1999;82(4):426–31.

19. Grines CL, Westerhausen DR Jr, Grines LL, et al. A randomized trial of transfer for primary angioplasty versus on-site thrombolysis in patients with high-risk myocardial infarction: the Air Primary Angioplasty in Myocardial Infarction study. J Am Coll Cardiol 2002;39(11):1713–9.

20. Andersen HR, Nielsen TT, Rasmussen K, et al. A comparison of coronary angioplasty with fibrinolytic therapy in acute myocardial infarction. N Engl J Med 2003;349(8):733–42.

21. Angeja BG, Gibson CM, Chin R, et al. Predictors of door-to-balloon delay in primary angioplasty. Am J Cardiol 2002;89(10):1156–61.

22. Nallamothu BK, Bates ER, Herrin J, et al. Times to treatment in transfer patients undergoing primary percutaneous coronary intervention in the United States: National Registry of Myocardial Infarction (NRMI)-3/4 analysis. Circulation 2005;111(6):761–7.

23. Magid DJ, Calonge BN, Rumsfeld JS, et al. Relation between hospital primary angioplasty volume and mortality for patients with acute MI treated with primary angioplasty vs thrombolytic therapy. JAMA 2000;284(24):3131–8.

24. Vakili BA, Kaplan R, Brown DL. Volume-outcome relation for physicians and hospitals performing angioplasty for acute myocardial infarction in New York state. Circulation 2001;104(18):2171–6.

25. Curtis JP, Portnay EL, Wang Y, et al. The prehospital electrocardiogram and time to reperfusion in patients with acute myocardial infarction, 2000-2002: findings from the National Registry of Myocardial Infarction-4. J Am Coll Cardiol 2006; 47(8):1544–52.

26. Foster DB, Dufendach JH, Barkdoll CM, et al. Prehospital recognition of AMI using independent nurse/paramedic 12-lead ECG evaluation: impact on in-hospital times to thrombolysis in a rural community hospital. Am J Emerg Med 1994;12(1): 25–31.

27. Karagounis L, Ipsen SK, Jessop MR, et al. Impact of field-transmitted electrocardiography on time to in-hospital thrombolytic therapy in acute myocardial infarction. Am J Cardiol 1990;66(10):786–91.

28. Kereiakes DJ, Gibler WB, Martin LH, et al. Relative importance of emergency medical system transport and the prehospital electrocardiogram on reducing hospital time delay to therapy for acute myocardial infarction: a preliminary report from the Cincinnati Heart Project. Am Heart J 1992; 123(4 Pt 1):835–40.

29. Bradley EH, Herrin J, Wang Y, et al. Strategies for reducing the door-to-balloon time in acute myocardial infarction. N Engl J Med 2006;355(22):2308–20.

30. Nallamothu BK, Bradley EH, Krumholz HM. Time to treatment in primary percutaneous coronary intervention. N Engl J Med 2007;357(16):1631–8.

31. Aufderheide TP, Hendley GE, Thakur RK, et al. The diagnostic impact of prehospital 12-lead electrocardiography. Ann Emerg Med 1990;19(11):1280–7.

32. Grim P, Feldman T, Martin M, et al. Cellular telephone transmission of 12-lead electrocardiograms from ambulance to hospital. Am J Cardiol 1987; 60(8):715–20.

33. Le May MR, Dionne R, Maloney J, et al. Diagnostic performance and potential clinical impact of advanced care paramedic interpretation of ST-segment elevation myocardial infarction in the field. CJEM 2006;8(6):401–7.

34. Le May MR, So DY, Dionne R, et al. A citywide protocol for primary PCI in ST-segment elevation myocardial infarction. N Engl J Med 2008;358(3): 231–40.

35. Le May MR, Wells GA, So DY, et al. Reduction in mortality as a result of direct transport from the field to a receiving center for primary percutaneous coronary intervention. J Am Coll Cardiol 2012; 60(14):1223–30.

36. Ting HH, Rihal CS, Gersh BJ, et al. Regional systems of care to optimize timeliness of reperfusion therapy for ST-elevation myocardial infarction: the Mayo Clinic STEMI Protocol. Circulation 2007; 116(7):729–36.

37. Henry TD, Sharkey SW, Burke MN, et al. A regional system to provide timely access to percutaneous coronary intervention for ST-elevation myocardial infarction. Circulation 2007;116(7):721–8.

38. Jollis JG, Roettig ML, Aluko AO, et al. Implementation of a statewide system for coronary reperfusion for ST-segment elevation myocardial infarction. JAMA 2007;298(20):2371–80.

39. Canto JG, Every NR, Magid DJ, et al. The volume of primary angioplasty procedures and survival after acute myocardial infarction. National Registry of Myocardial Infarction 2 Investigators. N Engl J Med 2000;342(21):1573–80.

40. Nallamothu BK, Normand SL, Wang Y, et al. Relation between door-to-balloon times and mortality after primary percutaneous coronary intervention over time: a retrospective study. Lancet 2015; 385(9973):1114–22.

41. Pinto DS, Kirtane AJ, Nallamothu BK, et al. Hospital delays in reperfusion for ST-elevation myocardial infarction: implications when selecting a reperfusion strategy. Circulation 2006;114(19):2019–25.

42. Boersma E. Does time matter? A pooled analysis of randomized clinical trials comparing primary percutaneous coronary intervention and in-hospital fibrinolysis in acute myocardial infarction patients. Eur Heart J 2006;27(7):779–88.

43. Steg PG, James SK, Atar D, et al. ESC Guidelines for the management of acute myocardial infarction in patients presenting with ST-segment elevation. Eur Heart J 2012;33(20):2569–619.

44. Wang TY, Nallamothu BK, Krumholz HM, et al. Association of door-in to door-out time with reperfusion delays and outcomes among patients transferred for primary percutaneous coronary intervention. JAMA 2011;305(24):2540–7.

45. Miedema MD, Newell MC, Duval S, et al. Causes of delay and associated mortality in patients transferred with ST-segment-elevation myocardial infarction. Circulation 2011;124(15):1636–44.

46. Vora AN, Holmes DN, Rokos I, et al. Fibrinolysis use among patients requiring interhospital transfer for ST-segment elevation myocardial infarction care: a report from the US National Cardiovascular Data Registry. JAMA Intern Med 2015;175(2): 207–15.

47. Swaminathan RV, Wang TY, Kaltenbach LA, et al. Nonsystem reasons for delay in door-to-balloon time and associated in-hospital mortality. a report from the National Cardiovascular Data Registry. J Am Coll Cardiol 2013;61(16):1688–95.

48. Cotoni DA, Roe MT, Li S, et al. Frequency of nonsystem delays in ST-elevation myocardial infarction patients undergoing primary percutaneous coronary intervention and implications for door-to-balloon time reporting (from the American Heart Association Mission: Lifeline program). Am J Cardiol 2014;114(1):24–8.

49. Menees DS, Peterson ED, Wang Y, et al. Door-to-balloon time and mortality among patients undergoing primary PCI. N Engl J Med 2013;369(10): 901–9.

50. Ryan TJ, Antman EM, Brooks NH, et al. 1999 update: ACC/AHA guidelines for the management of patients with acute myocardial infarction. A report of the American College of Cardiology/American Heart Association Task Force on Practice Guidelines (Committee on Management of Acute Myocardial Infarction). J Am Coll Cardiol 1999; 34(3):890–911.

51. Krumholz HM, Anderson JL, Bachelder BL, et al. ACC/AHA 2008 performance measures for adults with ST-elevation and non-ST-elevation myocardial infarction: a report of the American College of Cardiology/American Heart Association Task Force on Performance Measures (Writing Committee to Develop Performance Measures for ST-Elevation and Non-ST-Elevation Myocardial Infarction) Developed in Collaboration With the American Academy of Family Physicians and American College of Emergency Physicians Endorsed by the American Association of Cardiovascular and Pulmonary Rehabilitation, Society for Cardiovascular Angiography and Interventions, and Society of Hospital Medicine. J Am Coll Cardiol 2008;52(24):2046–99.

52. Bradley EH, Curry LA, Webster TR, et al. Achieving rapid door-to-balloon times: how top hospitals improve complex clinical systems. Circulation 2006;113(8):1079–85.

53. Antman EM, Hand M, Armstrong PW, et al. 2007 focused update of the ACC/AHA 2004 guidelines for the management of patients with ST-elevation myocardial infarction: a report of the American College of Cardiology/American Heart Association Task Force on Practice Guidelines. J Am Coll Cardiol 2008;51(2):210–47.

Reperfusion Options for ST Elevation Myocardial Infarction Patients with Expected Delays to Percutaneous Coronary Intervention

David M. Larson, MD[a,b,*], Peter McKavanagh, MD, PhD[c],
Timothy D. Henry, MD[d], Warren J. Cantor, MD[e,f]

KEYWORDS

- ST segment elevation myocardial infarction • Interhospital transfer • Pharmacoinvasive
- Percutaneous coronary intervention • Facilitated PCI • Rural

KEY POINTS

- Currently only one-third of US hospitals have the capability to perform primary percutaneous coronary intervention (PCI) 24/7.
- Patients with ST segment elevation myocardial infarction (STEMI) presenting to non-PCI hospitals should be transferred for primary PCI if it can be performed within 120 minutes of first medical contact.
- Unless there are contraindications, fibrinolysis should be administered to STEMI patients who present to non-PCI hospitals if anticipated time to PCI exceeds 120 minutes.
- STEMI patients who receive fibrinolysis should be transferred rapidly to PCI centers and undergo immediate rescue PCI if there is failed reperfusion or hemodynamic instability.
- Patients who have reperfused and are stable should undergo early routine coronary angiography and PCI within 24 hours of fibrinolysis.

INTRODUCTION

The primary goal in treating ST segment elevation myocardial infarction (STEMI) is rapid restoration of coronary arterial flow and reperfusion of the affected myocardium. In the 1980s, fibrinolysis was the only means to accomplish this. Over the last 2 decades, primary percutaneous coronary intervention (PCI) has emerged as the preferred reperfusion strategy if it can be performed in a timely manner by skilled operators. However, only about one-third of US hospitals currently have the capability to perform primary PCI 24/7.[1] This means that a substantial number of STEMI patients will need to either have the ambulance bypass the closest hospital or be transferred from non-PCI hospitals. Any

Author Disclosures: None of the contributing authors have financial disclosures or relationships with industry that pertain to this article.

[a] University of Minnesota Medical School, Minneapolis Heart Institute Foundation, Abbott Northwestern Hospital, 920 East 28th Street, Suite 100, Minneapolis, MN 55407, USA; [b] Division of Cardiology, Ridgeview Medical Center, 500 South Maple Street, Waconia, MN 55387, USA; [c] Division of Cardiology, St. Michael's Hospital, 30 Bond Street, Toronto, ON M5B 1W8, Canada; [d] Division of Cardiology, Cedars-Sinai Heart Institute, 127 South San Vicente Boulevard, Suite A3100, Los Angeles, CA 90048, USA; [e] Division of Cardiology, Southlake Regional Health Center, 596 Davis Drive, Newmarket, ON L3Y 2P9, Canada; [f] Department of Medicine, University of Toronto, 27 King's College Circle, Toronto, ON M5S, Canada

* Corresponding author. University of Minnesota Medical School, Minneapolis Heart Institute Foundation, Abbott Northwestern Hospital, 920 East 28th Street, Suite 100, Minneapolis, MN 55407, USA.
E-mail address: david.larson@ridgeviewmedical.org

Intervent Cardiol Clin 5 (2016) 439–450
http://dx.doi.org/10.1016/j.iccl.2016.06.004
2211-7458/16/$ – see front matter © 2016 Elsevier Inc. All rights reserved.

significant delays may negate the benefit of primary PCI over fibrinolysis. Current guidelines from the European Society of Cardiology and the American Heart Association/American College of Cardiology Foundation recommend fibrinolysis if PCI cannot be performed within 120 minutes from first medical contact.[2,3] Despite these recommendations, recent data from the US National Cardiovascular Data Registry showed that only 51% of STEMI patients transferred for Primary PCI achieved the recommended first door to balloon time of less than 120 minutes.[1] Data from Quebec,[4] where 65% of patients were transferred for primary PCI, found that 80% were not treated within the guideline recommended door to balloon time (90 minutes at that time) and that reperfusion delivered outside of guideline recommended delays was associated with significantly increased 30 day mortality. Likewise, in Denmark, which has an organized transfer system for STEMI, 65% of transferred STEMI patients experienced a system-related delay of greater than 120 minutes, which was associated independently with increased mortality.[5]

Several randomized controlled trials have evaluated strategies combining fibrinolysis and PCI, which has been termed "facilitated PCI" or "pharmacoinvasive strategy" (routine early PCI after fibrinolysis). This article reviews reperfusion options for STEMI patients who do not have timely access to primary PCI.

CASE PRESENTATION

A 51-year-old male with no prior history of cardiac disease had sudden onset of substernal chest pain at 1:30 AM. His wife drove him to a rural community hospital, located 100 miles from the nearest PCI capable hospital, arriving at 2:20 AM, nearly 1 hour after the onset of chest pain. His electrocardiograph showed anterolateral ST segment elevation (Fig. 1). What are the options for reperfusion therapy in this patient with a high-risk (anterolateral) myocardial infarction (MI) presenting early after the onset of symptoms (Box 1)?

REPERFUSION STRATEGIES
Full-Dose Fibrinolysis
Full-dose fibrinolysis remains the guideline recommended reperfusion strategy when PCI is not available within 120 minutes of first medical contact.[2,3] The advantages are accessibility and ease of administration, including the ability to be given in the prehospital setting. This strategy is most effective when administered early (especially within 1 hour of symptom onset) and in high-risk STEMI patients (eg, anterior MI). Unfortunately, only 50% to 60% of patients treated with fibrinolysis achieve restoration of TIMI (Thrombolysis in Myocardial Infarction) 3 flow.[6–8] And of course the other downside is the risk of bleeding, especially intracranial hemorrhage, which can occur in 1% to 3% of patients.

Transfer for Rescue Percutaneous Coronary Intervention After Fibrinolysis
For patients who receive fibrinolysis, randomized trials have shown a benefit to transfer for rescue PCI for failed reperfusion. The MERLIN (Middlesbrough Early Revascularization to Limit Infarction) trial, a randomized trial of rescue angioplasty versus a conservative approach for failed fibrinolysis, showed a reduction in 30- day revascularization (6.5% vs 20.1%; P<.1), but no difference in 30 day all-cause mortality (9.8% vs 11%; P = .7).[9] The REACT (Rescue Angioplasty after Failed Thrombolytic Therapy for Acute Myocardial Infarction) Trial was multicenter trial in the United Kingdom involving 427 STEMI patients comparing rescue PCI with repeat fibrinolysis or conservative treatment. The trial was stopped early owing to slow enrollment. The primary endpoint was a composite of death, reinfarction, stroke, or severe heart failure within 6 months. The rate of event-free survival for those treated with rescue PCI was 84.8% compared with 70.1% and 68.7% treated conservatively or with repeat fibrinolysis, respectively. There were no differences in all-cause mortality.[10] Subsequently, a metaanalysis published in 2007[11] showed no reduction in all-cause mortality, although there was a significant reduction in heart failure and reinfarction with rescue PCI compared with conservative therapy. One of the challenges with rescue PCI is the limited ability of noninvasive assessment based on chest pain and resolution of ST elevation to predict accurately whether reperfusion has been successful or not. Furthermore, waiting 60 to 90 minutes after fibrinolysis to see if reperfusion occurs before transfer of a patient will likely result in further delays and loss of an opportunity for myocardial salvage.

Transfer for Primary Percutaneous Coronary Intervention
More than 20 years ago, the PAMI trial first showed that immediate angioplasty resulted in restoration of TIMI 3 coronary flow in 90% of STEMI patients with a favorable decrease in short term mortality compared with patients

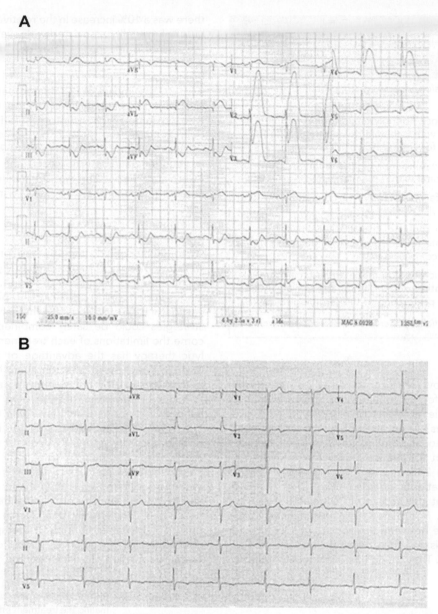

Fig. 1. (A) Initial electrocardiograph (ECG) obtained after arrival at the non-PCI hospital. (B) ECG after percutaneous coronary intervention.

treated with fibrinolysis (2.6 vs 6.5%; P = .06).[12] Subsequent randomized controlled trials and metaanalyses confirmed primary PCI as the preferred reperfusion strategy if it can be performed in a timely manner.[13,14] The main limitation with primary PCI as the reperfusion strategy for STEMI is limited availability and the logistic challenges, especially for transferred patients, leading to delayed reperfusion. Beginning around the turn of this century, several trials from Europe demonstrated superior outcomes in STEMI patients transferred for primary PCI compared with fibrinolysis.[15–18] These trials from the Czech Republic and Denmark enrolled patients who were in organized transfer systems with relatively short transfer times. Subsequently other observational studies from US centers with highly organized transfer systems demonstrated that transfer from non-PCI hospitals was feasible and safe with acceptable door to balloon times.[19,20] However, these results do not support the superiority of primary PCI over fibrinolytic therapy if delays exceed the guideline recommended door to balloon times.

So, how long of a delay to reperfusion to transfer a patient for primary PCI is acceptable in terms of mortality benefit over fibrinolysis? In an attempt to answer this question, Pinto and colleagues[21] analyzed registry data from the National Registry of Myocardial Infarction 2, 3, and 4, involving nearly 200,000 STEMI patients enrolled from 1994 to 2003, looking at the impact of PCI-related delays on mortality. PCI-related delay was defined as the difference between the door to needle time for fibrinolysis and the door to balloon time for primary PCI. They found that in the total population there was a 10% increase in the relative risk of in-hospital mortality associated with every 30-minute increase in the PCI related delay. The in-hospital survival benefit was lost when the PCI-related delay exceeded 114 minutes (Fig. 2). The impact of PCI-related delay on survival varied by patient characteristics. In patients who presented with symptom duration of less than 2 hours, the survival benefit of primary PCI was lost at a PCI-related delay of 94 minutes. In younger patients (<65 years), the maximum PCI-related delay time was 71 minutes and in anterior infarction the time was 115 minutes.

Combining Percutaneous Coronary Intervention and Fibrinolysis

Although fibrinolytic therapy and primary PCI were traditionally considered mutually exclusive and competing treatment strategies, the challenges in performing primary PCI rapidly led investigators to investigate whether these 2 strategies could be safely combined to overcome the limitations of each treatment. Fibrinolytic therapy has the advantage of availability (even in the prehospital setting) and is effective in establishing TIMI 3 flow if given early (within 2 hours of symptom onset).[22] On the other hand, PCI is not as readily available but is ultimately more effective in opening the infarct-related coronary artery. Two terms have been used to describe the process of combining fibrinolytic therapy with PCI into a single reperfusion therapy: facilitated PCI and pharmacoinvasive therapy (Table 1). The principle difference between the 2 is actually trial design, including timing of PCI after fibrinolytic therapy, use of clopidogrel as an adjunct to fibrinolysis, and target population. To illustrate the point, the

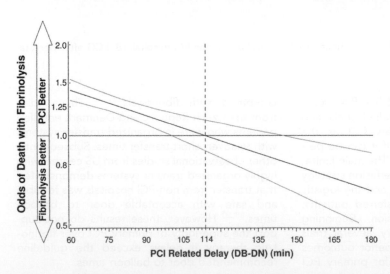

Fig. 2. Multivariable analysis estimating the treatment effect of reperfusion therapy with percutaneous coronary intervention (PCI) or fibrinolysis based on increasing PCI-related delay. After correction for patient- and hospital-based factors, the time at which odds of death with PCI were equal to those for fibrinolysis occurred when the PCI-related delay was approximately 114 minutes. DB-DN, door-to-ballon (DB)-door-to-needle (DN). (*From* Pinto DS, Kirtane AJ, Nallamothu BK, et al. Hospital delays in reperfusion for ST-elevation myocardial infarction: implications when selecting a reperfusion strategy. Circulation 2006;114(19): 2022; with permission.)

Table 1 Comparison between pharmacoinvasive and facilitated PCI trials		
Pharmacoinvasive vs Facilitated PCI Trials: What is the Difference?		
	Facilitated	Pharmacoinvasive
Trial design	Fibrinolytic + PCI vs PCI alone	Fibrinolytic + PCI vs conservative therapy (Ischemia guided PCI)
Enrollment	PCI hospitals, non-PCI hospitals and prehospital	Non-PCI hospitals and prehospital
Time to PCI	Shorter	Longer
Clopidogrel loading	No	Yes

CARESS-in-AMI (Combined Abciximab REte-plase Stent Study in Acute Myocardial Infarction) trial was described as a facilitated PCI trial in clinicaltrial.gov but a pharmacoinvasive trial when it was published.[23]

Facilitated Percutaneous Coronary Intervention

The original concept of facilitated PCI involved administration of pharmacotherapy (fibrinolytic agents and/or glycoprotein [GP]IIb/IIa inhibitors) to initiate reperfusion while the patient was en route to the catheterization laboratory. Several observational studies showed better outcomes in patients who had patent infarct arteries on arrival to the catheterization laboratory compared with patients with occluded arteries. It was therefore hypothesized that achieving pharmacologic reperfusion before PCI would improve clinical outcomes. Unfortunately, 2 large randomized trials did not show a benefit from a facilitated PCI strategy. The first trial, ASSENT-4 PCI (Assessment of the Safety and Efficacy of a New Treatment Strategy for Acute Myocardial Infarction), randomized patients to full-dose tenecteplase combined with PCI versus primary PCI. The trial was stopped early because of an increase in-hospital death in the facilitated PCI group (6% vs 3%; $P = .0105$).[24] The second was the FINESSE (Facilitated Intervention with Enhanced Reperfusion Speed to Stop Events) trial, which randomized STEMI patients presenting within 6 hours of symptom onset into 1 of 3 groups: abciximab alone with PCI, abciximab and half-dose reteplase with PCI, or primary PCI.[25] The trial was stopped prematurely owing to slow enrollment. The primary endpoint, a composite of all-cause death, ventricular fibrillation, cardiogenic shock, and congestive heart failure at 90 days, was not different in the 3 groups. Mortality rates at 90 days were 5.2% (abciximab + reteplase–

facilitated PCI), 5.5% (abciximab-facilitated PCI), and 4.5% (primary PCI; $P = .49$). A metaanalysis of facilitated PCI trials by Keeley and colleagues[26] (that did not include the FINESSE trial) showed no advantage of facilitated PCI compared with primary PCI and perhaps even harm. In response to this study and an accompanying editorial,[27] the enthusiasm for facilitated PCI rapidly waned.

However, a closer look at the data in the metaanalysis warrants further consideration. There were 17 randomized trials included in the analysis, of which 9 trials used only GP IIb/IIIa inhibitors and no fibrinolytics. In the 8 trials in which fibrinolytic therapy was used, most were small, and 75% did not allow antiplatelet agents including no P2Y12 inhibitors. In addition, one-half of the trials were before routine stenting and the majority of patients were enrolled either at a PCI hospital or a short distance transfer (Table 2). Therefore, these studies really were not designed to address the optimal strategy in patients with expected delays of greater than 120 minutes to PCI. In a reanalysis of the ASSENT-IV data, stratified by enrollment site, the highest mortality was in patients at the PCI hospital randomized to facilitated PCI (8.4%) compared with 6.5% at the non–PCI-capable hospital and 3.1% in patients randomized in the prehospital setting. The authors noted that few patients actually fit the target population for which facilitated PCI was designed.[28] Herrmann and colleagues[29] performed a retrospective analysis of the FINESSE trial stratified by enrollment site (hub vs spoke hospital), symptom onset to randomization time and TIMI risk score. Patients randomized at the non-PCI (spoke) hospital, with symptom to randomization time of <4 hours or longer and with a TIMI risk score of 3 or greater had a significant improvement in the 90-day composite endpoint (death, ventricular fibrillation at 48 hours, cardiogenic shock, or congestive heart failure) as well as 1-year survival with facilitated PCI.

Table 2
Trials in the Keeley metaanalysis that used a fibrinolytic

RCT Name	Year	Lytic	Antiplatelet (with Lytic)	Stents	Enrollment Location
SAMI (n = 58)	1992	STK	None	No	PCI hospital
LIMI (n = 74)	1999	tPA	None	No	Non-PCI hospital <30 miles
PRAGUE (n = 100)	1999	STK	None	No	Non-PCI hospital <45 miles
PACT (n = 302)	1999	tPA (1/2 dose)	None	26%	PCI hospital
GRACIA 2 (n = 104)	2003	TNK	None	Yes	PCI hospital, 67% Non-PCI hospital, 33%
BRAVE (n = 125)	2004	Reteplase (1/2 dose)	Abciximab	Yes	Non-PCI hospital <30 miles
ADVANCE MI (n = 69)	2005	TNK (1/2 dose)	Eptifibitide	Yes	
ASSENT-IV (n = 828)	2006	TNK	None	Yes	PCI hospital, 45% Non-PCI hospital, 35% Amb, 20%

Abbreviations: Amb, ambulance; PCI, percutaneous coronary intervention; TNK, tenectaplase; tPA, tissue plasminogen activator; STK, streptokinase.

With the exception of ASSENT-IV, most of these trials were small, about one-half did not use stents, 6 of the 8 did not use antiplatelets and most patients were randomized at or within short distances of the PCI center. ASSENT IV used full-dose TNK without antiplatelet and contributed >50% of the patients in this metaanalysis.

Pharmacoinvasive Percutaneous Coronary Intervention

Unlike the facilitated PCI trials that used fibrinolytic versus no fibrinolytic therapy for all STEMI patients en route to the catheterization laboratory, the pharmacoinvasive strategy trials focused on STEMI patients presenting to non-PCI hospitals who could not undergo timely primary PCI and therefore received fibrinolytic therapy as standard of care. Most of the trials

compared routine early PCI after fibrinolysis compared with a more conservative ischemia-guided approach (**Fig. 3**).

Two small randomized trials from Germany, SIAM-III (Southwest German Interventional Study in Acute Myocardial Infarction)[30] and Canada, CAPITAL AMI (Combined Angioplasty and Pharmacological Intervention versus Thrombolysis Alone in Acute Myocardial Infarction)[31] demonstrated benefit of immediate transfer for PCI

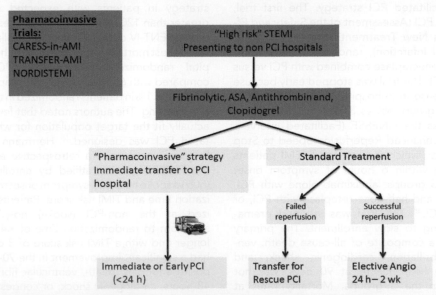

Fig. 3. Trial design of pharmacoinvasive percutaneous coronary intervention (PCI) trials.

after fibrinolysis without increased bleeding compared with fibrinolysis with rescue or delayed angioplasty. These were followed by several large randomized trials. The first of these trials was CARESS-in-AMI, which included high-risk STEMI patients who were admitted to non-PCI hospitals in France, Italy, or Poland.[23] All patients received half-dose reteplase, abciximab, heparin, and aspirin and were randomized to immediate transfer for PCI or admission to the non-PCI hospital with transfer for rescue PCI if needed. The primary outcome (composite of death, reinfarction, or refractory ischemia at 30 days) occurred in 4.4% of the immediate PCI group compared with 10.7% in the standard care/rescue PCI group (hazard ratio, 0.4%; 95% CI, 0.21–0.76; P = .004).

The TRANSFER-AMI (Trial of Routine Angioplasty and Stenting after Fibrinolysis to Enhance Reperfusion in Acute Myocardial Infarction) trial randomized high-risk STEMI patients presenting to non-PCI hospitals in Canada to full-dose tenectaplase and immediate transfer for PCI versus tenectaplase and transfer for rescue PCI if the patient had persistent ST segment elevation, chest pain, or hemodynamic instability.[32] The primary endpoint, a composite of death, reinfarction, recurrent ischemia, and new or worsening congestive heart failure or cardiogenic shock within 30 days, was significantly decreased in patients receiving pharmacoinvasive PCI (11%) compared with patients receiving standard care/ rescue PCI (17%; P = .004).

In the NORDISTEMI (NORwegian study on DIstrict treatment of ST-Elevation Myocardial Infarction) trial, 266 patients with acute STEMI living in rural areas with greater than 90-minute transfer times were treated with standard dose tenectaplase, aspirin, enoxaparin, and clopidogrel and then randomized to transfer for PCI or to standard treatment at the non-PCI hospital with transfer only if indicated for rescue PCI.[33] The primary endpoint, a composite of death, reinfarction, stroke, or new ischemia at 12 months, did not show a significant difference. However, a composite of death, reinfarction, or stroke at 12 months was significantly reduced in the early invasive group compared with the conservative group (6% vs 16%; hazard ratio, 0.36; 95% CI, 0.16–0.81; P = .01). There were no difference in bleeding (P = 0.68).

Subsequently, a metaanalysis of early routine PCI after fibrinolysis compared with standard therapy in STEMI patients demonstrated a significant reduction in reinfarction and recurrent ischemia at 30 days with no significant increase in major bleeding events (Fig. 4).[34] The benefits of early PCI were maintained at 6 to 12 months,

with persistent reduction in reinfarction (odds ratio [OR], 0.64; 95% CI, 0.040–0.98; P = .01) and combined death/reinfarction (OR, 0.71; 95% CI, 0.52–0.97; P = .03).

Prospective registry data from a large regional STEMI system (the Minneapolis Heart Institute Foundation, a Level 1 MI program), involving 2624 consecutive STEMI patients and 31 referring non-PCI hospitals demonstrated the safety and efficacy of a pharmacoinvasive reperfusion strategy in rural patients who had expected delays to PCI owing to long-distance transfers.[35] STEMI patients who were transferred from hospitals more than 60 miles from the PCI hospital received aspirin, clopidogrel, unfractionated heparin, and half-dose fibrinolytics were transferred for immediate PCI. There were no differences in 30-day mortality (5.5% vs 5.6%; P = .94), stroke (1.1% vs 1.3%; P = .66), major bleeding (1.5% vs 1.8%; P = .65), or reinfarction/ischemia (1.2% vs 2.5%; P = .088) in patients receiving a pharmacoinvasive strategy compared with patients presenting directly to the PCI center for primary PCI, despite a 93-minute longer door to balloon time.

The most recent pharmacoinvasive study was the STREAM (Strategic Reperfusion Early After Myocardial Infarction) trial, which was an international, multicenter study of STEMI patients who presented within 3 hours after symptom onset and who were unable to undergo primary PCI within 1 hour.[36] Patients were assigned randomly to undergo either primary PCI or receive tenectaplase, clopidogrel, and enoxaparin before transport to a PCI-capable hospital. Patients who received fibrinolysis had coronary angiography and PCI within 6 to 24 hours if there was resolution of ST elevation or rescue PCI if reperfusion failed to occur within 90 minutes. The primary endpoint, a composite of death, shock, congestive heart failure or reinfarction up to 30 days, occurred in 12.4% in the fibrinolysis group compared with 14.3% in the primary PCI group (relative risk, 0.86; 95% CI, 0.68–1.09; P = .21) There were more intracranial hemorrhages in the fibrinolysis group than in the primary PCI group overall (1% vs 0.2%; P = .04). However, after amendment of the protocol to a half-dose lytic in patients 75 year of age or older, the rates of intracranial hemorrhage was the same in both groups (0.5% vs 0.3%; P = .45). Despite the protocol specifying that patients were only to be included if they could not undergo PCI within 60 minutes of first medical contact, nearly one-third of patients had a PCI-related delay of less than 60 minutes. A prespecified substudy of the STREAM trial

Reinfarction, 30 d

Study	Early PCI Events	Total	Standard therapy Events	Total	Weight %	Odds ratio [M-H, Random, 95% CI]
CARESS-IN-AMI	4	299	6	301	10.1	0.67 [0.19, 2.39]
GRACIA-1	3	248	4	251	7.2	0.76 [0.17, 3.41]
CAPITAL-AMI	4	86	11	84	11.7	0.32 [0.10, 1.06]
SIAM-III	2	82	2	81	4.2	0.99 [0.14, 7.18]
TRANSFER-AMI	18	537	30	522	46.1	0.57 [0.31, 1.03]
WEST	6	104	9	100	14.3	0.62 [0.21, 1.81]
NORDISTEMI	2	134	7	132	6.5	0.27 [0.06, 1.33]
Total	39/1490 (2.6%)		69/1471 (4.7%)		100.0	0.55 [0.36, 0.82] NNT48[29-138]

Heterogeneity: $\tau^2 = 0.00$; $\chi^2 = 2.18$, df = 6 (P = .90); $I^2 = 0\%$
Test for overall effect: Z = 2.93 (P = .003)
Egger's regression test: P value 0.48

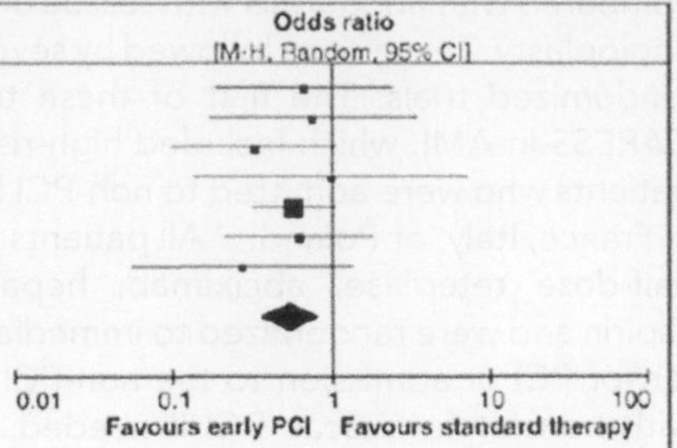

Odds ratio [M-H, Random, 95% CI]
0.01   0.1   1   10   100
Favours early PCI   Favours standard therapy

Reischemia, 30 d

Study	Early PCI Events	Total	Standard therapy Events	Total	Weight %	Odds ratio [M-H, Random, 95% CI]
CARESS-IN-AMI	1	299	12	301	8.1	0.08 [0.01, 0.63]
GRACIA-1	6	248	30	251	21.1	0.18 [0.07, 0.45]
CAPITAL-AMI	6	86	15	84	19.3	0.34 [0.13, 0.94]
SIAM-III	3	82	20	81	15.4	0.12 [0.03, 0.41]
TRANSFER-AMI	1	537	11	522	8.0	0.09 [0.01, 0.67]
WEST	3	104	0	100	6.8	2.94 [0.30, 28.7]
NORDISTEMI	8	134	16	132	21.3	0.46 [0.19, 1.12]
Total	28/1490 (1.9%)		104/1471 (7.1%)		100.0	0.25 [0.13, 0.49] NNT 19[15-27]

Heterogeneity: $\tau^2 = 0.33$; $\chi^2 = 10.93$, df = 6 (P = .09); $I^2 = 45\%$
Test for overall effect: Z = 4.10 (P < .001)
Egger's regression test: P value 0.50

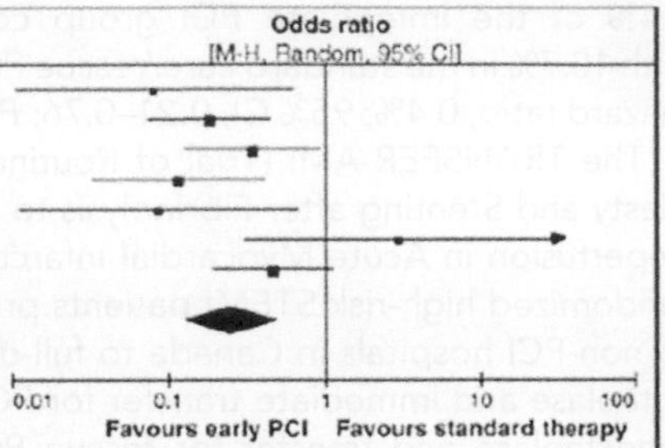

Odds ratio [M-H, Random, 95% CI]
0.01   0.1   1   10   100
Favours early PCI   Favours standard therapy

Fig. 4. Results from a metaanalysis of early routine percutaneous coronary intervention (PCI) after fibrinolysis versus standard therapy in ST-segment elevation myocardial infarction (STEMI). (*Adapted from* Borgia F, Goodman SG, Halvorsen S, et al. Early routine percutaneous coronary intervention after fibrinolysis vs standard therapy in ST-segment elevation myocardial infarction: a meta-analysis. Eur Heart J 2010;31(17):2161; with permission.)

examined 30 day clinical outcomes stratified according to PCI-related delay. They found that, as PCI-related delay increased, the outcomes (30-day death/congestive heart failure/shock/MI) for the pharmacoinvasive strategy became superior to primary PCI (Fig. 5).[37]

Pharmacoinvasive Strategy Controversies
Despite the guideline recommendations, many STEMI systems continue to do PCI despite the time delay. Unfortunately, there are no specific clinical trial data available to compare the 2 strategies in patients with a delay of greater than 120 min (although the subgroup analysis from FINESSE would support the pharmacoinvasive approach). It is clear that having a prespecified protocol in place is preferred over an "ad hoc" decision at 3:00 AM. Also, evidence suggests the availability of P2Y12 inhibitor has improved outcomes with the pharmacoinvasive approach. Two other controversies deserve discussion: the timing of PCI after fibrinolysis and the ideal fibrinolytic/antiplatelet regimen.

TIMING OF PERCUTANEOUS CORONARY INTERVENTION AFTER FIBRINOLYSIS

It is well-established that transferring patients to a PCI capable hospital within 6 hours after fibrinolysis is associated better outcomes.[32,33] However, the optimal timing of angiography and PCI postlytic therapy remains controversial. This question of PCI timing was recently assessed in a metaanalysis by Madan and colleagues,[38] who found that the time from fibrinolysis to angiography was not independently predictive of 30-day or 1-year death or reinfarction. Recurrent ischemia, however, was lower in patients undergoing angiography less than 4 hours after fibrinolysis (3.7% to 7.9%; P for trend = .02). Only symptom onset to angiography time was an independent predictor of 1-year death or reinfarction (HR, 1.07; 95% CI, 1.02–1.12; P = .01). Consistent with the Minneapolis Heart Institute experience, angiography postlysis less than 2 hours was not associated with an increased risk of 30-day death, reinfarction, or in-hospital major bleeding.

IDEAL PHARMACOLOGIC REGIMEN FOR PHARMACOINVASIVE PERCUTANEOUS CORONARY INTERVENTION

No trials have directly compared specific fibrinolytic agents in the pharmacoinvasive setting. The GRACIA-3 (Groupo De Analisis de la Cardiopata Isquemica) study compared the use of a combination of a tirofiban and tenectaplase with

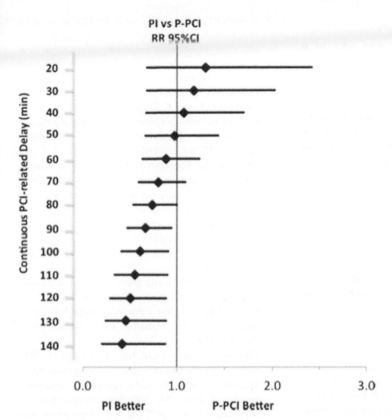

Fig. 5. Relative association of continuous PCI-related delay (minutes) and study treatment with 30-day death/congestive heart failure/shock/myocardial infarction. Relative risks and 95% CI are presented (PI vs P-PCI). PI, pharmacoinvasive; P-PCI, primary percutaneous coronary intervention. (*From* Gershlick AH, Westerhout CM, Armstrong PW, et al. Impact of a pharmacoinvasive strategy when delays to primary PCI are prolonged. Heart 2015;101(9):696; with permission.)

tenectaplase alone and found that addition of the GP IIb/IIIa inhibitor increased the risk of major bleed with no benefit on epicardial and myocardial perfusion.[39] As such, the routine use of the GP IIb/IIIa inhibitors with fibrinolytic therapy is not endorsed by guidelines.[2,3]

Fibrinolytic therapy enhances platelet activation and aggregation, which can be counteracted with oral antiplatelet therapy. Upfront clopidogrel loading with fibrinolytic therapy has been shown to improve clinical outcomes

in the CLARITY (Clopidogrel as Adjunctive Reperfusion Therapy) and COMMIT (ClOpidogrel and Metoprolol in Myocardial Infarction) trials.[40,41] None of the trials included in the Keeley metaanalysis used a P2Y12 inhibitor in contrast with CARESS-in-AMI, TRANSFER-AMI, and NORDISTEMI. There are limited data on the safety of newer oral P2Y12 inhibitors ticagrelor and prasugrel with fibrinolytic therapy, although large multicenter trials are in progress.

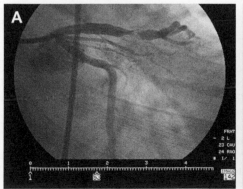
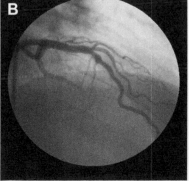

Fig. 6. (*A*) Initial coronary angiogram demonstrating TIMI 2 (thrombolysis in myocardial infarction) flow with a high-grade obstruction of the left anterior descending aorta. (*B*) Angiogram after percutaneous coronary intervention.

CASE RESOLUTION

The rural community hospital was part of a regional STEMI system and received the preestablished STEMI protocol (half-dose tenectaplase, aspirin, unfractionated heparin, and clopidogrel 600 mg at 2:45 AM; door to drug time of 25 minutes). The patient's pain improved with resolution of ST elevation by the time the helicopter had arrived for transport. On arrival to the PCI hospital, he was taken directly to the cardiac catheterization laboratory where he underwent successful PCI of a 99% proximal left anterior descending artery (TIMI 2 flow) using a drug-eluting stent (Fig. 6). The door to balloon time from the initial medical contact was 152 minutes (127 minutes after fibrinolysis). He was discharged home 2 days later with normal left ventricular ejection fraction; the post-PCI electrocardiograph is shown (see Fig. 1B).

SUMMARY

Primary PCI remains the optimal reperfusion strategy when it can be performed by an experienced team within 120 minutes of first medical contact. However, provided there are no contraindications present, fibrinolytic therapy should be administered when these timelines cannot be met. After fibrinolysis, patients should be rapidly transferred to a PCI center. Patients who arrive with evidence of failed reperfusion or hemodynamic instability should undergo emergent rescue PCI. Otherwise, patients should undergo routine early cardiac catheterization and PCI within 24 hours after fibrinolysis. Organized systems of care should be in place to ensure that patients can be transferred to PCI centers and undergo cardiac catheterization within these timelines.

REFERENCES

1. Vora AN, Holmes DN, Rokos I, et al. Fibrinolysis use among patients requiring interhospital transfer for ST-segment elevation myocardial infarction care: a report from the US National Cardiovascular Data Registry. JAMA Intern Med 2015;175(2): 207–15.

2. Task Force on the management of ST-segment elevation acute myocardial infarction of the European Society of Cardiology (ESC), Steg PG, James SK, et al. ESC guidelines for the management of acute myocardial infarction in patients presenting with ST-segment elevation. Eur Heart J 2012;33(20):2569–619.

3. O'Gara PT, Kushner FG, Ascheim DD, et al. 2013 ACCF/AHA guideline for the management of ST-elevation myocardial infarction: a report of the American College of Cardiology Foundation/ American Heart Association Task Force on Practice Guidelines. Circulation 2013;127(4):e362–425.

4. Lambert L, Brown K, Segal E, et al. Association between timeliness of reperfusion therapy and clinical outcomes in ST-elevation myocardial infarction. JAMA 2010;303(21):2148–55.

5. Terkelsen CJ, Sorensen JT, Maeng M, et al. System delay and mortality among patients with STEMI treated with primary percutaneous coronary intervention. JAMA 2010;304(7):763–71.

6. An international randomized trial comparing four thrombolytic strategies for acute myocardial infarction. The GUSTO investigators. N Engl J Med 1993; 329(10):673–82.

7. Granger CB, White HD, Bates ER, et al. A pooled analysis of coronary arterial patency and left ventricular function after intravenous thrombolysis for acute myocardial infarction. Am J Cardiol 1994; 74(12):1220–8.

8. Cannon CP, Gibson CM, McCabe CH, et al. TNK-tissue plasminogen activator compared with front-loaded alteplase in acute myocardial infarction: results of the TIMI 10B trial. Thrombolysis in Myocardial Infarction (TIMI) 10B Investigators. Circulation 1998;98(25):2805–14.

9. Sutton AG, Campbell PG, Graham R, et al. A randomized trial of rescue angioplasty versus a conservative approach for failed fibrinolysis in ST-segment elevation myocardial infarction: the Middlesbrough Early Revascularization to Limit INfarction (MERLIN) trial. J Am Coll Cardiol 2004; 44(2):287–96.

10. Gershlick AH, Stephens-Lloyd A, Hughes S, et al. Rescue angioplasty after failed thrombolytic therapy for acute myocardial infarction. N Engl J Med 2005;353(26):2758–68.

11. Wijeysundera HC, Vijayaraghavan R, Nallamothu BK, et al. Rescue angioplasty or repeat fibrinolysis after failed fibrinolytic therapy for ST-segment myocardial infarction: a meta-analysis of randomized trials. J Am Coll Cardiol 2007;49(4):422–30.

12. Grines CL, Browne KF, Marco J, et al. A comparison of immediate angioplasty with thrombolytic therapy for acute myocardial infarction. The Primary Angioplasty in Myocardial Infarction Study Group. N Engl J Med 1993;328(10):673–9.

13. Weaver WD, Simes RJ, Betriu A, et al. Comparison of primary coronary angioplasty and intravenous thrombolytic therapy for acute myocardial infarction: a quantitative review. JAMA 1997;278(23): 2093–8.

14. Keeley EC, Boura JA, Grines CL. Primary angioplasty versus intravenous thrombolytic therapy for

acute myocardial infarction: a quantitative review of 23 randomised trials. Lancet 2003;361(9351):13–20.

15. Widimsky P, Groch L, Zelizko M, et al. Multicentre randomized trial comparing transport to primary angioplasty vs immediate thrombolysis vs combined strategy for patients with acute myocardial infarction presenting to a community hospital without a catheterization laboratory. The PRAGUE study. Eur Heart J 2000;21(10):823–31.

16. Widimsky P, Budesinsky T, Vorac D, et al. Long distance transport for primary angioplasty vs immediate thrombolysis in acute myocardial infarction. Final results of the randomized national multicentre trial–PRAGUE-2. Eur Heart J 2003;24(1):94–104.

17. Andersen HR, Nielsen TT, Rasmussen K, et al. A comparison of coronary angioplasty with fibrinolytic therapy in acute myocardial infarction. N Engl J Med 2003;349(8):733–42.

18. Dalby M, Bouzamondo A, Lechat P, et al. Transfer for primary angioplasty versus immediate thrombolysis in acute myocardial infarction: a meta-analysis. Circulation 2003;108(15):1809–14.

19. Henry TD, Sharkey SW, Burke MN, et al. A regional system to provide timely access to percutaneous coronary intervention for ST-elevation myocardial infarction. Circulation 2007;116(7):721–8.

20. Jollis JG, Roettig ML, Aluko AO, et al. Implementation of a statewide system for coronary reperfusion for ST-segment elevation myocardial infarction. JAMA 2007;298(20):2371–80.

21. Pinto DS, Kirtane AJ, Nallamothu BK, et al. Hospital delays in reperfusion for ST-elevation myocardial infarction: implications when selecting a reperfusion strategy. Circulation 2006;114(19):2019–25.

22. Weaver WD, Cerqueira M, Hallstrom AP, et al. Prehospital-initiated vs hospital-initiated thrombolytic therapy. The myocardial infarction triage and intervention trial. JAMA 1993;270(10):1211–6.

23. Di Mario C, Dudek D, Piscione F, et al. Immediate angioplasty versus standard therapy with rescue angioplasty after thrombolysis in the Combined Abciximab REteplase Stent Study in Acute Myocardial Infarction (CARESS-in-AMI): an open, prospective, randomised, multicentre trial. Lancet 2008; 371(9612):559–68.

24. Assessment of the Safety and Efficacy of a New Treatment Strategy with Percutaneous Coronary Intervention (ASSENT-4 PCI) investigators. Primary versus tenectaplase-facilitated percutaneous coronary intervention in patients with ST-segment elevation acute myocardial infarction (ASSENT-4 PCI): randomised trial. Lancet 2006;367(9510): 569–78.

25. Ellis SG, Armstrong P, Betriu A, et al. Facilitated percutaneous coronary intervention versus primary percutaneous coronary intervention: design and rationale of the Facilitated Intervention with Enhanced Reperfusion Speed to Stop Events (FINESSE) trial. Am Heart J 2004;147(4):E16.

26. Keeley EC, Boura JA, Grines CL. Comparison of primary and facilitated percutaneous coronary interventions for ST-elevation myocardial infarction: quantitative review of randomised trials. Lancet 2006;367(9510):579–88.

27. Stone GW, Gersh BJ. Facilitated angioplasty: paradise lost. Lancet 2006;367(9510):543–6.

28. Ross AM, Huber K, Zeymer U, et al. The impact of place of enrollment and delay to reperfusion on 90-day post-infarction mortality in the ASSENT-4 PCI trial: assessment of the safety and efficacy of a new treatment strategy with percutaneous coronary intervention. JACC Cardiovasc Interv 2009; 2(10):925–30.

29. Herrmann HC, Lu J, Brodie BR, et al. Benefit of facilitated percutaneous coronary intervention in high-risk ST-segment elevation myocardial infarction patients presenting to nonpercutaneous coronary intervention hospitals. JACC Cardiovasc Interv 2009;2(10):917–24.

30. Scheller B, Hennen B, Hammer B, et al. Beneficial effects of immediate stenting after thrombolysis in acute myocardial infarction. J Am Coll Cardiol 2003;42(4):634–41.

31. Le May MR, Wells GA, Labinaz M, et al. Combined angioplasty and pharmacological intervention versus thrombolysis alone in acute myocardial infarction (CAPITAL AMI study). J Am Coll Cardiol 2005;46(3):417–24.

32. Cantor WJ, Fitchett D, Borgundvaag B, et al. Routine early angioplasty after fibrinolysis for acute myocardial infarction. N Engl J Med 2009;360(26): 2705–18.

33. Bohmer E, Hoffmann P, Abdelnoor M, et al. Efficacy and safety of immediate angioplasty versus ischemia-guided management after thrombolysis in acute myocardial infarction in areas with very long transfer distances results of the NORDISTEMI (NORwegian study on DIstrict treatment of ST-elevation myocardial infarction). J Am Coll Cardiol 2010;55(2):102–10.

34. Borgia F, Goodman SG, Halvorsen S, et al. Early routine percutaneous coronary intervention after fibrinolysis vs. standard therapy in ST-segment elevation myocardial infarction: a meta-analysis Eur Heart J 2010;31(17):2156–69.

35. Larson DM, Duval S, Sharkey SW, et al. Safety and efficacy of a pharmacoinvasive reperfusion strategy in rural ST-elevation myocardial infarction patients with expected delays due to long-distance transfers. Eur Heart J 2012;33(10):1232–40.

36. Armstrong PW, Gershlick AH, Goldstein P, et al. Fibrinolysis or primary PCI in ST-segment elevation myocardial infarction. N Engl J Med 2013;368(15): 1379–87.

37. Gershlick AH, Westerhout CM, Armstrong PW, et al. Impact of a pharmacoinvasive strategy when delays to primary PCI are prolonged. Heart 2015; 101(9):692–8.

38. Madan M, Halvorsen S, Di Mario C, et al. Relationship between time to invasive assessment and clinical outcomes of patients undergoing an early invasive strategy after fibrinolysis for ST-segment elevation myocardial infarction: a patient-level analysis of the randomized early routine invasive clinical trials. JACC Cardiovasc Interv 2015;8(1 Pt B):166–74.

39. Sanchez PL, Gimeno F, Ancillo P, et al. Role of the paclitaxel-eluting stent and tirofiban in patients with ST-elevation myocardial infarction undergoing postfibrinolysis angioplasty: the GRACIA-3 randomized clinical trial. Circ Cardiovasc Interv 2010; 3(4):297–307.

40. Sabatine MS, Cannon CP, Gibson CM, et al. Effect of clopidogrel pretreatment before percutaneous coronary intervention in patients with ST-elevation myocardial infarction treated with fibrinolytics: the PCI-CLARITY study. JAMA 2005; 294(10):1224–32.

41. Chen ZM, Jiang LX, Chen YP, et al. Addition of clopidogrel to aspirin in 45,852 patients with acute myocardial infarction: randomised placebo-controlled trial. Lancet 2005;366(9497):1607–21.

False Activations for ST-Segment Elevation Myocardial Infarction

David C. Lange, MD[a], Ivan C. Rokos, MD[b],
J. Lee Garvey, MD[c], David M. Larson, MD[d],
Timothy D. Henry, MD[a],*

KEYWORDS

- ST-elevation myocardial infarction • False activation
- Primary percutaneous coronary intervention • Systems of care • Quality improvement
- Quality outcomes • Assessment

KEY POINTS

- Although first-medical-contact-to-device times and clinical outcomes for ST-elevation myocardial infarction (STEMI) have markedly improved, false activation of the cardiac catheterization laboratory (CCL) has become an increasing problem.
- False-activation rates vary widely across STEMI systems because of differences in definition, emergency medical service training, and CCL-activation work flow.
- False activations are costly to the medical system for a variety of reasons: patient satisfaction and trust, CCL morale and economics, and health care resource utilization.
- Universal definitions for false activations are necessary to define the scope of the problem.
- Efforts to reduce false activation rates must target process improvement but CANNOT lead to increased rates of missed STEMIs. Specificity of CCL activation for STEMI must be optimized without sacrificing the sensitivity.

INTRODUCTION

Approximately 500,000 patients have an acute ST-elevation myocardial infarction (STEMI) each year in the United States. A decade ago, roughly 30% of patients with STEMI were not receiving any form of reperfusion therapy (primary percutaneous coronary intervention [PPCI] or fibrinolysis). Furthermore, only 40% of those who received PPCI were treated within the recommended time frame (first-medical-contact-to-device [FMC2D] time ≤ 90 minutes).[1,2] These shortcomings in FMC2D stimulated the development of the American College of Cardiology Door-to-Balloon (D2B) Alliance and the American Heart Association (AHA) Mission: Lifeline Program. Along with regional STEMI systems of care, these programs have dramatically changed the approach to health care delivery for STEMI, providing timely access to PPCI for an increasing proportion of the population while decreasing the eligible but untreated population. These advances have resulted in marked improvements in time-to-treatment (**Fig. 1**) and

---

Author Disclosures: Dr L. Garvey has had research support and has served as an advisory board member to Phillips Healthcare (Koninklijke Philips N.V. Amsterdam, Netherlands). None of the other contributing authors have financial disclosures or relationships with industry that pertain to this study.

[a] Division of Cardiology, Cedars-Sinai Heart Institute, Los Angeles, CA, USA; [b] Department of Emergency Medicine, University of California, Los Angeles, Los Angeles, CA, USA; [c] Department of Emergency Medicine, Carolinas Medical Center, Charlotte, NC, USA; [d] Minneapolis Heart Institute Foundation, Abbott Northwestern Hospital, Minneapolis, MN, USA

* Corresponding author. 127 South San Vicente Boulevard, Suite A3100, Los Angeles, CA 90048.
E-mail address: henryt@cshs.org

Intervent Cardiol Clin 5 (2016) 451–469
http://dx.doi.org/10.1016/j.iccl.2016.06.002

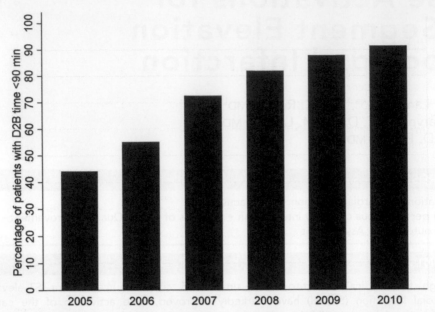

Fig. 1. Marked improvement in the percentage of patients with D2B time less than 90 minutes from 2005 to 2010. (*From* Krumholz H, Herrin J, Miller LE, et al. Improvements in door-to-balloon time in the United States, 2005 to 2010. Circulation 2011;124:1044; with permission.)

cardiovascular outcomes (Fig. 2).[1,3–7] However, inappropriate, overcall, or false-positive cardiac catheterization laboratory (CCL) activations have become a challenging problem.

False activations have several adverse consequences. First, false activations can cause patient confusion, frustration, and perhaps even distrust in the medical providers. Secondly, false

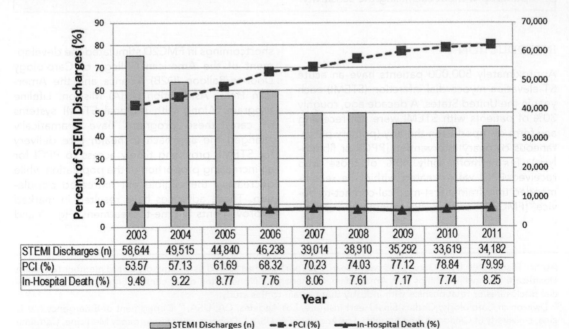

	2003	2004	2005	2006	2007	2008	2009	2010	2011
STEMI Discharges (n)	58,644	49,515	44,840	46,238	39,014	38,910	35,292	33,619	34,182
PCI (%)	53.57	57.13	61.69	68.32	70.23	74.03	77.12	78.84	79.99
In-Hospital Death (%)	9.49	9.22	8.77	7.76	8.06	7.61	7.17	7.74	8.25

Year

☐ STEMI Discharges (n)   ■ PCI (%)   ▲ In-Hospital Death (%)

Fig. 2. Trends in US STEMI care 2003 to 2011. Note the percent of discharged patients with STEMI who received, percutaneous coronary intervention (PCI) increased to 80% (*blue line*), whereas mortality decreased (*red line*). Number of STEMI discharges and rates of PCI and in-hospital death in the United States, 2003 to 2011. (*From* Shah RU, Henry TD, Rutten-Ramos S, et al. Increasing percutaneous coronary interventions for ST-segment elevation myocardial infarction in the United States. JACC Cardiovasc Interv 2015;8:141; with permission.)

activations can cause CCL staff fatigue, burnout, and loss of productivity. Finally, false activations are costly to the medical system, as staff is often paid overtime wages to take call and respond to CCL activations, regardless of whether or not patients receive emergent coronary angiography.

The authors begin with an overview of several core concepts for STEMI systems. The second section summarizes the current literature on false activations, and the final section introduces several quality improvement (QI) metrics that may help reduce false activations and improve the efficiency of STEMI systems (Table 1).

ST-Elevation Myocardial Infarction Process Versus Procedure

Successful treatment of patients with STEMI can be divided into 2 separate but intertwined operations: the STEMI *procedure* and the STEMI *process* (Fig. 3). The STEMI *procedure* is the actual revascularization via PPCI once patients arrive in the CCL and may occasionally require coronary artery bypass grafting (CABG) surgery. The STEMI *process* includes all of the events and personnel outside of the CCL that work to deliver patients to the CCL. The STEMI *process* begins with patients who experience chest pain (or some symptom of myocardial ischemia) and seek medical attention. This action triggers a rapid and coordinated series of evaluations, including triage and treatment strategies by various medical providers (9-1-1 dispatchers, first-responders, emergency physicians and nurses, among others), frontline support staff (hospital registration clerks, laboratory personnel, page operators, and others), and postevent administrators and QI personnel. Whenever possible, parallel processing is encouraged to minimize time to reperfusion.

At the center of an efficient STEMI process is the appropriate diagnosis of STEMI based on a 12-lead electrocardiogram (ECG). The ECG must effectively stratify the large group of patients who experience ischemic symptoms into 2 distinct groups: those who are likely experiencing an STEMI (<5% of chest pain patients) versus those who are not experiencing an STEMI (~95% of patients with chest pain who present with non ST-Segment Elevation Myocardial Infarction (NSTEMI), unstable angina, or noncardiac chest pain). The ECG is an excellent but still imperfect tool for diagnosing STEMI, and a variety of conditions may mimic STEMI that do not require PPCI (Table 2).[8,9]

When a patient has activated 9-1-1, the STEMI process is initiated by emergency medical service (EMS) providers via prehospital-ECG (PH-ECG) acquisition. If the PH-ECG is consistent with

STEMI, EMS then activates an STEMI alert and triages the patient to the closest appropriate STEMI receiving center (SRC) for PPCI, even if it means bypassing non-PPCI capable hospitals en route. The prehospital STEMI alert may not always result in CCL activation. EMS can transport a patient to an SRC based on their initial PH-ECG assessment, even if some uncertainty about the diagnosis and/or CCL activation exists. Once STEMI is confirmed and the patient is deemed an appropriate candidate for cardiac catheterization, a Code STEMI should be activated and the CCL team should begin preparation for emergent coronary angiography ± PPCI. Thus, transport to an appropriate SRC and CCL activation at the SRC are 2 distinct steps in the STEMI process.

The Code STEMI initiates a series of predefined hospital operations in preparation for the STEMI procedure, which include (1) notification of all CCL staff to prepare for emergent coronary angiography ± PPCI (2) establishment of intravenous access and ascertainment of key laboratory values (hemoglobin, platelets, creatinine, potassium, and so forth); (3) administration of guideline-directed medical therapies (aspirin, $P2Y_{12}$ inhibitors, antithrombin therapy, statin, and so forth); (4) consenting patients for emergent coronary angiography; and (5) stabilization and monitoring during transportation to the CCL (see Fig. 3). Standardized protocols that streamline these efforts with patient-centered care is the guiding principle for the STEMI process. However, protocols must have the flexibility to address the individual needs of patients and staff.

The individuals responsible for initiating the Code STEMI may vary across STEMI systems. In general, FMC2D times are shorter with upstream CCL activation from EMS or emergency physicians; the guidelines do not recommend cardiology consultation before CCL activation. Upstream activation is especially important when STEMI is clearly diagnosed by PH-ECG.[10,11] However, consulting the on-duty interventional cardiologist *before* activation of the CCL team may be required for a small subset of patients with complex clinical scenarios, equivocal ECG findings, and so forth.

EMS is not always involved in patients presenting with chest pain. Indeed, population studies have demonstrated that up to 70% of patients with chest pain do not use EMS, particularly in rural communities.[12] For patients who self-present to non–PPCI-capable hospitals (ie, referral hospitals), emergency departments should have protocols to rapidly obtain and interpret the ECG and then initiate the Code STEMI process including transfer to a PPCI center. Likewise, SRCs capable

Table 1
Definitions for standardized terminology regarding false activations

	Definitions
False activation	It is any activation of the CCL staff for a patient who does not require or has contraindications to cardiac catheterization. Synonyms: overactivation, false-positive CCL activation, inappropriate CCL activation, CCL cancellation
No culprit	It is any activation of the CCL staff that results in a coronary angiogram with no identifiable culprit lesion. Please note, no culprit is NOT synonymous with false activation; these are separate entities. For example, a patient with ECG criteria for STEMI and positive cardiac biomarkers but no culprit on cardiac catheterization (eg, takotsubo cardiomyopathy) should NOT be classified as a false activation. The goal for an efficient STEMI system should be between 10% and 20%.
STEMI procedure	It is the act of revascularization for STEMI via PPCI (or occasionally via surgery after cardiac catheterization).
STEMI process	It is all of the events and personnel outside of the CCL that result in the delivery of patients to the CCL.
STEMI alert	It is the EMS-based initiation of the STEMI process wherein STEMI is suspected based on clinical presentation and prehospital ECG findings. EMS then triages patients to the closest STEMI receiving center for PPCI, even if it means bypassing non–PPCI-capable hospitals en route.
Code STEMI (also called CCL activation)	It is the hospital-based initiation or continuation of the STEMI process wherein STEMI is confirmed and the CCL team should begin preparation for emergent coronary angiography ± PPCI.
CCL activation index	It is the number of CCL activation patients who receive emergent coronary angiography divided by the total number of CCL activations. The goal is ≥90% to 95%.
Revascularization index	It is the number of PPCI + number of CABG procedures divided by the number of CCL activation patients that receive emergent coronary angiography. The goal is 80% to 90%. Revascularization index >90% likely indicates too few emergent coronary angiography procedures. Revascularization index <80% likely indicates too many emergent coronary angiography procedures.
Missed STEMI	It is patients with symptoms consistent with acute coronary syndrome and ECG findings consistent with STEMI who do not receive emergent cardiac catheterization in the absence of contraindications. Synonyms are false-negative CCL activation and inappropriate CCL cancellation. The goal is <1%.
STEMI process efficiency	It is the number of appropriate cardiac catheterizations divided by the total number of CCL activations. The goal for an efficient STEMI system should be ≥90%.
Avoidable cardiac catheterization	It is cardiac catheterization performed on patients who have no culprit lesion and negative cardiac biomarkers. These patients are the most difficult to recognize up front and can only be definitively identified on retrospective analysis, once the angiogram and cardiac enzymes have resulted. These patients should represent most of the false activations for an efficient STEMI system.

of PPCI should have standardized protocols for their own emergency departments to rapidly diagnose and triage patients with STEMI to the CCL. All systems should have standardized protocols for posthospital care of their patients with STEMI, whether follow-up care is provided at a referral center or at the SRC.

Time is Myocardium

Diversity in geography, politics, and sociodemographics across the United States, and throughout the world, necessitate a wide variety of STEMI processes. Current guidelines from the American College of Cardiology Foundation/ AHA and European Society of Cardiology

STEMI Process

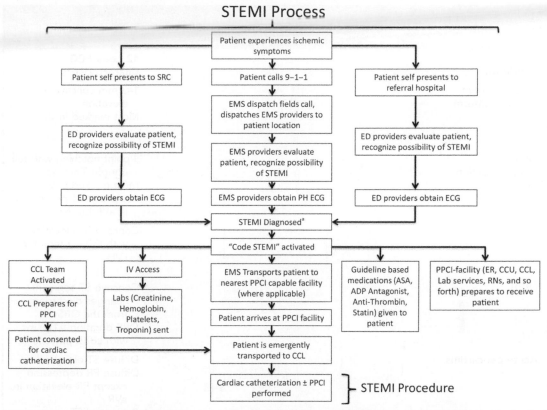

Fig. 3. Example of the important distinction of the STEMI process and STEMI procedure. STEMI *process* is all of the events and personnel outside of the CCL that result in the delivery of patients to the CCL, whereas the STEMI *procedure* is the act of revascularization for STEMI via PPCI (or occasionally via surgery after cardiac catheterization). ECG, electrocardiogram; EMS, emergency medical service; ER, emergency room; IV, intravenous; RNs, registered nurses.

recommend PPCI as the preferred therapy for STEMI, provided it can be performed in a timely manner by an experienced operator.[10,11] Guidelines also recommend an ideal FMC2D time goal of less than 90 minutes.[10,11] For patients presenting to a non–PPCI-capable hospital, immediate transfer to an SRC for PPCI is the recommended reperfusion strategy with a goal FMC2D time of less than 120 minutes.[10,11] For these reasons, PPCI remains one of the most complex, multidisciplinary, and time-sensitive therapeutic interventions in medicine today: the process is measured in minutes, whereas the outcomes are measured in terms of significant morbidity and mortality. Teamwork, coordination of care, and smooth transitions along every step of the process are critically important.[13,14]

The Role of Emergency Medical Services for Diagnosis and Treatment of ST-Elevation Myocardial Infarction

EMS providers have 3 crucial roles in the STEMI process. First, EMS must assess and stabilize patients, which includes recognizing and treating malignant arrhythmias, such as ventricular tachycardia and ventricular fibrillation, with defibrillation when necessary and managing any respiratory distress associated with STEMI. Assessment and stabilization must be performed as quickly as possible to ensure appropriate and timely transport.

Second, EMS providers must be capable of diagnosing STEMI using a PH-ECG. The ability to obtain a high-fidelity PH-ECG and correctly interpret ECG patterns consistent with STEMI is a crucial step to initiating the STEMI process. Ideally, EMS expedites the STEMI process by issuing an STEMI alert and prepares patients for transport to an SRC.

Finally, EMS providers must have predefined destination protocols that allow EMS to transport any identified patients with STEMI to the closest appropriate PPCI-capable hospital, even if it means bypassing non–PPCI-capable hospitals en route. In some systems, EMS may also provide rapid interhospital transport to

Table 2
Causes of ST-segment elevation on 12-lead electrocardiogram that are ST elevation myocardial infarction mimics

Condition		12 Lead ECG Characteristics
Normal variant (male pattern)		1–3 mm concave ST elevation Most marked in V_2
Early repolarization		J point notching with tall upright T waves Most marked in V_4 Reciprocal ST depression in aVR but NOT aVL
LVH		Concave ST elevation with ECG criteria for LVH
LBBB		Concave ST segment changes discordant from the QRS QRS duration >120 ms with LBBB pattern
Acute pericarditis		Diffuse ST elevation Diffuse PR depression except PR elevation in aVR Reciprocal ST depression in aVR but NOT aVL ST Elevation rarely >5 mm
Hyperkalemia		Tall peaked (tented) T waves QRS widening PR prolongation Low amplitude or absent P waves ST segment usually downsloping
Brugada syndrome		rSR′ in V_1 and V_2 ST segment elevation in V_1 and V_2 typically downsloping
Postcardioversion		Marked ST elevation, often >10 mm that resolves within minutes of cardioversion
Prinzmetal angina		Transient ischemic ST elevation in a coronary distribution ± reciprocal depressions that resolves spontaneously

(continued on next page)

Condition		12 Lead ECG Characteristics
Prior myocardial infarction/ aneurysm	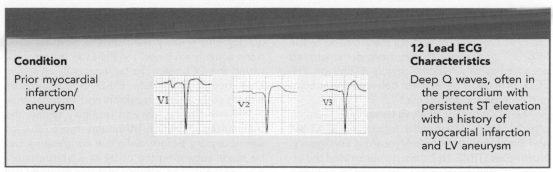	Deep Q waves, often in the precordium with persistent ST elevation with a history of myocardial infarction and LV aneurysm

Abbreviations: LBBB, left bundle branch block; LVH, left ventricular hypertrophy.

minimize time to reperfusion for patients who initially self-present to a non-PPCI hospital.

Prehospital-Electrocardiogram Interpretation and Transmission

It is desirable to maximize the rate of appropriate CCL activations following the PH-ECG.[15] Time to revascularization can be substantially reduced with a PH-ECG–based CCL activation strategy.[16,17] However, emergent coronary angiography ± PPCI is a precious resource, particularly after working hours and on weekends when CCL staff are not on site. Therefore, the rate of appropriate CCL activation is an important quality measure that should be tracked and reported.

Structured interpretation of the PH-ECG can help to mitigate the frequency of false activations by using 3 different approaches: (1) computer algorithm reading, (2) EMS interpretation, or (3) wireless transmission for off-site interpretation. Each strategy has potential strengths and drawbacks, but all rely on EMS-initiated PH-ECG acquisition (Table 3).[18] Thus, training and adherence to standardized protocols are important. Some STEMI systems may rely solely on one of these strategies, whereas others may use a combination to optimize diagnostic accuracy. All STEMI systems should try to maximize the specificity of their CCL activation system without sacrificing the sensitivity: an occasional false activation is far more acceptable than a missed STEMI.

Table 3
Strengths and weaknesses of various prehospital-electrocardiogram interpretation strategies

Method of PH-ECG Interpretation	Strengths	Weaknesses
Computer algorithm interpretation	Rapid, easy No specific transmission capabilities or agreements necessary	Higher rates of inappropriate CCL activation Higher rates of missed STEMIs (?)
EMS Interpretation	Rapid, easy No specific transmission capabilities or agreements necessary	Requires intensive training and education, ongoing quality assurance Variable PH-ECG interpretation capabilities, compliance, and so forth resulting from multiple EMS agencies serving a given geographic location
Wireless transmission and physician interpretation	Lower rates of inappropriate CCL activation and missed STEMIs Medical oversight can provide oversight on destination hospital and treatment en route	Wireless transmission capabilities and training for EMS providers and hospitals Predefined receiver station Predefined responsible party for over-read Subject to transmission failures

Multiple studies have demonstrated decreased time to revascularization on implementation of the PH-ECG, with or without transmission to the SRC.[13,15–35] Several studies have demonstrated paramedics can reliably identify STEMI on PH-ECG, with good agreement between paramedics and emergency physicians.[22,32–34]

The ST-Segment Analysis Using Wire Technology in Acute Myocardial Infarction (STAT-MI) and Timely Intervention in Myocardial Emergency, North-East (TIME-NE) trials demonstrated the efficacy of transmission for over-read in reducing D2B times. The STAT-MI study examined 80 consecutive suspected STEMIs based on a PH-ECG, which was transmitted over a wireless network. Compared with historical controls, they found significant improvements in mean D2B times (80.1 minutes with transmission vs 145.6 minutes before transmission, P<.0001).[28] The TIME-NE trial enrolled with STEMI to a single PPCI facility during the rollout of PH-ECG transmission. Successful PH-ECG transmission patients (n = 24) were compared with self-presenting and unsuccessful PH-ECG transmission patients. The investigators found that the successful PH-ECG transmission group had the shortest D2B times of any of the groups (D2B 50 minutes in successful transmission vs 96 minutes for self-presenting patients vs 78 minutes for failed transmission, P<.0001).[30] In these studies, the major limitation of the transmission strategy was failed transmission due to suboptimal technological infrastructure.[28,30] Advances in technology, wireless network coverage, and smart-phone devices will likely mitigate these shortcomings. Of note, these studies were small and had markedly prolonged revascularization times in the comparison groups. Currently data comparing the efficacy, diagnostic accuracy, or time to reperfusion of paramedic and/or computer interpretation to a transmission for over-read strategy are lacking.

Davis and colleagues[31] compared the positive predictive value (PPV) of paramedic interpretation versus transmission to emergency physicians for over-reading in consecutive phases of a PH-ECG trial and demonstrated improved PPV during the transmission phase of their trial. More recently, Bosson and colleagues[35] compared PH-ECG computer read versus PH-ECG transmission in Los Angeles County by determining the rates of false-positive CCL activations (defined in this study as CCL activation that did not result in PPCI or CABG). They found that transmission reduced the rates of false activations by only 6% (95% confidence interval [CI] −3% to 9%), which was not statistically significant. Limitations of this study include the

inability to determine how quickly transmission occurred after PH-ECG acquisition and how quickly and reliably the frontline hospital clinicians actually reviewed the PH-ECG before activating the CCL team. To be maximally effective, EMS needs to initiate PH-ECG transmission immediately after acquisition and hospital providers need to rapidly and routinely review the transmitted PH-ECG. Although more studies are necessary before definitive conclusions can be made regarding the utility of a transmission, it is reasonable to assume that this strategy will further evolve with ongoing improvements in digital technology.

CURRENT LITERATURE ON FALSE-POSITIVE CARDIAC CATHETERIZATION LABORATORY ACTIVATIONS

False activations occur in almost every STEMI system. However, the frequency and reasons for false activations vary substantially. Larson and colleagues[36] performed the first extensive study of false activations in 2007, using a prospective registry from the Minneapolis Heart Institute level 1 regional STEMI system in Minneapolis, Minnesota. False activations were defined as no culprit lesion on coronary angiography and negative cardiac biomarkers. Of the 1345 patients included in the study, 187 (14%, 95% CI 12.2%–16.0%) patients had no culprit lesion but 64 of the 187 patients (34.2%) had positive biomarkers. These 64 patients had ischemic symptoms, ST elevation, and positive biomarkers, therefore, meeting the universal definition of STEMI despite no clear culprit artery.[37] Therefore, the actual false-activation rate was 123 of 1345 (9.2%).

Of note, only 10 of the 1345 (0.8%) CCL activations in this study did not receive emergent coronary angiography; 5 patients died before angiography; 3 patients had renal failure; and nondiagnostic ECGs accounted for the final 2 patients (Fig. 4). Mortality was not significantly different between patients with culprit lesions versus those without.[36]

Also in 2007, Khot and colleagues[38] reported differences in D2B times based on a serial processing CCL activation model, whereby the cardiologist was responsible for CCL activation versus parallel processing CCL activation, whereby the emergency physicians initiated CCL activation (Fig. 5). False activation was not a prespecified end point and was not subjected to rigorous statistical analyses. Additionally, biomarkers were not reported. In the serial processing arm, 3 of 68 patients (4.4%) had normal or mild coronary artery disease (CAD) compared

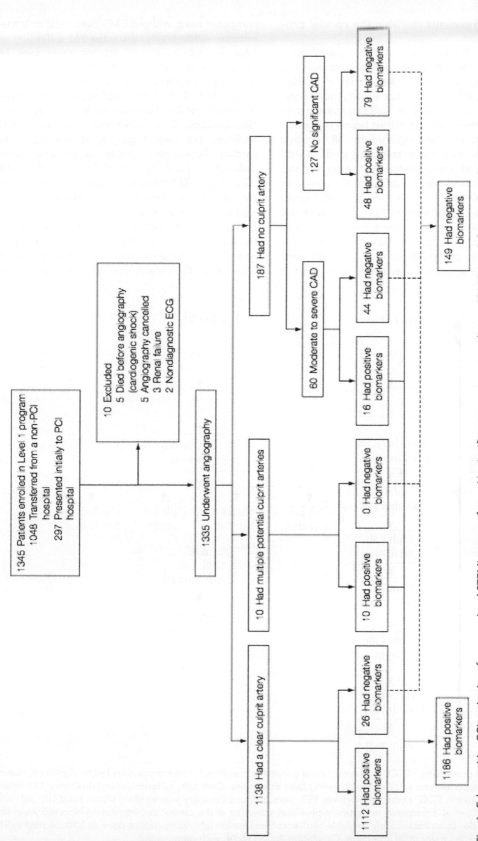

Fig. 4. False-positive CCL activations from a regional STEMI system of care. No significant coronary artery disease (CAD) was defined as less than 50% stenosis in any coronary artery; moderate to severe CAD was defined as 50% or greater stenosis in 1 or more coronary arteries. PCI, percutaneous coronary intervention. (*From* Larson DM, Menssen KM, Sharkey SW, et al. "False-positive" cardiac catheterization activation among patients with suspected ST-elevation myocardial infarction. JAMA 2007;298:2757; with permission.)

with 5 of 95 patients (5.2%) in the parallel processing arm.[38]

In 2008, Youngquist and colleagues[39] performed a retrospective analysis comparing false-positive activation rates from PH-ECG–based CCL activation versus emergency physician–based CCL activation. False activation was defined as absence of a culprit lesion or significant CAD on coronary angiography OR negative cardiac enzymes in the presence of an ECG with ST-segment elevation explained by an alternative cause. There was a significant difference in false-activation rates, with 9 of 23 (39%) false-positive activations from the PH-ECG arm versus 3 of 33 (9%) false activations from the emergency physician arm (P = .02).[39] Important caveats include the small numbers in both arms and PH-ECG activation was based solely on the

computer read, without EMS over-read or transmission. Additionally, the either/or definition of false activations allows retrospective bias to select false activations while limiting the study's generalizability to real-life practice.

In 2010, Kontos and colleagues[40] reported the results of 249 consecutive emergency physician–initiated CCL activations, including ECG findings, coronary angiography findings, and cardiac biomarkers. False activations were defined as patients with ECGs that met the criteria for STEMI but were ultimately ruled out by cardiac biomarkers and coronary angiography. They also reviewed patients with ECG findings that did not meet STEMI criteria when the CCL was not activated (called the no STEMI group) and patients who had CCL activation without ECG criteria for STEMI (called the

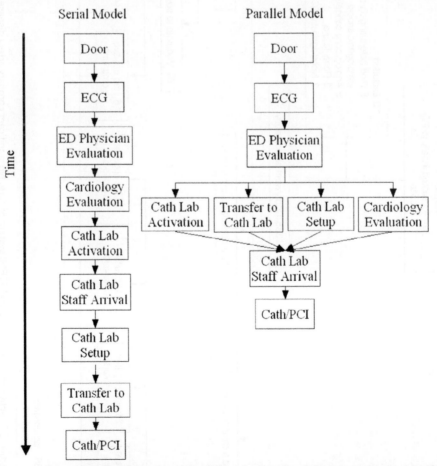

Fig. 5. Serial processing of CCL activation versus parallel processing. Parallel processing led to significant reductions in D2B time without significantly changing false activations. Cath Lab, catheterization laboratory; ED, emergency department; ECG, electrocardiogram; PCI, percutaneous coronary intervention. (*From* Khot UK, Johnson ML, Ramsey C, et al. Emergency department physician activation of the cardiac catheterization laboratory and immediate transfer to an immediately available cardiac catheterization laboratory reduce door-to-balloon time in ST-segment elevation myocardial infarction. Circulation 2007;116:74; with permission.)

unnecessary CCL activation group). Based on these definitions, 37 of 249 (14.9%) were false-positive CCL activations, 11 (4.4%) were no STEMI, and 13 (5.2%) were unnecessary CCL activations. Therefore, a total of 61 patients (24.5%) did not have an STEMI in this cohort, including 39 of 234 patients who received emergent coronary angiography (16.7%) but had no culprit and negative enzymes (**Fig. 6**).[40] Although the investigators reported the cardiac biomarker levels for the true STEMI group and the no STEMI group, they were not specifically reported for the false-positive STEMI or unnecessary CCL activation groups. No outcome measures were reported, and the investigators noted the subjectivity in deciding appropriate versus unnecessary CCL activation as a limitation.

The Reperfusion of Acute Myocardial Infarction in North Carolina Emergency Departments (RACE) program is a statewide STEMI system that relies on PH-ECG–triggered CCL activation. In 2012, the RACE investigators reported on 3973 consecutive CCL activations and defined appropriate CCL activations as activations that resulted in emergent coronary angiography or those canceled because of a change in clinical status (resolution of

symptoms, resolution of ST segment changes on ECG, or death). Inappropriate CCL activations were defined as CCL activations that were canceled because of ECG reinterpretation or contraindications to emergent coronary angiography. Using these definitions, 3377 (85%) CCL activations were deemed appropriate, whereas 596 (15%) were deemed inappropriate. Of note, 364 (9.1%) of the appropriate CCL activations had no culprit artery on emergent coronary angiography and an additional 145 (4.3%) of appropriate CCL activations did not receive emergent coronary angiography because of a change in clinical status (**Fig. 7**). If these two patient groups were to be reclassified as inappropriate CCL activations, the rate would increase to 18.7% (741 of 3973 CCL activations).[41] Cardiac biomarkers and clinical outcome data were not included.

Also in 2012, Mixon and colleagues[42] performed a retrospective analysis of 345 consecutive CCL activations from an STEMI system in central Texas. A blinded review of the ECG that triggered the CCL activation was performed by 2 cardiologists to determine whether the CCL activation was appropriate or inappropriate. STEMI was confirmed by the combination of a culprit vessel on emergent coronary

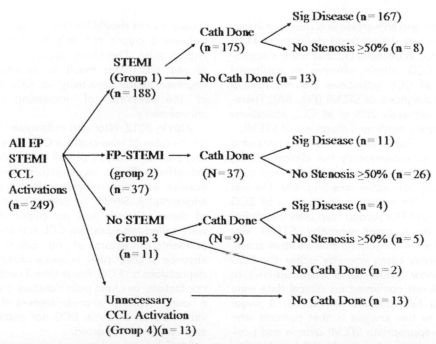

Fig. 6. Study diagram from Kontos and colleagues.[40] Cath, catheterization. EP, emergency physician; FP, false positive; Sig, significant. (*From* Kontos MC, Kurz MC, Roberts CS, et al. An evaluation of the accuracy of emergency physician activation of the cardiac catheterization laboratory for patients with suspected ST-segment elevation myocardial infarction. Ann Emerg Med 2010;55:425; with permission.)

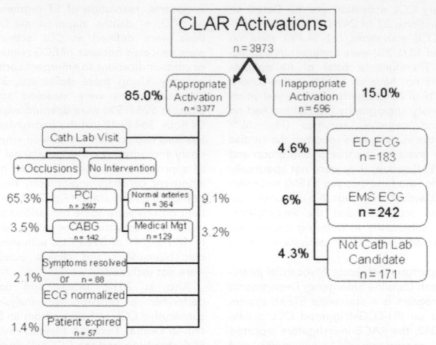

Fig. 7. CCL activations from the North Carolina RACE registry. Cath Lab, catheterization laboratory; ED, emergency department; Mgt, management; PCI, percutaneous coronary intervention. CLAR, catheterization laboratory activation registry. (*Adapted from* Garvey JL, Monk L, Granger CB, et al. Rates of cardiac catheterization cancellation for ST-segment elevation myocardial infarction after activation by emergency medical services or emergency physicians: results from the North Carolina catheterization laboratory activation registry. Circulation 2012;125:310; with permission.)

angiography and an increase and decrease in cardiac biomarkers. Using these definitions, 44 of the 345 CCL activations (12.8%) were inappropriate by ECG criteria, whereas an additional 15.6% of all CCL activations did not have a confirmed diagnosis of STEMI (Fig. 8A). Therefore, approximately 28% of all CCL activations failed to have a confirmed diagnosis of STEMI.[42] Based on this tiered approach of first reviewing the ECG and subsequently the clinical course, the investigators proposed a 2-step approach to classifying false activations (Fig. 8B). The first step asks, is the activation appropriate by ECG criteria or not? The second step uses the clinical outcome data; cases whereby STEMI was confirmed were considered true-positive activations, whereas cases whereby either the ECG did not show STEMI (ECG inappropriate) or STEMI was not confirmed on clinical data were considered false-positive activations. A major limitation to this analysis is that patients who have ECG-appropriate STEMI criteria and positive cardiac biomarkers could still be classified as false-positive activations if there was no culprit, even though these patients fulfill the definition of STEMI.[37] Certainly CCL activation for

these patients should be considered appropriate because a culprit can only be determined by angiography. Therefore, applying this scheme to real life might result in an unacceptable decrease in the sensitivity for CCL activations in the interest of increasing specificity unnecessarily.

Also in 2012, Nfor and colleagues[43] reported on the rates of false-positive CCL activations in a single-center analysis of 489 consecutive STEMI activations. These investigators defined false positive as no identifiable culprit on coronary angiography. Similar to previous reports, 11% of these subjects had no culprit lesion and were called false-positive CCL activations. Independent predictors of no culprit included absence of chest pain, absence of reciprocal ST depressions on ECG, fewer than 3 cardiovascular risk factors, or chest pain duration greater than 6 hours.[43] Neither appropriateness of CCL activation based on initial ECG nor outcome measures were not reported.

McCabe and colleagues[44] reviewed data from the Activate-SF registry to determine the rate of false activations. In this study, false activation was defined as no culprit or by assessment of

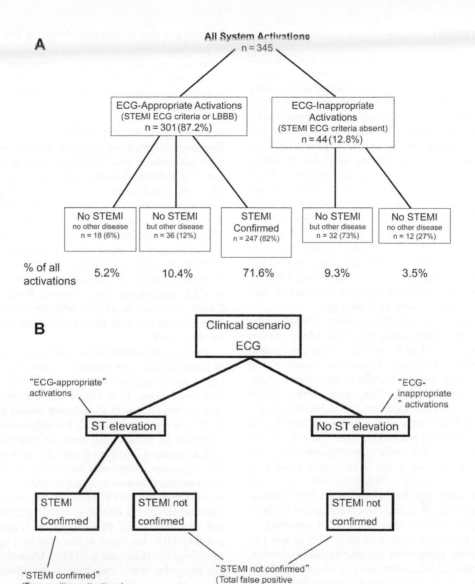

Fig. 8. (A) Classification scheme of CCL activations by Mixon and colleagues.[42] (B) Proposed false-activation classification scheme by Mixon and colleagues. LBBB, left bundle branch block. (From Mixon TA, Suhr E, Caldwell G, et al. Retrospective description and analysis of consecutive catheterization ST-segment elevation myocardial infarction activations with proposal, rationale and use of a new classification scheme. Circ Cardiovasc Qual Outcomes 2012;5:65 and 67; with permission.)

clinical, ECG, and biomarker data (In patients who did not receive emergent coronary angiography). They reported 146 of 411 (36%) patients were false activations by this criteria. At angiography, 101 of the 352 (28.7%) patients had no culprit; but this included 62 patients with CAD and 37 with elevation of their cardiac biomarkers. As noted earlier, patients with ischemic symptoms, ST-elevation, and elevated biomarkers fulfill the universal definition for

STEMI.[37] Therefore, it is difficult to consider these patients (who may have takotsubo, coronary spasm, coronary thrombus with resolution, and so forth) false activations. Additionally, 16 of 59 patients who did not receive coronary angiography (27%) had elevated cardiac biomarkers, 14 (23.7%) had clinical criteria consistent with STEMI, and 4 (6.7%) had ECG criteria consistent with STEMI raising the possibility of missed STEMIs in this cohort.[44]

DISCUSSION

Several important insights can be made based on the available literature. First, false-activation rates vary widely, from as low as approximately 5% to as high as approximately 40%. Secondly, this wide range in false-activation prevalence is, in part, due to the variability in definitions for overcall, false-positive, or inappropriate CCL activations. Common themes used for deciding which CCL activations are appropriate versus those that are inappropriate or false positive include ECG criteria, cardiac biomarkers, and/or findings on emergent coronary angiography. Individual patient goals of care, medical comorbidities, and contraindications to cardiac catheterization further complicate the matter of defining appropriate and inappropriate CCL activations. These issues highlight the need for universal definitions and terminology.

A third lesson is that the reasons for false activation are incompletely reported. Many studies cite incorrect ECG interpretation as the reason for false-positive CCL activations; however, the specific reasons (ie, bundle branch block, early repolarization, pericarditis, and other STEMI mimics) are not reported. In a recent single-center subset study of the RACE registry based on 231 PH-ECG activations over 3 years, bundle branch block, left ventricular hypertrophy, and nonwhite race were the 3 strongest predictors of false activations.[45] No other literature exists on the topic. The final observation from reviewing the literature is that clinical outcomes for false activation patients have rarely been reported.

The universal definition of STEMI is any patient with symptoms of myocardial ischemia, characteristic ECG changes ($\geq$1 mm of ST elevation on $\geq$2 contiguous leads, except lead V2-V3 whereby 2 mm is the threshold), and a typical increase and decrease in cardiac biomarkers.[37] The definition does not depend on angiographic findings; therefore, no culprit patients that fit the definition of STEMI should be considered appropriate CCL activations.

The authors think that the terms *inappropriate*, *false activations*, and *overactivation* are synonymous and represent a patient population that for reasons related to ECG findings, clinical scenarios, goals of care, or medical comorbidities *do not warrant emergent coronary angiography*. Three important principles must be kept in mind when considering novel metrics:

1. What population are we trying to define and for what purpose?

2. How can the information improve the STEMI process?
3. What are the risks or consequences of altering the STEMI process to try to minimize false activations (ie, maximizing the CCL activation index)?

Basic Metrics: Simple and Objective

The authors propose 2 novel metrics to track false activations and STEMI systems efficiency: the *CCL activation index* and the *revascularization index*. Both are relatively simple to calculate and remain objective because they track the occurrence of specific events. The authors think STEMI systems should begin to consistently track the total number of CCL activations, the number of CCL activations that proceed to emergent coronary angiography, the number of CCL activations that receive PPCI and/or CABG, the number of CCL activations with positive biomarkers, and clinical outcome measures for all patients.

The CCL activation index is defined as the ratio of patients receiving emergent coronary angiography as compared with the total number of CCL activations. In a highly functioning STEMI system, the CCL activation index should be 90% to 95% or greater. PH-ECG transmission has the potential to reduce the rates of inappropriate CCL activations, increasing the CCL Activation Index. However, clear roles for where the PH-ECG is transmitted and who is responsible for quickly interpreting the PH-ECG must be defined for transmission to be effective. A CCL activation index goal of 90% to 95% or greater is attainable but CANNOT be done at the cost of a systems' sensitivity for diagnosing STEMI. Missed STEMIs are likely far more detrimental for clinical outcomes than an unnecessary coronary angiogram. Rapid preactivation by EMS and emergency department staff should be the norm for most patients with STEMI, whereas on-duty interventional cardiology consultation may be required *before* activation in patients with equivocal ECGs or complex clinical scenarios.

The *revascularization index* is defined as the number of emergent PPCI + CABG performed divided by the total number of emergent coronary angiography procedures. A reasonable goal for the revascularization index is 80% to 90%. The literature indicates 5% to 20% of STEMI activations will have no culprit on coronary angiography.[36,38–44] Therefore, if the revascularization index is greater than 90%, it is likely that too few patients with probable STEMI are being taken for emergent coronary angiography.

In contrast, a revascularization index less than 00% likely indicates an overly aggressive system that performs too many emergent coronary angiography procedures. Improved screening of patients for common STEMI mimics or abnormal baseline ECGs are reasonable strategies to increase the revascularization index in these instances.

Fig. 9 illustrates a highly efficient STEMI system with high CCL activation index and an appropriate revascularization index (see Fig. 9A), an inefficient STEMI system with a low CCL activation index and high revascularization index (see Fig. 9B), an inefficient STEMI system with a low CCL activation index and an appropriate revascularization index (see Fig. 9C), and an inefficient STEMI system with a high CCL activation index and a low revascularization index (see Fig. 9D).

Advanced Metrics More Complex and Subjective

STEMI systems should also track and report more advanced metrics. For example, STEMI systems should make every effort to identify and minimize the occurrence of missed STEMIs. A missed STEMI is defined as a patient with myocardial ischemic symptoms and ECG findings consistent with STEMI who does not receive emergent cardiac catheterization in the absence of contraindications. Missed STEMIs may include patients with borderline or equivocal ECG changes, patients with left bundle branch block (LBBB), and so forth that are more evident with the advantage of retrospective review. Cross-referencing national registries, such as the National Cardiovascular Data Registry, the CathPCI Registry, or the Joint Commission Reporting may help to identify these patients.[46] The rate of missed STEMIs has been

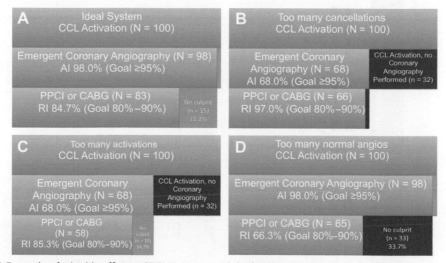

Fig. 9. (A) Example of a highly efficient STEMI system with high CCL activation index and an appropriate revascularization index. CCL activation index = 98.0% (98 of 100). Goal of 95% or greater. Revascularization index = 84.7% (83 of 98). Goal of 80% to 90%. (B) Example of an inefficient STEMI system with a low CCL activation index and an inappropriately high revascularization index. This is an example of a system that is, overly selective in determining what patients receive emergent coronary angiography. In this system, the CCL-team is frequently activated without performing emergent coronary angiography. However, nearly every emergent coronary angiography procedure results in a revascularization. Being overly selective in determining which patients receive emergent coronary angiography subjects the system to missed STEMIs. CCL activation index = 68.0% (68 of 100). Goal of 95% or greater. Revascularization index = 97.0% (66 of 68). Goal of 80% to 90%. (C) Example of an inefficient STEMI system with a low CCL activation index and an appropriate revascularization index. This system is an example of a system that is overly aggressive in CCL activation. Although relatively few CCL activations result in emergent coronary angiography, the appropriate revascularization indicates that neither too few nor too many emergent coronary angiograms are being performed. This high CCL activation rate with low CCL activation index represents an unnecessary utilization of a precious resource within an STEMI system and something that on-duty frontline EMS and emergency department staff should work to minimize by carefully evaluating patients and scrutinizing the PH-ECG. CCL activation index = 68.0% (68 of 100). Goal of 95% or greater. Revascularization index = 85.3% (58 of 68). Goal of 80% to 90%. (D) Example of an overly aggressive STEMI system with a high CCL activation index and a low revascularization index. This system is an example of a system that is not being selective enough in who receives emergent coronary angiography. CCL activation index = 98.0% (98 of 100). Goal of 95% or greater. Revascularization index = 66.3% (65 of 98). Goal of 80% to 90%. AI, angiographic index; RI, revascularization index.

Table 4
Reclassification of false-positive activations according to the proposed universal definitions

	(+) ECG, CI to Cath (n, %)	(+) ECG, No Culprit, (−) Enzymes (n, %)	(−) ECG, (+) Enzymes (n, %)	(−) ECG, (−) Enzymes (n, %)	Total False Activations (n, %)	CCL Activation Index (No. Emergent Coronary Angiograms/ No. of CCL Activations)	Revascularization Index (No. PPCI + No. CABG/ No. Emergent Coronary Angiograms)
Larson et al,[36] 2007 (n = 1335)	3 (0.2)	123 (9.2)	?1 (0.1)	?1 (0.1)	128 (9.6)	1335 of 1345 (99.2%)	1148 of 1335 (86.0%)
Khot et al,[38] 2007 (n = 164)	???	?10 (6.1)	???	???	???	163 of 164 (99.3%)	149 of 163 (91.4%)
Youngquist et al,[39] 2008 (n = 56)	???	???	?12 (21.4)	???	???	???	???
Kontos et al,[40] 2010 (n = 249)	13 (5.2)	37 (14.9)	?6 (2.4)	?20 (8.0)	?74 (29.7)	221 of 249 (88.8%)	?182 of 221 (82.4%)
Garvey et al,[41] 2012 (n = 3973)	171 (4.3)	?364 (9.1)	???	?425 (10.7)	960 (24.2)	3232 of 3377 (95.7%)	2739 of 3232 (84.7%)
Mixon et al,[42] 2012 (n = 345)	???	?54 (15.7)	?21 (6.1)	?23 (6.7)	?98 (28.4)	???	???
Nfor et al,[43] 2012 (n = 489)	???	???	???	?21 (4.3)	???	?489 of 489 (100%)	435 of 489 (88.9%)
McCabe et al,[44] 2012 (n = 411)	14 (5.8)	24 (5.8)	9 (2.2)	35 (8.5)	82 (20.0)	352 of 411 (85.6%)	251 of 352 (71.3%)

Abbreviation: Cath, catheterization.

reported as high as 8% in a large retrospective cohort study.[47] However, in highly functioning STEMI systems, missed STEMIs should be rare (<2% of all STEMIs).

SRCs should also consider tracking the CCL activation to STEMI alert ratio, defined as the number of EMS initiated CCL activations divided by the total number of patients who are triaged by EMS to the SRC. A clear goal is challenging as there is considerable variation from region to region regarding what triggers an STEMI alert. Some regions have strict criteria that maximize specificity, whereas others have many more STEMI alerts. However, tracking these data would give a sense of the traffic within an STEMI system as well as an additional measure of system efficiency.

SRCs that receive interhospital transfers from non-PPCI facilities should track a CCL activation to transfer ratio. This ratio, defined as the number of CCL activations that arrive via transfer divided by the total number of STEMI alert transfers from a given non-PPCI facility. Ideally, this ratio should approach 1; however, there may be some variability from system to system. This ratio allows for identification of highly functioning non-PPCI centers and inefficient non-PPCI centers within a given STEMI system. Identification of non-PPCI centers with particularly low CCL activation to transfer ratios allows for feedback and cooperative development of process improvement initiatives by the various stakeholders to optimize this ratio.

Finally, a proportion of false activations that do not receive emergent coronary angiography may receive elective coronary angiography during the same hospitalization, for example, patients with clear STEMIs but medical contraindications to cardiac catheterization requiring treatment or stabilization, NSTEMIs that inappropriately triggered CCL activation, or changes in patient goals of care. Although there is very little literature on this population, tracking these patients, including the circumstances of CCL activation, reasons for CCL cancellation, and clinical outcomes, will help to identify targets for process improvement within an SRC.

The rates of false activations based on these new definitions and the available data are shown in Table 4. In the studies that provided the relevant information, false-activation rates varied from 9.6% to 28.4%. Important take-home messages from this table include

1. Many of these studies did not provide sufficient data to allow for proper classification of false activations according to this scheme.

2. In the most efficient systems, most of the false activations should result from patients who meet ECG criteria for STEMI and receive emergent coronary angiography but are found to have no culprit lesion and negative cardiac enzymes, which may constitute up to 10% of patients and is likely unavoidable because of challenging clinical scenarios, such as LBBB, previous myocardial infarction, and other STEMI mimics.

3. Highly efficient STEMI systems, such as those reported by Larson and colleagues,[36] Garvey and colleagues,[41] and Nfor and colleagues,[43] can achieve a CCL activation index of 95% or greater and a revascularization index between 80% and 90%.

FUTURE DIRECTIONS

False activations should be defined as patients who triggered CCL activation but did not require emergent coronary angiography. There are limited data in the literature according to this definition, highlighting the need for further studies. Additionally, studies are needed to better understand the reasons for false activations. Clinical outcome data are necessary to better understand the predictors for false activations, findings on coronary angiography, cardiac enzyme levels and short- and long-term mortality.

Lessons learned from these studies can be applied to refine the STEMI process in the interest of optimizing efficiency. Each STEMI system should collect ongoing data to determine the effect of STEMI process changes on clinical outcomes and resource utilization. Finally, it is of the utmost importance that changes to the STEMI process that attempt to optimize efficiency do not detract from the sensitivity for detecting and diagnosing STEMI. Every effort must be made to minimize missed STEMIs, as these represent eligible but untreated patients who could benefit greatly from PPCI.

Winston Churchill[48] once said, "to improve is to change; to be perfect is to change often." False-positive CCL activations are an area ripe for improvement; however, a better understanding of the scope, causes, and consequences of this clinical conundrum is necessary before improvement can be obtained.

REFERENCES

1. Krumholz H, Herrin J, Miller LE, et al. Improvements in door-to-balloon time in the United States, 2005 to 2010. Circulation 2011;124:1038–45.

2. American Heart Association Mission: Lifeline. 2015. Available at: http://www.heart.org/HEART ORG/HealthcareResearch/MissionLifelineHomePage/ LearnAboutMissionLifeline/STEMI-Systems-of-Care_ UCM_439065_SubHomePage.jsp. Accessed January 2016. Accessed January 27, 2016.

3. Menees DS, Peterson ED, Wang Y, et al. Door-to-balloon time and mortality among patients undergoing primary PCI. N Engl J Med 2013;369:901–9.

4. Bates ER, Jacobs AK. Time to treatment in patients with STEMI. N Engl J Med 2013;369:889–92.

5. Nallamothu BK, Normand ST, Wang Y, et al. Relation between door-to-balloon times and mortality after percutaneous coronary intervention over time: a retrospective study. Lancet 2015;385: 1114–22.

6. Masoudi FA, Ponirakis A, Yeh RW, et al. Cardiovascular care facts: a report from the national cardiovascular data registry: 2011. J Am Coll Cardiol 2013;62(21):1931–47.

7. Shah RU, Henry TD, Rutten-Ramos S, et al. Increasing percutaneous coronary interventions for ST-segment elevation myocardial infarction in the United States. JACC Cardiovasc Interv 2015;8:139–46.

8. Muller D, Schnitzer L, Brandt J, et al. The accuracy of an out-of-hospital 12-lead ECG for the detection of ST-elevation myocardial infarction immediately after resuscitation. Ann Emerg Med 2008;52: 658–64.

9. Wang K, Asinger R, Marriott H. ST-segment elevation in conditions other than acute myocardial infarction. N Engl J Med 2003;349:2128–35.

10. O'Gara PT, Kushner FG, Ascheim DD, et al. 2013 ACCF/AHA guideline for the management of ST-elevation myocardial infarction: a report from the American College of Cardiology Foundation/ American Heart Association Task Force on Practice Guidelines. J Am Coll Cardiol 2013;61(4):e78–140.

11. Steg PG, James SK, Atar D, et al. ESC guidelines for the management of acute myocardial infarction in patients presenting with ST-segment elevation. Eur Heart J 2012;33:2569–619.

12. Luepker RV, Raczynski JM, Osganian S, et al. Effect of a community intervention on patient delay and emergency medical service use in acute coronary heart disease: the rapid early action for coronary treatment (REACT) trial. JAMA 2000;284:60–7.

13. Rokos IC, French WJ, Koenig WJ, et al. Integration of pre-hospital electrocardiograms and ST-elevation myocardial infarction receiving center (SRC) networks: impact on door-to-balloon times across 10 independent regions. JACC Cardiovasc Interv 2009;2:339–46.

14. Henry TD. From concept to reality: a decade of progress in regional ST-segment elevation myocardial infarction systems. Circulation 2012; 126:166–8.

15. Rokos IC, French WJ, Mattu A, et al. Appropriate cardiac cath lab activation: optimizing electrocardiogram interpretation and clinical decision-making for acute ST-elevation myocardial infarction. Am Heart J 2010;160:995–1003, 1003.e1-8.

16. Le May MR, Dionne R, Maloney J, et al. Diagnostic performance and potential clinical impact of advanced care paramedic interpretation of ST-segment elevation myocardial infarction in the field. CJEM 2006;8:401–7.

17. Kereiakes DJ, Gibler WB, Martin LH, et al. Relative importance of emergency medical system transport and the prehospital electrocardiogram on reducing hospital time delay to therapy for acute myocardial infarction: a preliminary report from the Cincinnati heart project. Am Heart J 1992;123: 835–40.

18. Ting HH, Krumholz HM, Bradley EH, et al. Implementation and integration of prehospital ECGs into systems of care for acute coronary syndrome: a statement from the American Heart Association. Circulation 2008;118:1066–79.

19. Curtis JP, Portnay EL, Wang Y, et al. The pre-hospital electrocardiogram and time to reperfusion in patients with acute myocardial infarction, 2000-2002: findings from the National Registry of Myocardial Infarction-4. J Am Coll Cardiol 2006; 47:1544–52.

20. Weaver WD, Cerqueira M, Hallstrom AP, et al. Pre-hospital-initiated vs hospital-initiated thrombolytic therapy: the myocardial infarction triage and intervention trial. JAMA 1993;270:1211–6.

21. Foster DB, Dufendach JH, Barkdoll CM, et al. Prehospital recognition of AMI using independent nurse/paramedic 12-lead ECG evaluation: impact on in-hospital times to thrombolysis in a rural community hospital. Am J Emerg Med 1994;12:25–31.

22. Ioannidis JP, Salem D, Chew PW, et al. Accuracy and clinical effect of out-of-hospital electrocardiography in the diagnosis of acute cardiac ischemia: a meta-analysis. Ann Emerg Med 2001;37:461–70.

23. Morrow DA, Antman EM, Sayah A, et al. Evaluation of the time saved by pre-hospital initiation of reteplase for ST-elevation myocardial infarction: results of the early retavase-thrombolysis in myocardial infarction (ER-TIMI) 19 trial. J Am Coll Cardiol 2002;40:71–7.

24. Pedley DK, Bissett K, Connolly EM, et al. Prospective observational cohort study of time saved by prehospital thrombolysis for ST elevation myocardial infarction delivered by paramedics. BMJ 2003;327:22–6.

25. Terkelsen CJ, Lassen JF, Nørgaard BL, et al. Reduction of treatment delay in patients with ST-elevation myocardial infarction: impact of pre-hospital diagnosis and direct referral to primary

percutaneous coronary intervention. Eur Heart J 2005;26:770–7.

26. Brainard AH, Raynovich W, Tandberg D, et al. The prehospital 12-lead electrocardiogram's effect on time to initiation of reperfusion therapy: a systematic review and meta-analysis of existing literature. Am J Emerg Med 2005;23:351–6.

27. Brown JP, Mahmud E, Dunford JV, et al. Effect of prehospital 12-lead electrocardiogram on activation of the cardiac catheterization laboratory and door-to-balloon time in ST-segment elevation acute myocardial infarction. Am J Cardiol 2008;101:158–61.

28. Dhruva VN, Abdelhadi SI, Anis A, et al. ST-segment analysis using wireless technology in acute myocardial infarction (STAT-MI) trial. J Am Coll Cardiol 2007;50:509–13.

29. Terkelsen CJ, Nørgaard BL, Lassen JF, et al. Telemedicine used for remote prehospital diagnosing in patients suspected of acute myocardial infarction. J Intern Med 2002;252:412–20.

30. Adams GL, Campbell PT, Adams JM, et al. Effectiveness of prehospital wireless transmission of electrocardiograms to a cardiologist via handheld device for patients with acute myocardial infarction (from the Timely Intervention in Myocardial Emergency, NorthEast Experience [TIME-NE]). Am J Cardiol 2006;98:1160–4.

31. Davis DP, Graydon C, Stein R, et al. The positive predictive value of paramedic versus emergency physician interpretation of the prehospital 12-lead electrocardiogram. Prehosp Emerg Care 2007;11:399–402.

32. Whitbread M, Leah V, Bell T, et al. Recognition of ST elevation by paramedics. Emerg Med J 2002;19:66–7.

33. Keeling P, Hughes D, Price L, et al. Safety and feasibility of prehospital fibrinolysis carried out by paramedics. BMJ 2003;327:27–8.

34. Feldman JA, Brinsfield K, Bernard S, et al. Real-time paramedic compared with blinded physician identification of ST-segment elevation myocardial infarction: results of an observational study. Am J Emerg Med 2005;23:443–8.

35. Bosson N, Kaji AH, Niemann JT, et al. The utility of prehospital ECG transmission in a large EMS system. Prehosp Emerg Care 2015;19:496–503.

36. Larson DM, Menssen KM, Sharkey SW, et al. "False-positive" cardiac catheterization activation among patients with suspected ST-elevation myocardial infarction. JAMA 2007;298:2754–60.

37. Thygesen K, Alpert JS, Jaffe AS, et al. ESC/ACCF/AHA/WHF expert consensus document: third universal definition of myocardial infarction. Circulation 2012;126:2020–35.

38. Khot UK, Johnson ML, Ramsey C, et al. Emergency department physician activation of the cardiac catheterization laboratory and immediate transfer to an immediately available cardiac catheterization laboratory reduce door-to-balloon time in ST-segment elevation myocardial infarction. Circulation 2007;116:67–76.

39. Youngquist ST, Shah AP, Niemann JT, et al. A comparison of door-to-balloon times and false-positive activations between emergency department and out-of-hospital activation of the coronary catheterization team. Acad Emerg Med 2008;15:784–7.

40. Kontos MC, Kurz MC, Roberts CS, et al. An evaluation of the accuracy of emergency physician activation of the cardiac catheterization laboratory for patients with suspected ST-segment elevation myocardial infarction. Ann Emerg Med 2010;55:423–30.

41. Garvey JL, Monk L, Granger CB, et al. Rates of cardiac catheterization cancellation for ST-segment elevation myocardial infarction after activation by emergency medical services or emergency physicians: results from the North Carolina catheterization laboratory activation registry. Circulation 2012;125:308–13.

42. Mixon TA, Suhr E, Caldwell G, et al. Retrospective description and analysis of consecutive catheterization ST-segment elevation myocardial infarction activations with proposal, rationale and use of a new classification scheme. Circ Cardiovasc Qual Outcomes 2012;5:62–9.

43. Nfor T, Kostopoulos L, Hashim H, et al. Identifying false-positive ST-elevation myocardial infarction in emergency department patients. J Emerg Med 2012;43:561–7.

44. McCabe JM, Armstrong EJ, Kulkarni A, et al. Prevalence and factors associated with false-positive ST-segment elevation myocardial infarction diagnoses at primary percutaneous coronary intervention-capable centers: a report from the ACTIVAT-SF registry. Arch Intern Med 2012;172:864–71.

45. Musey PI, Studnek JR, Garvey L. Characteristics of ST-elevation myocardial infarction patients who do not undergo percutaneous coronary intervention after prehospital cardiac catheterization activation. Crit Pathw Cardiol 2016;15:16–21.

46. Campbell AR, Satran D, Larson DM, et al. ST-elevation myocardial infarction: which patients do quality assurance programs include? Circ Cardiovasc Qual Outcomes 2009;2:648–55.

47. Tricomi AJ, Magid DJ, Rumsfeld JS, et al. Missed opportunities for reperfusion therapy for ST-segment elevation myocardial infarction: results of the emergency department quality in myocardial infarction (EDQMI) study. Am Heart J 2008;155:471–7.

48. Wikiquote. Available at: https://en.wikiquote.org/wiki/Winston_Churchill. Accessed July 8, 2016.

In-Hospital ST Elevation Myocardial Infarction

Clinical Characteristics, Management Challenges, and Outcome

Xuming Dai, MD, PhD[a],*, Ross F. Garberich, MS[b],
Brian E. Jaski, MD[c], Sidney C. Smith Jr, MD[a],
Timothy D. Henry, MD[d]

KEYWORDS

- Myocardial infarction • In-hospital STEMI • Delivery of care • Standardized protocol

---

KEY POINTS

- Patients who develop ST elevation myocardial infarction (STEMI) while admitted to the hospital are a complex patient population who are typically excluded from clinical trials and registries.
- They are known to be older with more comorbidities, have delayed recognition times, and longer times to reperfusion.
- The implementation of a standardized protocol has been shown to improve recognition and outcomes.
- Still, given the heterogeneity and complexity of the patient population with in-hospital STEMI, complex clinical decisions are required.

Contemporary treatment of ST elevation myocardial infarction (STEMI) emphasizes timely reperfusion therapy. Established systems of care for STEMI start with a patient who develops ischemic symptoms in the community and enters the healthcare system either by calling emergency medical service (EMS) or presenting to an emergency department (ED). This system of care integrates EMS, ED, cardiology, cardiac catheterization laboratory (CCL) and interhospital transfers to establish a chain of survival for these patients. Recently, some studies have focused attention on patients who develop STEMIs while already hospitalized in an acute care facility. Because in-hospital STEMIs are typically excluded from clinical trials, registries, and quality reporting, there are limited and incomplete

data available. However, it has been consistently shown that in-hospital STEMIs are a heterogeneous group with unique clinical characteristics and worse outcomes when compared with outpatient STEMIs. This article summarizes our current understanding of in-hospital STEMI, specifically in comparison with the more familiar outpatient STEMI, identifies opportunities for quality improvement, and proposes strategies to improve care for these patients and future directions for in-hospital STEMI guidelines.

OUTPTAIENT VERSUS IN-HOSPITAL ST ELEVATION MYOCARDIAL INFARCTION

The widely accepted open-artery theory considers an STEMI to be the result of acute

---

[a] Division of Cardiology, University of North Carolina at Chapel Hill, 160 Dental Circle, Chapel Hill, NC 27599, USA; [b] Minneapolis Heart Institute Foundation, Abbott Northwestern Hospital, 920 East 28th Street, Suite 100, Minneapolis, MN 55407, USA; [c] San Diego Cardiac Center, Sharp Healthcare, 3131 Berger Avenue, San Diego, CA 92123, USA; [d] Cedars-Sinai Heart Institute, 127 South San Vicente Boulevard, Suite A3100, Los Angeles, CA 90048, USA
* Corresponding author. Division of Cardiology, University of North Carolina at Chapel Hill, Chapel Hill, NC 27514.
E-mail address: xuming_dai@med.unc.edu

Intervent Cardiol Clin 5 (2016) 471–480
http://dx.doi.org/10.1016/j.iccl.2016.06.005

occlusion of a coronary artery leading to myocardial ischemia.[1] Timely reperfusion therapy, in particular, by primary percutaneous coronary intervention (PCI) minimizes myocardial damage, reduces complications, and improves survival.[2] Large randomized clinical studies, national and regional quality improvement initiatives, and public education have promoted the establishment of STEMI systems of care across the country. An STEMI system of care is an integrated group of entities, including EMS, ED, cardiology, critical care units, nursing, hospital administration, and other supportive staff, who share the same goal of providing timely reperfusion therapy for STEMI. As a result of these efforts, the last decade has witnessed significant improvements in door-to-balloon time and STEMI survival across the world.[3,4] However, all these efforts target patients who develop symptoms outside of a hospital (outpatient STEMI) and subsequently enter the health care system either by presenting to the ED or urgent care facility or by calling EMS to the scene. The STEMI chain of survival starts with an early recognition of STEMI achieved by high awareness, early acquisition and interpretation of an electrocardiogram (ECG) by a trained ED or EMS team, followed by a highly specialized cardiology care team proceeding with timely primary PCI (Fig. 1, top panel).

In the era of primary PCI and STEMI systems of care, recent studies have identified a unique subset of patients whose STEMI develops while hospitalized for a variety of conditions (in-hospital or inpatient STEMI). Their primary reasons for admission are often not related to coronary artery disease (CAD). These patients are frequently under direct care of physicians, whose expertise may not pertain to the diagnosis and management of CAD or STEMI. Patients with in-hospital STEMIs have unique clinical features,

a less-well-defined chain of management process, and unfavorable outcomes. Better understanding of the risk factors, outcome predictors, and methods to improve the system of care for in-hospital STEMI is the next challenge of STEMI care.

EPIDEMIOLOGY OF IN-HOSPITAL ST ELEVATION MYOCARDIAL INFARCTION
Incidence Rate

Since 2007, the US Center for Medicare and Medicaid Services (CMS) has required a present-on-admission indicator for all diagnoses in CMS claims. This policy has been adopted by most private payers and state inpatient databases and provides an opportunity to identify whether an acute myocardial infarction (AMI) including STEMI was present or not on admission. Based on clinical practice, in-hospital STEMI is not uncommon; but its incident rate in our health care system is controversial due to incomplete data. Dai and colleagues[5] reported 3.4 confirmed in-hospital STEMIs per 10,000 adult discharges in a single tertiary university-based teaching hospital in the period of 2007 to 2011. A California State Inpatient Database (CA-SID) analysis reported 2.7 in-hospital STEMIs per 10,000 hospitalizations in the period of 2008 to 2011.[6] According to the American Hospital Association's data, there were 36 million adult admissions in United States in 2013. Based on this information, the authors estimate an incidence of approximately 10,000 in-hospital STEMI cases in the United States in 2013. Compared with the reported incidence rate of outpatient STEMI in older adults living in the community,[7,8] the incident rate of in-hospital STEMI is actually 40 to 50 fold higher.[9]

Acute care facilities concentrate individuals with various illness, injuries, or stresses requiring medical or surgical attention. Compared with

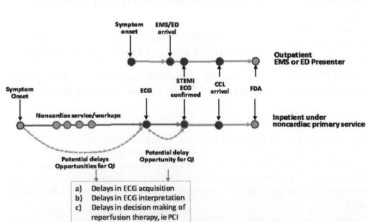

Fig. 1. Comparison of current processes managing patients with outpatient and in-hospital STEMIs and potential delays in the latter. FDA, Food and Drug Administration; QI, quality improvement.

the general population, hospitalized patients are older and have higher levels of anxiety, stress, inflammation, and, by definition, high-risk conditions. These patients are often undergoing or experiencing (1) medication changes, including interruptions of antiplatelet and anticoagulation therapies; (2) metabolic and hemostatic derangements; (3) hemodynamic instabilities; and (4) physical and/or emotional stress. A high incidence of AMI during the preoperative and postoperative periods is well recognized.[10–12] Current AMI pathophysiology theory predicts a higher risk of AMI (including STEMI) for hospitalized individuals than adults in the general public in the community, consistent with the estimates discussed earlier. However, the proportion of reported patients with in-hospital STEMI to total patients with STEMI varies dramatically from 1% to 20% (Table 1) depending on the data source and definitions for inclusion of in-hospital STEMI or AMI. For example, Erne and colleagues[16] reported only 126 of 19,359 patients with STEMI are in-hospital STEMI (0.6%) in the National Registry of Acute Myocardial Infarction in Switzerland (AMIS Plus) from 2002 to 2014, including 34% hospitalized for various internal medicine diseases, 49.2% for surgery, and 16.9% for diagnostic procedures. Dai and colleagues[5] reported 48 out of 275 (17%) STEMIs from 2007 to 2011 were in-hospital STEMIs. Garberich and colleagues[14] found 83 out of 990 (8.4%) patients had their STEMI occur while in the hospital. Richmond and colleagues[15] reported the onset of 35 out of 172 (20%) patients with STEMI were inpatients (see Table 1).

Clinical Outcomes

Clinical outcomes of patients with in-hospital STEMI are worse than that of outpatient STEMI, including a 2- to 10-fold higher in-hospital mortality (Fig. 2). Thirty-day and 1-year mortality are also higher for in-hospital STEMI according to the Garberich and colleagues[14] and Richmond and colleagues[15] studies. The higher mortality reported in these patients is not surprising. Patients with in-hospital STEMI are older, with more comorbidities and complex underlying primary admission conditions. Additionally, cardiogenic shock and cardiac arrest are also more frequent for patients with in-hospital STEMI.[14] All of these factors lead to increased resource utilization as reflected by greater lengths of hospital stay and increased total hospital charges.[6,15,17] Variations in the reported in-hospital mortality are at least partially due to the data source used to identify patients with

in-hospital STEMI and if patients who are primarily admitted for other CAD-related conditions are included. Lower in-hospital mortality of inpatient STEMI was observed in patients who were admitted for cardiac conditions, including unstable angina or non-STEMI progressing to STEMI, as well as patients who were undergoing stress testing or post-PCI stent thrombosis.[14,15] Studies that include only individuals with inpatient STEMI who underwent cardiac catheterization or PCI also reported lower rates of mortality, as opposed to studies that include all in-hospital STEMIs identified from medical records or inpatient databases regardless of cardiac catheterization or PCI. These observations support the notion that invasive therapy reduces mortality of in-hospital STEMI. Kaul and colleagues[6] analyzed patients with in-hospital STEMI in the CA-SID and found that individuals with in-hospital STEMI who received PCI had higher survival in all quartiles of risk profiles stratified by Elixhauser comorbidity criteria.

Garberich and colleagues reported the reason for initial admission directly affected outcomes for in-hospital STEMI. Patients admitted for noncardiac reasons (eg, after surgery, respiratory failure, cancer) had increased morality rates in-hospital at 30 days and 1 year compared with patients admitted for a cardiac reason (eg, acute coronary syndrome, stress testing, after PCI). Additionally, patients initially admitted for noncardiac reasons had longer times from initial admission to diagnostic ECG times, longer diagnostic to ECG to balloon times, and longer lengths of stay when compared with patients admitted for cardiac reasons.[14,18,19]

CLINICAL CHARACTERISTICS OF IN-HOSPITAL ST ELEVATION MYOCARDIAL INFARCTION

Demographic Features

Compared with outpatient STEMI, multiple studies have reported that patients with in-hospital STEMI are older, more often female, and have higher rates of comorbid conditions, in particular, chronic kidney disease, prior cerebrovascular events, and known history of CAD and peripheral artery disease. Additionally, patients with in-hospital STEMI have a higher prevalence of hypertension, diabetes with chronic complications, chronic lung disease, cerebrovascular accident, intracranial hemorrhage, respiratory failure, and congestive heart failure. They are less likely to be current smokers but more likely to be former smokers compared with those who have outpatient STEMI. Patients with in-hospital STEMI also present more

Table 1
Summary of published studies on in-hospital ST elevation myocardial infarction

Studies	Study Period	Study Design	Data Source	No. of Subjects (In-Hospital vs Total STEMIs)	In-Hospital Mortality (In-Hospital vs Outpatient STEMIs)	PCI Utilization (In-Hospital vs Outpatient STEMIs)
Zahn et al,[13] 2000	1994–1997	Retrospective	MITRA registry	403 vs 5888; 6.8%	27.3% vs 13.9%	57.6% vs 59.3%
Dai et al,[5] 2013	2007–2011	Retrospective	Medical records	48 vs 275; 17%	40.0% vs 4.0%	56.0% vs 100%
Garberich et al,[14] 2014	2003–2013	Retrospective	Local PCI registry	83 vs 990; 8.4%	8.4% vs 4.6%	100% vs 100%
Kaul et al,[6] 2014	2008–2011	Retrospective	Inpatient database	3068 vs 62,021; 4.9%	33.6% vs 10.4%	21.6% vs 65.0%
Richmond et al,[15] 2015	2004–2010	Retrospective	Local PCI registry	35 vs 172; 20%	14.0% vs 5.8%	100% vs 100%
Jaski et al,[23] 2016	2009–2015	Retrospective	Medical records/registry	71 vs 1774; 40%	42.3% vs 23.0%	52.1% vs 87.5%

Abbreviation: MITRA, Maximal Individual Therapy in Acute Myocardial Infarction.

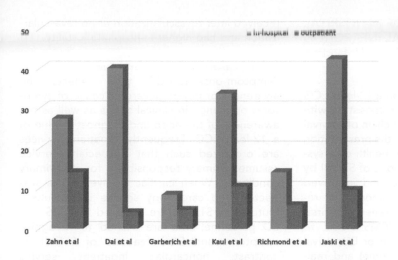

frequently with cardiac arrest and cardiogenic shock.

Risk Profile

Beyond a high prevalence of comorbidities, hospitalized patients may experience interruptions of dual antiplatelet or anticoagulation therapy, that is, in the setting of hemorrhage or surgery. Interruptions of antiplatelet and anticoagulation therapy in patients with CAD or previous stent procedures may predispose patients to stent thrombosis and/or occlusion of a coronary artery. In addition, a variety of inpatient conditions, including surgery, predispose patients to a prothrombotic state or increased platelet aggregation.[20] Anecdotal experiences suggest that recovery from thrombocytopenia in oncological patients from chemotherapy or patients receiving effective therapy for thrombocytopenia may experience dramatic increases in functional platelets. Hemodynamic challenges in patients with known CAD also predispose to the development of acute coronary syndrome, including STEMI.

Presentation and Symptoms

Preoperative and postoperative AMI is well recognized to have more insidious or atypical symptoms with delayed recognition than outpatient STEMI.[10–12,21] Three studies have analyzed clinical presentation of in-hospital STEMI. Compared with patients with outpatient STEMIs, inpatients present with fewer typical ischemic symptoms, including retrosternal chest pain, neck pain, or shoulder pain; fewer typical associated symptoms, such as nausea and diaphoresis; and fewer exertional symptoms.[5,17,22] Dai and colleagues[5] examined the events or symptoms that triggered the

performance of an index ECG leading to the diagnosis of in-hospital STEMIs and found that the most common trigger (up to 60% of cases) was a change of clinical status as observed and documented by the caring staff (ie, altered mental status, hypotension, and respiratory distress). Less frequently, an ECG was obtained in response to patient complaints, such as chest pain, dyspnea, and/or palpitation, or changes on telemetry. Unique to in-hospital STEMI, index ECGs were performed after the report of elevated cardiac biomarkers in nearly 20% of in-hospital STEMI cases.[5,17] These atypical symptoms and alternate modes of recognition are related to multiple factors: (1) hospitalized patients have symptoms related to their primary admitting conditions that may complicate their interpretation and perception; (2) a high use of analgesics and other medications may compromise symptom presentation; (3) female and elderly patients have more atypical symptoms of AMI; (4) postoperative and poststroke patients as well as intubated patients with respiratory failure frequently have altered levels of consciousness. Computational analysis of the cohort in the CA-SID found both procedural and patient-level factors were associated with the onset of STEMI in hospitalized patients.[6] Patients who underwent any surgical procedure as part of their hospitalization had a higher risk of in-hospital STEMI, compared with those who did not. The risk of in-hospital STEMI was lowest in patients with no procedures and highest in patients undergoing cardiac surgery. Congestive heart failure, coagulopathy, low-risk surgery, valvular disease, and peripheral artery disease were also variables associated with the development of in-hospital STEMI.

CLINICAL MANAGEMENT OF IN-HOSPITAL ST ELEVATION MYOCARDIAL INFARCTION

In-Hospital ST Elevation Myocardial Infarction Recognition

Electrocardiogram acquisition

The diagnosis of STEMI relies on a 12-lead ECG in addition to clinical symptoms consistent with myocardial ischemia. An STEMI chain of survival for outpatient STEMI starts with the presentation of symptomatic patients to the health care system, via EMS or ED, and diagnosis of STEMI by a 12-ECG. Systematic training and improved awareness of potential STEMI among first responders (EMS, ED) have shortened the first-medical-contact-to-ECG time (EMS arrival to completion of 12-lead ECG time or ED arrival to completion of 12-lead ECG time) and real-time ECG interpretation. Maynard and colleagues[17] reported that the first troponin value obtained for in-hospital AMIs was more often elevated, indicating a delay in diagnosis. Dai and colleagues[5] reviewed medical records of 48 in-hospital STEMI cases and found that the time between onset of the ischemic event and the performance of the index ECG varied dramatically, from a few minutes to more than 48 hours. The median time to obtain an ECG was 41 (10, 660) minutes in patients whose symptom onset time was documented compared with the median door-to-ECG time for ED presentation outpatients of 5 (2, 10) minutes ($P<.001$). Detailed analysis of how symptom-to-ECG time of in-hospital STEMI was associated with subsequent management and outcome (Fig. 3) revealed that individuals with in-hospital STEMIs who received early revascularization (within 2 hours of diagnostic ECG) all had an ECG performed within 1 hour of symptom onset. Triggers for the ECG acquisition were ischemic symptoms rather than observed changes of clinical status in those who had an ECG performed within 1 hour (61% vs 8%; $P<.001$). Individuals who had an ECG done 2 hours or more after symptom onset received later revascularization or no revascularization and had higher in-hospital mortality.

Electrocardiogram interpretation

Symptom-onset-to-ECG time reflects the awareness of potential cardiac cause of symptoms or change in clinical status as well as the awareness of the need and diagnostic value of a 12-lead ECG. Frequently, inpatient services are organized such that a specialty service assumes primary responsibility for its primary conditions. When cardiac involvement is suspected, the cardiology service is consulted. Outpatient STEMIs are received by EMS and ED personnel who are trained to recognize symptoms and ECG features of STEMI. In contrast, noncardiac inpatient service personnel may be less well equipped to recognize STEMI. The existing STEMI systems of care (see Fig. 1 upper panel) may not be applicable to in-hospital STEMI because these patients do not present to the EMS or ED, but rather the primary caregiver will be the initial front line for diagnosis and management. Although it is difficult to retrospectively identify the time when a diagnostic ECG was recognized as an STEMI, the time from ECG to the activation of cardiac catheterization laboratory or first device activation is a surrogate benchmark for door-to-balloon time or first-medical-contact-to-first-device-activation time. This ECG to CCL activation time also reflects the elapsed time from performing an ECG to recognizing STEMI, at least in those PCI-eligible patients. Although both Dai and colleagues[5] and Garberich and colleagues[14] reported comparable CCL performance (CCL-arrival-to-first-device time) between in-hospital and outpatient STEMI, prolonged ECG-to-first-device-activation time for in-hospital versus outpatient STEMI indicates that longer time elapsed from the performance of an ECG to the arrival at the CCL. This finding is likely due to the prolonged time for an ECG to be interpreted and STEMI to be diagnosed.

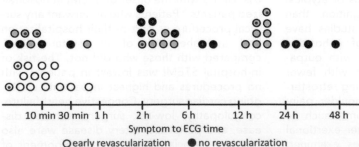

Fig. 3. Case analysis of 48 consecutive patients with in-hospital STEMIs revealing the distribution of symptom-to-ECG time, revascularization, and in-hospital death.

Treatment of In-Hospital ST Elevation Myocardial Infarction

Whereas effective guideline-directed medical and reperfusion therapy strategies have been well established for patients with STEMI, medical therapy for patients with in-hospital STEMIs has been less well studied. Erne and colleagues[16] reported that patients with in-hospital non-ST segment elevation myocardial infarction (NSTEMI) and STEMIs were less likely to receive immediate therapy with aspirin, P2Y12 inhibitor, heparin, beta-blocker, angiotensin-converting enzyme inhibitor/angiotensin-receptor blocker, and statin compared with outpatient AMI and to be less likely to be discharged with these medications.

Primary PCI is well known to be the most effective guideline-recommended reperfusion treatment of STEMI. Both patient-level and database analyses have found that PCI revascularization of in-hospital STEMI is associated with improved survival in all quartiles of comorbidity risk profiles. Studies that identify in-hospital STEMI from medical records or databases reveal low rates of primary PCI in treating in-hospital STEMI (see Table 1). Older age, complex comorbid conditions, concurrent primary illness or recent surgery, or terminal illness in hospitalized patients likely contribute to the lower revascularization rates and increased in-hospital mortality for inpatient STEMI. Delayed ECG acquisition and interpretation could also contribute to the low rates of revascularization.

Analyses of patients with in-hospital STEMIs who underwent invasive evaluation and revascularization found no significant difference of the distribution of infarct-related coronary territories. The absence of differences between patients with PCI-eligible in-hospital and outpatient STEMIs for the CCL team to achieve reperfusion (CCL-arrival-to-first-device-activation time), with comparable rates of successful revascularization after diagnostic coronary angiography, suggests that once in-hospital STEMIs enter the chain of survival, the subsequent treatment should follow standard STEMI guidelines.

STRATEGIES FOR QUALITY IMPROVEMENT
Potential Causes of Mortality

The high mortality observed for patients with in-hospital STEMIs is likely to be multifactorial. The reasons include (1) significantly higher rate of comorbidities, including higher rates of surgical procedures; (2) delayed recognition of the ischemic conditions; and (3) low utilization rates of proven beneficial therapeutic strategies, in particular, primary PCI as the revascularization approach. Further studies may enable the clinician to identify high-risk patients earlier and use appropriate reperfusion and adjunctive therapies to reduce the incidence rate overall.

Opportunities and Strategies for Quality Improvement

Previous studies have identified opportunities for quality improvement and successful strategies to improve quality of care for in-hospital STEMI. The cornerstone of STEMI treatment is timely reperfusion, ideally with primary PCI. Substantial delay of diagnosis and treatment of in-hospital STEMI and low rate of utilization of PCI have a negative effect on outcomes. Comparing the systems of care for patients with in-hospital STEMIs and patients with outpatient STEMIs reveals significant differences in many steps (Table 2). There are at least 3 sources of delay: (1) delays in ECG acquisition, (2) delays in ECG interpretation, and (3) delays in risk stratification and activation of existing STEMI system of care (Table 3).

Garberich and colleagues[14] reported their experience of the implementation of a "Level 1 MI program," a standardized STEMI protocol for in-hospital STEMI that resulted in a moderate decrease in median reperfusion times and an important reduction in in-hospital mortality. The authors have instituted a health care system–wide educational program to improve awareness of in-hospital STEMI among all levels of health care staff and an in-hospital STEMI response protocol to standardize the education, response, and rapid reperfusion process. Preliminary data convincingly demonstrate a significant improvement of STEMI care benchmarks, such as symptom-to-ECG time and ECG-to-first-device time.[9]

FUTURE DIRECTION

- Studies to model risk profiles of in-hospital STEMI for prediction risk and outcome
- Multicenter quality improvement program to gather evidence whether a quality improvement program improves outcome (ongoing)
- Development of guidelines to advise acute care facilities implementing practice protocols to facilitate early recognition and response for in-hospital STEMIs and to encourage reperfusion therapy as defined by guidelines

Table 2
Comparison of system of care for in-hospital versus outpatient ST elevation myocardial infarction

	In-Hospital STEMIs	Outpatient STEMIs
Location at symptom onset	Within a health care facility	In the community
Surrounding of the individual	Under care and monitor of staff and primary team	+/− Bystanders
Symptoms and presentation	Often atypical, less-specific complaints, rely more on observations	More often typical and specific complaints
First responders	In-hospital primary care team	EMS or ED staff
Responder's readiness for STEMI	Often not trained, not familiar with, or alert to STEMI	High alert, well trained, organized for STEMI
ECG acquisition	Often delayed in acquisition, primary condition or other comorbidities may mask ischemic symptoms	Protocol driven, often obtained and interpreted within 10 min
ECG interpretation	Possible delay due to less-well-trained staff and providers as primary team and lack of protocol	Protocol driven, immediate interpretation by trained personnel
Activation of STEMI team	Often require cardiology consultation, lack of protocol	Protocol driven, single-pager activation by EMS or ED as designated
Decision-making for reperfusion	Often complicated by primary reason for hospitalization and other comorbidities	Less complicated

Controversies for In-Hospital ST Elevation Myocardial Infarction Management

All studies previously mentioned acknowledge that patients with in-hospital STEMI are a heterogeneous and complex group of patients. Because many are already admitted to the hospital for illnesses that are not cardiac related, there are delays in recognition, transfer, and

Table 3
Potential delays and causes in in-hospital ST elevation myocardial infarction management and strategies for quality improvement

Delays	Potential Cause	QI Strategies
ECG acquisition	1. Atypical presentation 2. Complicated comorbid and primary conditions 3. Use of analgesics and sedatives 4. Less alertness and awareness among primary providers and staff	1. Education to improve awareness alertness 2. Clearly define criteria for ECG acquisition 3. RN perform/order ECG as needed
ECG interpretation	1. Less familiar with ECG by primary team 2. Ineffective system for rapid ECG interpretation within hospitals	1. Policy for STAT ECG physician interpretation 2. Cardiology response to interpret ECG
Risk stratification and activation of STEMI system	1. Lack of urgency of timely STEMI management among primary team 2. Unfamiliar with medical treatment of STEMI 3. Unfamiliar with the benefit and timeliness of reperfusion therapy and associated risks	1. Education to improve awareness and knowledge 2. Clinical protocol to direct involve cardiology team and facilitate communication with primary team

Abbreviations: QI, quality improvement; RN, registered nurse; STAT, statim.

treatment. In addition to these issues, complex decisions arise regarding which patients are suitable for immediate PCI and in which patients do the risks outweigh the benefits. Early postoperative patients, including neurosurgery or patients with intracerebral bleeds, may be too high risk for anticoagulation. Although which patients should be immediately referred or transferred for PCI and which are at too great of a risk may be controversial at times, having a standardized protocol for rapid diagnosis should not be controversial. Having a protocol and response team in place give the cardiovascular physician and staff the option to discuss any controversies through early recognition, quick referral or transfer, and standardized care, even when the decisions are complex.

In summary, patients with in-hospital STEMIs are a high-risk and complex patient population. These patients have increased comorbidities and have delays in recognition and reperfusion. However, the implementation of a standardized protocol for patients who develop STEMIs after admission to the hospital may improve recognition, decrease time to reperfusion, and subsequently improve clinical outcomes, including mortality.

REFERENCES

1. DeWood MA, Spores J, Notske R, et al. Prevalence of total coronary occlusion during the early hours of transmural myocardial infarction. N Engl J Med 1980;303(16):897–902.

2. O'Gara PT, Kushner FG, Ascheim DD, et al. 2013 ACCF/AHA guideline for the management of ST-elevation myocardial infarction: executive summary: a report of the American College of Cardiology Foundation/American Heart Association Task Force on Practice Guidelines. J Am Coll Cardiol 2013;61(4):485–510.

3. Krumholz HM, Herrin J, Miller LE, et al. Improvements in door-to-balloon time in the United States, 2005 to 2010. Circulation 2011;124(9):1038–45.

4. Rokos IC, French WJ, Koenig WJ, et al. Integration of pre-hospital electrocardiograms and ST-elevation myocardial infarction receiving center (SRC) networks: impact on door-to-balloon times across 10 independent regions. JACC Cardiovasc Interv 2009;2(4):339–46.

5. Dai X, Bumgarner J, Spangler A, et al. Acute ST-elevation myocardial infarction in patients hospitalized for noncardiac conditions. J Am Heart Assoc 2013;2(2):e000004.

6. Kaul P, Federspiel JJ, Dai X, et al. Association of inpatient vs outpatient onset of ST-elevation myocardial infarction with treatment and clinical outcomes. JAMA 2014;312(19):1999–2007.

7. Yeh RW, Sidney S, Chandra M, et al. Population trends in the incidence and outcomes of acute myocardial infarction. N Engl J Med 2010;362(23): 2155–65.

8. Go AS, Mozaffarian D, Roger VL, et al. Heart disease and stroke statistics–2014 update: a report from the American Heart Association. Circulation 2014;129(3):e28–292.

9. Dai X, Kaul P, Smith SC Jr, et al. Predictors, treatment, and outcomes of STEMI occurring in hospitalized patients. Nat Rev Cardiol 2015;13(3):148–54.

10. Goldman L, Caldera DL, Nussbaum SR, et al. Multifactorial index of cardiac risk in noncardiac surgical procedures. N Engl J Med 1977;297(16):845–50.

11. Devereaux PJ, Bradley D, Chan MT, et al. An international prospective cohort study evaluating major vascular complications among patients undergoing noncardiac surgery: the VISION Pilot Study. Open Med 2011;5(4):e193–200.

12. Goldman L. Multifactorial index of cardiac risk in noncardiac surgery: ten-year status report. J Cardiothorac Anesth 1987;1(3):237–44.

13. Zahn R, Schiele R, Seidl K, et al. Acute myocardial infarction occurring in versus out of the hospital: patient characteristics and clinical outcome. Maximal Individual TheRapy in Acute Myocardial Infarction (MITRA) Study Group. J Am Coll Cardiol 2000;35(7):1820–6.

14. Garberich RF, Traverse JH, Claussen MT, et al. ST-elevation myocardial infarction diagnosed after hospital admission. Circulation 2014;129(11):1225–32.

15. Richmond T, Holoshitz N, Haryani A, et al. Adverse outcomes in hospitalized patients who develop ST-elevation myocardial infarction. Crit Pathw Cardiol 2014;13(2):62–5.

16. Erne P, Bertel O, Urban P, et al. Inpatient versus outpatient onsets of acute myocardial infarction. Eur J Intern Med 2015;26(6):414–9.

17. Maynard C, Lowy E, Rumsfeld J, et al. The prevalence and outcomes of in-hospital acute myocardial infarction in the Department of Veterans Affairs Health System. Arch Intern Med 2006;166(13):1410–6.

18. Dai X, Kaul P, Stouffer GA. Letter by Dai et al regarding article, "ST-elevation myocardial infarction diagnosed after hospital admission". Circulation 2015;131(1):e6.

19. Garberich RF, Traverse JH, Claussen MT, et al. Response to letter regarding article, "ST-elevation myocardial infarction diagnosed after hospital admission". Circulation 2015;131(1):e7.

20. Genereux P, Rutledge DR, Palmerini T, et al. Stent thrombosis and dual antiplatelet therapy interruption with everolimus-eluting stents: insights from the Xience V coronary stent system trials. Circ Cardiovasc Interv 2015;8(5):1–10.

21. Devereaux PJ, Xavier D, Pogue J, et al. Characteristics and short-term prognosis of perioperative myocardial infarction in patients undergoing noncardiac surgery: a cohort study. Ann Intern Med 2011;154(8):523–8.

22. Zmyslinski RW, Lackland DT, Keil JE, et al. Increased fatality and difficult diagnosis of in-hospital acute myocardial infarction: comparison to lower mortality and more easily recognized pre-hospital infarction. Am Heart J 1981;101(5):586–92.

23. Jaski BE, Grigoriadis CE, Dai X, et al. Factors associated with ineligibility for PCI differ between inpatient and outpatient ST-elevation myocardial infarction. J Interv Cardiol 2016. [Epub ahead of print].

Optimal Antiplatelet Therapy In ST-Segment Elevation Myocardial Infarction

Rafael Harari, MD, Usman Baber, MD, MS*

KEYWORDS

- Antiplatelet agents • ST-segment elevation myocardial infarction • STEMI • P2Y$_{12}$ inhibitors
- GP IIb/IIIa inhibitors

KEY POINTS

- Antiplatelet therapy remains the cornerstone of treatment of myocardial infarction (MI).
- Advances in antiplatelet agents have resulted in improved outcomes for patients with ST-segment elevation MI (STEMI).
- Guideline recommendations for the use of antiplatelet agents in STEMI are discussed.
- Landmark clinical trials are reviewed.

INTRODUCTION

Cardiovascular disease is the leading cause of death worldwide, with an estimated 1 in every 3 deaths in 2012 attributed to this condition.[1] In the United States, heart disease has remained the leading cause of death since 1935, resulting in approximately 611,105 deaths and 735,000 MIs in 2013.[2] Coronary heart disease death rates in the United States have fallen steadily since 1968, with approximately 21% of this decrease attributed to initial treatments of MI and secondary preventive therapies.[3] Similarly, the case fatality of STEMI continues to decrease.[4–6]

Coronary artery disease is a chronic inflammatory vasculopathy characterized by endothelial dysfunction, smooth muscle cell proliferation, and the development of an atheromatous plaque within the intimal layer of coronary arteries.[7] STEMI most commonly occurs as a result of plaque rupture or endothelial erosion, leading to thrombus formation within the arterial lumen that impedes blood flow.[8] Since the 1960s, platelets have been recognized as playing a central role in the pathogenesis of MI by forming a thrombus and releasing chemical mediators

(serotonin, ADP, AMP, collagen, and thrombin) that perpetuate the hemostatic cascade.[9] For this reason, antiplatelet therapy remains the cornerstone in the medical management of acute coronary syndromes (ACSs), particularly in patients presenting with STEMI and undergoing percutaneous coronary intervention (PCI).

Current American College of Cardiology Foundation (ACCF)/American Heart Association (AHA) guidelines present 3 different classes of antiplatelet agents that are approved for use in patients with STEMI (Table 1): cyclooxygenase (COX) inhibitors (aspirin), P2Y$_{12}$ receptor antagonists (clopidogrel, prasugrel, and ticagrelor), and glycoprotein (GP) IIb/IIIa inhibitors (abciximab, eptifibatide, and tirofiban). This article provides an overview of these agents as well as the evidence supporting their use in STEMI.

CYCLOOXYGENASE INHIBITOR: ASPIRIN

Arachidonic acid is converted to thromboxane in a chemical reaction catalyzed by the COX enzyme (Fig. 1). Thromboxane is a potent vasoconstrictor and promotes platelet activation and

---

Conflicts of Interest: None.
Funding Support: None.
Department of Cardiology, The Mount Sinai Hospital, One Gustave L. Levy Place, New York, NY 10029-6574, USA
* Corresponding author.
E-mail address: usman.baber@mountsinai.org

Intervent Cardiol Clin 5 (2016) 481–495
http://dx.doi.org/10.1016/j.iccl.2016.06.007

Table 1
2013 American College of Chest Physicians/American Heart Association guideline for the management of ST-segment elevation myocardial infarction: antiplatelet therapy to support percutaneous coronary intervention in ST-segment elevation myocardial infarction

	Level of Evidence
Class I	
Aspirin, 162–325 mg, before primary PCI	B
Aspirin, 81–325 mg, daily should be continued indefinitely after PCI	A
A loading dose of a $P1Y_{12}$ inhibitor should be given as early as possible or at time of primary PCI	
Clopidogrel, 600 mg	B
Prasugrel, 60 mg	B
Ticagrelor, 180 mg	B
$P2Y_{12}$ inhibitor therapy, in addition to aspirin, should be given for 1 y to patients who receive a stent (BMS or DES) during primary PCI	
Clopidogrel, 75 mg daily	B
Prasugrel, 10 mg daily	B
Ticagrelor, 90 mg twice a day	B
Class IIa	
It is reasonable to use aspirin, 81 mg daily, over higher doses after primary PCI	B
It is reasonable to use intravenous GP IIb/IIIa receptor antagonist at time of primary PCI in selected patients who are receiving unfractionated heparin	
Abciximab	A
High-bolus-dose tirofiban	B
Double-bolus eptifibatide	B
Class IIb	
It may be reasonable to administer intravenous GP IIb/IIIa receptor antagonist in the precatheterization laboratory setting (ambulance or emergency department) to patients with STEMI for whom primary PCI is intended	B
It may be reasonable to administer intracoronary abciximab to patients with STEMI undergoing primary PCI	B
Continuation of $P2Y_{12}$ inhibitor beyond 1 y may be considered in patients undergoing DES placement	C
Class III	
Prasugrel should not be administered to patients with a history of stroke or TIA	B

Abbreviations: BMS, bare metal stents; DES, drug eluting stents.
Data from O'Gara PT, Kushner FG, Ascheim DD, et al. 2013 ACCF/AHA guideline for the management of ST-elevation myocardial infarction: a report of the American College of Cardiology Foundation/American Heart Association Task Force on Practice Guidelines. Circulation 2013;127(4):e362–425.

aggregation.[10–13] Aspirin irreversibly inhibits the COX enzyme, thereby impairing the platelet hemostatic response to plaque rupture and thrombus formation in a coronary artery.

The efficacy of aspirin in STEMI was initially described in the Second International Study of Infarct Survival (ISIS-2). In this study, 17,187 patients were randomized to streptokinase infusion, aspirin (162 mg for 1 month), both treatments, or neither after the onset of suspected acute MI. Aspirin resulted in 23% reduction in vascular mortality at 5 weeks compared

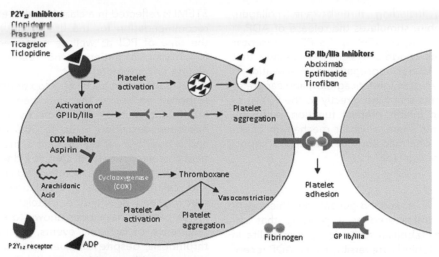

Fig. 1. Site of action of approved antiplatelet agents.

with placebo.[14] Secondary endpoints included nonfatal reinfarction and nonfatal stroke and were also statistically significant in favor of aspirin at 5 weeks. Subsequent studies have replicated the results from the ISIS-2 trial.[15,16] The early survival benefit conferred by 1 month of aspirin therapy after acute MI persisted for at least 10 years.[17]

Multiple studies have examined the dose of aspirin that would confer the greatest benefit without an unreasonably high risk of bleeding complications. The Global Utilization of Streptokinase and Tissue Plasminogen Activator for Occluded Coronary Arteries (GUSTO I) and GUSTO III randomized trials enrolled 31,575 and 12,893 patients, respectively, who presented with STEMI within 6 hours of symptom onset. A subsequent analysis of these trials concluded that there was no significant difference between aspirin, 162 mg, and aspirin, 325 mg, with respect to risk of death, MI, or stroke at 30 days.[18] Similar findings were reported in subsequent landmark studies. In the CURRENT-OASIS 7 trial, 25,086 patients, of whom approximately 37% presented with STEMI, were randomized in a 2-by-2 factorial design to double-dose versus standard-dose clopidogrel and high-dose (300–325 mg daily) or low-dose (75–100 mg daily) aspirin. The study found no significant difference with respect to the primary outcome of cardiovascular death, MI, or stroke at 30 days (4.2% vs 4.4%, hazard ratio [HR] 0.97; 95% CI, 0.86–1.09; $P = .61$).[19] An analysis of the HORIZONS-AMI trial reported the outcomes in patients with STEMI who were discharged from the hospital on low-dose ($\leq$200 mg daily) or high-dose (>200 mg daily)

aspirin. At 3 years, there was no difference in mortality, mortality/reinfarction, and major adverse cardiac events (MACE); mortality; reinfarction; ischemic target vessel revascularization (TVR); or stroke between the 2 groups.[20] Low-dose aspirin (81 mg) is equally efficacious as high-dose aspirin for secondary prevention of cardiovascular events after STEMI, resulting in a class IIa level of evidence B recommendation (see Table 1).

The safety of high-dose aspirin, however, remains controversial. The HORIZONS-AMI trial analysis demonstrated that high-dose aspirin was an independent predictor of major bleeding (HR 2.8; 95% CI, 1.31–5.99; $P = .008$).[20] Similarly, Serebruany and colleagues[21] conducted a meta-analysis of 31 randomized trials involving 192,036 patients and also concluded that aspirin doses of less than or equal to 200 mg daily (equivalent to 81 mg in the United States) were associated with fewer major bleeding events, when compared with aspirin greater than 200 mg (equivalent to 325 mg in the United States). Similar findings were reported in the BRAVO trial and post hoc analysis of the CURE trial.[20,22] This conflicts with the findings of the CURRENT-OASIS 7 trial, which showed no significant difference in major bleeding at 30 days between high-dose and low-dose aspirin arms, although a small increase in the incidence of major gastrointestinal bleeding among patients randomized to high-dose aspirin was noted (0.4% vs 0.2%, $P = .04$).[19]

P2Y12 INHIBITORS

ADP is stored in high concentrations in platelet granules. Activation of platelets by other mediators, including thromboxane, collagen, and thrombin, stimulates the release of ADP.[23] In turn, binding of ADP to the $P2Y_{12}$ receptor on platelets triggers a signaling cascade that amplifies platelet aggregation and activation.[24] Clopidogrel, prasugrel, ticagrelor, and cangrelor are all agents that bind directly to the $P2Y_{12}$ receptor and inhibit platelet function. Although these agents share a similar mechanism of action, their pharmacology demonstrates important differences (Table 2).[25]

Clopidogrel

Clopidogrel, a second-generation thienopyridine, is administered as a prodrug that undergoes metabolism to its active metabolite in the liver.[26] It binds irreversibly to the ADP receptor and, therefore, inhibits the ADP receptor for the lifespan of the platelet.[27] The CAPRIE trial was a landmark study that established the efficacy and safety of clopidogrel.[28] In this trial 19,185 patients with a history of ischemic stroke, MI, or peripheral arterial disease were randomized to either aspirin, 325 mg, or clopidogrel, 75 mg, daily. The primary outcome was an aggregate of ischemic stroke, MI, and vascular death. Event rates in the aspirin and clopidogrel arms were 5.83% and 5.23% ($P = .043$), respectively, yielding a modest relative reduction of 8.7% favoring clopidogrel use. In terms of safety, a statistically significant difference with respect to gastrointestinal bleeding favoring clopidogrel was found (1.99% vs 2.66%, $P<.002$). Numerous subsequent large trials established the efficacy of clopidogrel in STEMI (Table 3). The indisputable evidence supporting the use of clopidogrel in addition to aspirin in patients presenting with STEMI is reflected in a class I level of evidence B recommendation for the use of clopidogrel at the time of PCI as well as continued therapy for 1 year in patients who receive a drug-eluting or bare-metal stent.[29]

A major drawback of clopidogrel is the response variability that has been observed. Insufficient platelet inhibition by clopidogrel has been described in up to 30% of patients and is due to a variety of factors, including patient characteristics (age, chronic kidney disease, and diabetes), genetic factors, drug interactions, and cellular factors (up-regulation of $P2Y_{12}$ pathway and accelerated platelet turnover).[30] These patients have been shown to experience recurrence of ischemic events, including stent thrombosis, despite adequate dual antiplatelet therapy with aspirin and clopidogrel.[31,32] Despite such associations, tailoring the intensity of $P2Y_{12}$ inhibition based on results of genetic or platelet function tests has not shown any benefit in several randomized studies.[33-35] Accordingly, platelet function testing received a class II level of evidence B recommendation by the 2011 ACCF/AHA/Society for Cardiovascular Angiography and Interventions guideline for percutaneous coronary intervention, indicating that further studies are needed to support its routine use.[36]

Prasugrel

Prasugrel is an orally administered third-generation thienopyridine that irreversibly inhibits the $P2Y_{12}$ receptor. Similar to clopidogrel, it is administered as a prodrug that undergoes conversion to its active metabolite in the liver.[37] When compared with clopidogrel, prasugrel is a

Table 2
Pharmacologic properties of the $P2Y_{12}$ receptor inhibitors

	Route	Half-life	Prodrug	Receptor Inhibition	Onset of Action
Clopidogrel	PO	C 6 h AM 30 min	Yes[a]	Irreversible	2–8 h
Prasugrel	PO	P 7 h AM 44–68 h	Yes[b]	Irreversible	30 min to 4 h
Ticagrelor	PO	7 h AM 8.5 h	No	Reversible[c]	30 min to 4 h
Cangrelor	IV	3–5 min	No	Reversible[d]	2 min

Abbreviations: AM, active metabolite; c, clopidogrel; IV, intravenous; P, prasugrel.
[a] Clopidogrel is administered as a prodrug that is converted to its active metabolite in the liver.
[b] Prasugrel is administered as a prodrug that is converted to its active metabolite in a 2-step process mediated by esterases and liver enzymes.
[c] Ticagrelor is a reversible inhibitor of the $P2Y_{12}$ receptor that binds at a site different from the ADP binding site. The degree of receptor inhibition is dependent on the concentration of ticagrelor.
[d] Cangrelor in an ADP analog that binds reversibly to the ADP binding site.

Table 3
Landmark clinical trials evaluating the efficacy of approved P2Y$_{12}$ inhibitors in ST-segment elevation myocardial infarction

	CLARITY-TIMI 28	COMMIT	CURRENT-OASIS 7	TRITON-TIMI 38	PLATO
N	3491	45,852	25,086	13,608	18,624
Comparison	A + F + CL vs A + F + placebo	A + placebo vs A + CL	CL, 600 mg, + HDA vs CL, 600 mg, + LDA vs CL, 300 mg, + HDA vs CL, 300 mg, + LDA	A + prasugrel vs A + CL	A + ticagrelor vs A + CL
Study population	STEMI	STEMI (87%)	STEMI (37%)	STEMI (26%)	STEMI (37%)
Primary endpoint	OIRA, death, or recurrent MI at 30 d	1. Death, reinfarction or stroke[a] 2. Death from any cause[a]	Cardiovascular death, MI or stroke at 30 d	Death from cardiovascular causes, nonfatal MI, nonfatal stroke	Death from cardiovascular causes, MI, or stroke at 12 mo
Results	15% vs 21.7% (P<.001)	1. 9.2% vs 10.1% (P = .002) 2. 7.5% vs 8.1% (P = .03)	CL, 600 mg: 3.9% CL, 300 mg: 4.5% (P = .039)	CL, 12.1% Prasugrel, 9.9% (P<.001)	CL, 11.7% Ticagrelor, 9.8% (P<.001)

Abbreviations: A, aspirin; CL, clopidogrel; F, fibrinolytics; HDA, high-dose aspirin (300–325 mg); LDA, low-dose aspirin (75–100 mg); OIRA, occluded infarct-related artery.
[a] At discharge or 4 weeks.

more potent platelet inhibitor, displays a onset of action, and is associated with a more predictable response.[38]

The TRITON-TIMI 38 trial evaluated the efficacy and safety of prasugrel in patients with ACSs, of whom 26% presented with STEMI.[39] It randomized 13,608 patients to prasugrel (60-mg loading dose and 10-mg daily maintenance dose) versus clopidogrel (300-mg loading dose and 75-mg daily maintenance dose). The primary efficacy endpoint was death from cardiovascular causes, nonfatal MI, or nonfatal stroke at 1 year. Prasugrel was shown to significantly reduce the primary efficacy outcome compared with clopidogrel (see Table 2). The benefit conferred by prasugrel was counteracted, however, by an increased risk of major bleeding, including fatal bleeding (2.4% vs 1.8%, $P = .03$). The efficacy of prasugrel was driven by nonfatal MI (7.3% vs 9.5%, $P<.001$). Additionally, rates of definite or probable stent thrombosis were significantly lower in the prasugrel group (1.1% vs 2.4%; $P<.001$; HR 0.48 [0.36–0.64]) (Fig. 2).[39] A subgroup analysis of the STEMI patients from the TRITON-TIMI 38 concluded that prasugrel offered statistically significant benefits with regard to cardiovascular death, MI, or stroke at 15 months, irrespective of whether these patients underwent PCI within 12 hours of presentation (primary PCI) or between 12 hours and 14 days of presentation (secondary PCI).[40]

Lastly, 3 subgroups merit special consideration: patients greater than or equal to 75 years, patients weighing less than or equal to 60 kg, and patients with a history of stroke or transient ischemic attack (TIA). The latter population experienced harm from prasugrel, as evidence by a higher rate of ischemic events as well as bleeding events, including hemorrhagic stroke.[41] Prasugrel is, therefore, contraindicated in these patients. No net benefit was observed in patients greater than or equal to 75 years or weighing less than or equal to 60 kg, in whom a decrease in ischemic events was balance by a higher risk of bleeding.[41]

Ticagrelor
Ticagrelor is an orally administered cyclopentyl-triazolopyrimidine that reversibly inhibits the $P2Y_{12}$ receptor. Unlike clopidogrel and prasugrel, it is administered as an active compound that does not require activation by hepatic metabolism.[42] Compared with clopidogrel, ticagrelor demonstrates faster onset of action and more potent inhibition of platelet aggregation.[43]

The PLATO trial evaluated the efficacy and safety of ticagrelor in patients with ACSs; 18,624 patients, of whom approximately 37% presented with STEMI, were randomized to ticagrelor (180-mg loading dose, 90-mg twice-daily maintenance dose) or clopidogrel (300–600-mg loading dose, 75-mg maintenance dose). Compared with clopidogrel, ticagrelor was shown to reduce the rate of death from vascular

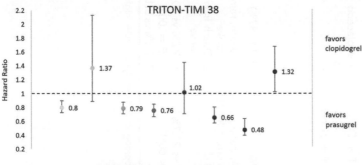

Fig. 2. Results of the TRITON-TIMI 38 trial: clopidogrel versus prasugrel. (*Adapted from* Rafique A, Nayyar P, Baber U, et al. Optimal P2Y12 inhibitor in patients with ST segment elevation myocardial infarction undergoing primary percutaneous coronary intervention: a network meta-analysis. J Am Coll Cardiol 2016;67(13_S):212-212; with permission.)

causes, MI, or stroke at 12 months (9.8% vs 11.7%, P<.001) (Fig. 3).[44] There are several additional conclusions from the PLATO trial:

1. Ticagrelor showed statistically significant lower rates of definite stent thrombosis compared with clopidogrel (1.2% vs 1.9%, P = .009).
2. The benefit of ticagrelor over clopidogrel was observed in patients with ACSs who underwent PCI as well as those who received noninvasive management.[45]
3. There was no difference with respect to protocol-defined major bleeding between groups although non–coronary artery bypass graft (CABG) Thrombolysis in Myocardial Infarction (TIMI) major bleeding was higher in the ticagrelor arm. Although uncommon, fatal intracranial bleeding was more frequent in the ticagrelor group (0.1% vs 0.01%, P = .02).
4. After the PLATO trial, no subgroups with a higher bleeding potential were identified, including patients with a history of TIA or stroke.

A subgroup analysis of STEMI patients in the PLATO trial showed reduction in a composite of death from vascular causes, MI, or stroke (HR 0.87; 95% CI, 0.75–1.01; P = .07), consistent with the results from the PLATO trial.[46] In addition, ticagrelor was associated with a higher rate of stroke (1.7% vs 1.0%, P = .02), without a significant increase in the rate of major bleeding (9.0% vs 9.2%, P = .76).[46]

Cangrelor

Cangrelor is a novel, intravenously administered ATP analog that reversibly inhibits the $P2Y_{12}$ receptor.[47] Compared with the orally administered P2Y12 inhibitors, cangrelor offers several advantageous pharmacologic properties[47,48]:

1. Linear, dose-dependent, pharmacokinetic profile, resulting in predictable plasma levels
2. Immediate inhibition of platelet aggregation when given as a bolus followed by an infusion
3. Short half-life (3–5 minutes), resulting in normalization of platelet function within 30 to 90 minutes after discontinuation of the infusion.

Two landmark trials investigated the efficacy and safety of cangrelor in patients with ACSs undergoing PCI. The CHAMPION-PCI trial randomized 8877 patients with ACS (11% STEMI) to 600 mg of clopidogrel or cangrelor before PCI. The primary efficacy endpoint evaluated was a composite of death, MI, or ischemia-driven revascularization at 48 hours. Cangrelor was not superior to clopidogrel with respect to the primary endpoint at 48 hours (7.5% vs 7.1%, P = .59) and at 30 days (8.7% vs 8.5%, P = .73).[49] In terms of safety, the investigators reported bleeding rates according to different criteria, including ACUITY, GUSTO, and TIMI criteria. There was no statistical difference with respect to major bleeding, but cangrelor was associated with statistically significant higher minor bleeding rates according to ACUITY and GUSTO criteria.[49]

In the CHAMPION-PHOENIX trial, 11,145 patients presenting with ACS (approximately 18% STEMI) were randomized to cangrelor (bolus followed by infusion) or a clopidogrel loading dose (300 mg–600 mg) at the time of PCI. The primary efficacy endpoint was a composite of death from any cause, ischemia-driven revascularization, or stent thrombosis at 48 hours. The cangrelor

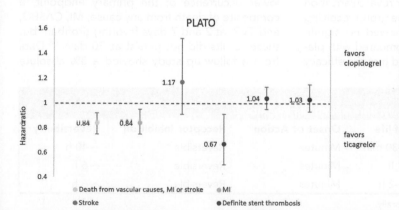

Fig. 3. Results of the PLATO trial: clopidogrel versus ticagrelor. (Adapted from Rafique A, Nayyar P, Baber U, et al. Optimal P2Y12 inhibitor in patients with ST segment elevation myocardial infarction undergoing primary percutaneous coronary intervention: a network meta-analysis. J Am Coll Cardiol 2016;67(13_S):212-212; with permission.)

arm of the study experienced a significant lower rate of the primary efficacy endpoint compared with the clopidogrel arm (4.7% vs 5.9%, P = .005).[50] Stent thrombosis, a secondary efficacy endpoint, was also lower in the cangrelor arm at 48 hours (0.8% vs 1.4, P = .01).[50] With regard to safety, cangrelor was not associated with significantly higher risk of GUSTO-defined severe bleeding.[50]

Cangrelor is not included in the current ACCF/AHA guidelines for the management of ST-elevation myocardial infarction. In light of the evidence demonstrating the efficacy and safety of cangrelor, however, the Food and Drug Administration approved its use in 2015 in patients with STEMI undergoing PCI in 2015.

GLYCOPROTEIN IIB/IIIA INHIBITORS

The GP IIb/IIIa molecule is expressed on the cell surface of platelets. It is an adhesion receptor that mediates platelet aggregation by binding to fibrinogen[51] but is only able to bind its ligand in activated platelets.[52] GP IIb/IIIa inhibitors prevent binding of fibrinogen to the receptor, thereby antagonizing platelet aggregation. Three GP IIb/IIIa inhibitors are approved for use in patients with STEMI undergoing PCI: abciximab, eptifibatide, and tirofiban (Table 4).

Abciximab
The EPIC trial was the first to investigate the efficacy of abciximab in patients undergoing PCI. In this trial, 2099 patients at high risk of vessel closure undergoing PCI were randomized to placebo, abciximab bolus, or abciximab bolus plus infusion. At 30 days, the abciximab bolus plus infusion group experienced a 35% reduction in the primary endpoint; a composite of death from any cause, nonfatal MI, or revascularization (8.3% vs 12.8%, P = .008).[53] The group receiving the bolus-only intervention showed no significant difference in outcomes compared with placebo. A follow-up study showed that the efficacy

of abciximab remained statistically significant at 3 years.[54] Three major subsequent studies examined the efficacy of abciximab in patients with STEMI (Table 5).[55–57]

Although the RAPPORT trial showed no significant difference between placebo and abciximab, the abciximab group showed statistically lower rates of urgent TVR at 7 days, 30 days, and 6 months as well as lower rates of death or repeat MI at 7 days. With regard to safety, the RAPPORT trial showed higher risk of major bleeding associated with abciximab use (16.6% vs 9.5%, P = .02).[55]

Eptifibatide
Several trials have demonstrated the efficacy of eptifibatide in PCI.[58–61] The data for eptifibatide in STEMI are more limited. Three trials have shown favorable angiographic outcomes associated with eptifibatide (Table 6).[62–64] These outcomes did not translate into clinical benefits, because no difference in death, reinfarction, stroke, or major bleeding was observed in these trials.

The largest registry study conducted of eptifibatide in the setting of STEMI evaluated outcomes in 11,479 patients undergoing PCI for STEMI who received abciximab or eptifibatide. The primary endpoint, death or MI at 1 year, occurred in 15% of patients who received eptifibatide and 15.7% of patients who received abciximab (odds ratio 0.94; CI, 0.84–1.08).[65] Death and MI, taken as separate secondary endpoints, also demonstrated noniferiority of eptifibatide.

Tirofiban
The RESTORE trial randomized 2212 patients with ACSs to tirofiban bolus and infusion versus placebo. The trial showed statistically significant lower occurrence of the primary endpoint, a composite of death from any cause, MI, CASBG, and TVR, at 2 and 7 days favoring tirofiban, but these results did not persist at 30 days.[66] Data from a follow-up study showed a 3% absolute

Table 4
Pharmacologic properties of glycoprotein IIb/IIIa inhibitors

	Route	Half-life	Onset of Action[a]	Receptor Inhibition	Reversibility[b]
Abciximab	IV	20–30 min	Minutes	Reversible	~40 h
Eptifibatide	IV	2–3 h	Minutes	Reversible	~6 h
Tirofiban	IV	1.5–2 h	Minutes	Reversible	~6 h

Abbreviations: IV, intravenous; PO, orally.
[a] Onset of action defined as approximately greater than 80% inhibition of platelet aggregation.
[b] Reversibility defined as return approximately greater than 80% of baseline platelet aggregation.
Data from Coller BS. Glycoprotein IIb/IIIa antagonists: development of abciximab and pharmacology of select agents. 1999;67–89.

Table 5
Clinical trials evaluating the efficacy of abciximab in ST-segment elevation myocardial infarction

	RAPPORT	ADMIRAL	CADILLAC
N	483	300	2082
Comparison	PCI + abciximab vs PCI + placebo	PCI + abciximab bolus + infusion vs PCI + placebo	PTCA alone vs PTCA + abciximab therapy vs Stenting alone vs Stenting + abciximab therapy
Study population	STEMI or new LBBB	STEMI	STEMI or new LBBB
Primary endpoint	Composite of death, reinfarction or TVR at 6 mo	Composite of death, reinfarction, or urgent TVR at 30 d	Composite of death from any cause, reinfarction, disabling stroke or TVR at 6 mo
Results	28.1% vs 28.2% ($P = .97$)	6% vs 14.6% ($P = .01$)	20% PTCA 16.5% PTCA + abciximab 11.5% Stenting 10.2% Stenting + abciximab $P<.001$

Abbreviations: LBBB, left bundle branch block; PTCA, percutaneous transluminal coronary angioplasty.

reduction in the incidence of the primary endpoint at 6 months, which was also not statistically significant.[67] In the ON-TIME 2 trial, 984 patients with STEMI were randomized 984 patients to high-bolus dose tirofiban versus placebo. Tirofiban was associated with significantly lower ST-segment deviation 1 hour after PCI compared with placebo (10.9 mm vs 12.1 mm, $P = .028$).[68] A secondary efficacy endpoint, including a composite of death, recurrent MI, urgent TVR, or thrombotic bailout at 30 days, also favored tirofiban (32.9% vs 26%, $P = .020$).[68] Tirofiban was not associated with a higher risk of major bleeding.

CONTEMPORARY USE OF ANTIPLATELET THERAPY IN ST-SEGMENT ELEVATION MYOCARDIAL INFARCTION

Recent studies that examined current trends in the use of antiplatelet agents have shown interesting results. Despite strong evidence supporting the use of newer, more potent P2Y$_{12}$ inhibitors, like prasugrel and ticagrelor, clopidogrel remains the most commonly used P2Y$_{12}$ inhibitor.[69] Two factors that may result in this practice are patients' comorbidities and their bleeding risk. Prasugrel is favored in low-risk patients, who tend to be younger and have fewer comorbidities like

Table 6
Clinical trials evaluating the efficacy of eptifibatide in ST-segment elevation myocardial infarction

	IMPACT-AMI	INTAMI	TITAN-TIMI 34
N	132	102	343
Comparison	Eptifibatide vs placebo	Early eptifibatide (ED) vs Optional eptifibatide at time of PCI	Early eptifibatide (ED) vs Late eptifibatide (after diagnostic angiography)
Study population	STEMI or new LBBB	STEMI or new LBBB	STEMI or new LBBB
Primary endpoint	TIMI flow 3 at 90 min	Patency of infarct vessel before PCI	Corrected TIMI frame count before PCI
Results	39% vs 66% ($P = .006$)	34% vs 10% ($P = .01\%$)	75.3 ± 32.1, early 84.4 ± 30.7, late $P = .021$

Abbreviation: ED, emergency department.

hypertension, hyperlipidemia, diabetes, or a history of prior MI[70] (Fig. 4B). Prasugrel use also decreases in patients with an increased risk of bleeding[70] (see Fig. 4A). Similar trends emerged from a study of contemporary use of ticagrelor in Sweden, where ticagrelor was more often used in patients with lower GRACE and CRUSADE scores, indicating lower mortality and bleeding risks.[71] Prasugrel is also favored over ticagrelor in low-risk patients, with lower risk of bleeding.[72]

Another plausible explanation for the observed trends is the cost associated with these agents, particularly at a time when generic clopidogrel is available in the United States. Cost-effectiveness studies of the TRITON-TIMI 38 and the PLATO trials have shown that prasugrel and ticagrelor offer economically viable alternatives to clopidogrel.[73,74] The initial higher cost of these agents compared with clopidogrel is balanced by gains in quality-adjusted life years, life expectancy, and reduced rates of hospitalization.[75] It is possible, however, that physicians are more likely to prescribe clopidogrel due to the financial burden that prasugrel or ticagrelor may have on many patients.

Lastly, familiarity with clopidogrel may also influence the choice of antiplatelet agent used in ACS. The underutilization of prasugrel and ticagrelor may be explained by a temporal delay between guideline updates and clinical practice. A few years after its approval for use in ACS, clopidogrel was underutilized.[76] A similar phenomenon may account for the current underutilization of prasugrel and ticagrelor, which may disappear in the coming years as the medical field gains experience with their use.

CONTROVERSIES IN ANTIPLATELET THERAPY IN STEMI

Although there is a wealth of evidence derived mostly from randomized clinical trials that evaluated antiplatelet agents in ACS, several gaps in knowledge persist. A prime example of this is the lack of a randomized trial comparing prasugrel and ticagrelor in STEMI. An indirect comparison study of these agents in patients with ACSs concluded the following[77]:

1. Prasugrel and ticagrelor are superior to clopidogrel with respect to all-cause mortality.
2. The efficacy of prasugrel and ticagrelor is comparable.
3. Prasugrel is associated with a lower risk of stent thrombosis, which did not have an impact on the other endpoints.
4. Ticagrelor is associated with lower risk of any major bleeding.

Similar results were reported from a network meta-analysis of 14 randomized clinical trials.[78] A recently published meta-analysis of 37 studies, including 88,402 patients, concluded that prasugrel seems superior to ticagrelor in STEMI patients undergoing primary PCI.[79] An ongoing head-to-head comparison of prasugrel and ticagrelor in STEMI might yield insights in this area.[80] In the absence of a randomized trial comparing these 2 agents, the optimal $P2Y_{12}$ inhibitor remains an issue of much debate. Similarly, the role cangrelor in patients with STEMI undergoing PCI remains unclear. Its immediate platelet inhibition, very short half-life, and predictable pharmacokinetics

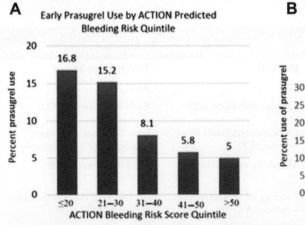

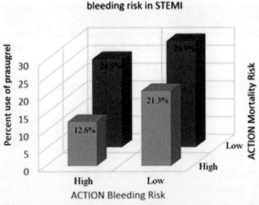

Fig. 4. Prasugrel use by ACTION (Acute Coronary Treatment and Intervention Outcomes Network) predicted bleeding risk and mortality. (*Adapted from* Sherwood MW, Wiviott SD, Peng SA, et al. Early clopidogrel versus prasugrel use among contemporary STEMI and NSTEMI patients in the US: insights from the National Cardiovascular Data Registry. J Am Heart Assoc 2014;3(2):e000849; with permission.)

are appealing properties of this novel intravenous P2Y$_{12}$ inhibitor. These features may be particularly relevant in the setting of impaired gastric absorption and delayed onset of action for oral P2Y$_{12}$ inhibitors among STEMI patients.[81] At this point, randomized trials have only compared it to clopidogrel, again providing an opportunity to further study this agent and determine which patients would derive the greatest benefit from its use.

Another contentious issue is the role of GP IIb/IIIa inhibitors in an era when revascularization is most often undertaken in patients with STEMI. A meta-analysis of 6 trials involving 32,402 patients with ACS concluded that GP IIb/IIIa inhibitors reduce the rate of death or MI in patients with ACS who are not routinely scheduled for early revascularization.[82] In addition, most major randomized clinical trials that established the efficacy of GP IIb/IIIa inhibitors were conducted in the 1990s, raising the possibility that the results observed in those trials may not be replicated in an era where potent P2Y$_{12}$ inhibitors along with PCI are the standard of care of STEMI. The recent INFUSE-AMI trial showed a small but significant reduction in infarct size in STEMI patients after intracoronary administration of abciximab, but further studies are needed to support this practice.[83]

Finally, an area that merits further study is pretreatment with P2Y$_{12}$ inhibitors prior to diagnostic angiography in STEMI patients. Studies evaluating pretreatment with clopidogrel had conflicting results, and major trials powered to provide definite conclusions are lacking.[84] For ticagrelor, the ATLANTIC trial concluded that prehospital treatment with ticagrelor did not affect reperfusion of the culprit vessel but was associated with a lower risk of stent thrombosis.[85] This is in contrast to a small study that showed improved angiographic reperfusion in STEMI patients pretreated with prasugrel.[86] Current ACCF/AHA guidelines state that P2Y$_{12}$ inhibitors should be administered "as early as possible or at time of PCI," lacking further indication as to whether prehospital administration of these agents offers an additional benefit.

SUMMARY

Antiplatelet therapy has been used for the treatment of cardiovascular disease for the past several decades, resulting in significant improvement in clinical outcomes. These agents remain the cornerstone of treatment of STEMI and have shown clear benefits as adjunct therapy at the time of primary PCI as well as secondary preventive therapy after STEMI.

Recent advances have led to the discovery of P2Y$_{12}$ inhibitors, prasugrel and ticagrelor, which offer a favorable pharmacologic profile over clopidogrel and proved efficacy and safety. Genotyping and phenotyping may lead to individualized therapy that would benefit certain patients. Ongoing investigation should address persistent gaps in the evidence base, such as the comparative efficacy and safety of different potent P2Y$_{12}$ inhibitors, refining the role of GP IIb/IIIa inhibitors in the contemporary era of revascularization and potent antiplatelet pharmacotherapy and the utility and timing of upstream pretreatment. Understanding the evidence and guideline recommendations for antiplatelet therapy in STEMI is fundamental as the field is constantly evolving and offers a promising future with regards to lowering the mortality and morbidity of STEMI.

REFERENCES

1. World Health Organization. Available at: http://www.who.int/en/.
2. Centers for Disease Control and Prevention. Available at: http://www.cdc.gov/.
3. Mozaffarian D, Benjamin EJ, Go AS, et al. Heart disease and stroke statistics–2015 update: a report from the American Heart Association. Circulation 2015;131(4):e29–322.
4. Newman JD, Shimbo D, Baggett C, et al. Trends in myocardial infarction rates and case fatality by anatomical location in four United States communities, 1987 to 2008 (from the Atherosclerosis Risk in Communities Study). Am J Cardiol 2013; 112(11):1714–9.
5. Rogers WJ, Canto JG, Lambrew CT, et al. Temporal trends in the treatment of over 1.5 million patients with myocardial infarction in the US from 1990 through 1999: the National Registry of Myocardial Infarction 1, 2 and 3. J Am Coll Cardiol 2000;36(7):2056–63.
6. McManus DD, Gore J, Yarzebski J, et al. Recent trends in the incidence, treatment, and outcomes of patients with STEMI and NSTEMI. Am J Med 2011;124(1):40–7.
7. Nabel EG, Braunwald E. A tale of coronary artery disease and myocardial infarction. N Engl J Med 2012;366(1):54–63.
8. Hansson GK. Inflammation, atherosclerosis, and coronary artery disease. N Engl J Med 2005; 352(16):1685–95.
9. Page IH. Atherosclerosis. Circulation 1968;38(6): 1164–72.
10. Needleman P, Minkes M, Raz A. Thromboxanes: selective biosynthesis and distinct biological properties. Science 1976;193(4248):163–5.

11. Svensson J, Hamberg M, Samuelsson B. On the formation and effects of thromboxane A2 in human platelets. Acta Physiol Scand 1976;98(3):285–94.

12. Ellis EF, Oelz O, Roberts LJ 2nd, et al. Coronary arterial smooth muscle contraction by a substance released from platelets: evidence that it is thromboxane A2. Science 1976;193(4258):1135–7.

13. Davi G, Patrono C. Platelet activation and atherothrombosis. N Engl J Med 2007;357(24):2482–94.

14. Randomised trial of intravenous streptokinase, oral aspirin, both, or neither among 17,187 cases of suspected acute myocardial infarction: ISIS-2. ISIS-2 (Second International Study of Infarct Survival) Collaborative Group. Lancet 1988;2(8607):349–60.

15. Antithrombotic Trialists Collaboration. Collaborative meta-analysis of randomised trials of antiplatelet therapy for prevention of death, myocardial infarction, and stroke in high risk patients. BMJ 2002;324(7329):71–86.

16. Mehta SR, Tanguay JF, Eikelboom JW, et al. Double-dose versus standard-dose clopidogrel and high-dose versus low-dose aspirin in individuals undergoing percutaneous coronary intervention for acute coronary syndromes (CURRENT-OASIS 7): a randomised factorial trial. Lancet 2010;376(9748): 1233–43.

17. Baigent C, Collins R, Appleby P, et al. ISIS-2: 10 year survival among patients with suspected acute myocardial infarction in randomised comparison of intravenous streptokinase, oral aspirin, both, or neither. The ISIS-2 (Second International Study of Infarct Survival) Collaborative Group. BMJ 1998; 316(7141):1337–43.

18. Berger JS, Stebbins A, Granger CB, et al. Initial aspirin dose and outcome among ST-elevation myocardial infarction patients treated with fibrinolytic therapy. Circulation 2008;117(2):192–9.

19. CURRENT-OASIS 7 Investigators, Mehta SR, Bassand JP, et al. Dose comparisons of clopidogrel and aspirin in acute coronary syndromes. N Engl J Med 2010;363(10):930–42.

20. Yu J, Mehran R, Dangas GD, et al. Safety and efficacy of high- versus low-dose aspirin after primary percutaneous coronary intervention in ST-segment elevation myocardial infarction: the HORIZONS-AMI (Harmonizing Outcomes With Revascularization and Stents in Acute Myocardial Infarction) trial. JACC Cardiovasc Interv 2012; 5(12):1231–8.

21. Serebruany VL, Steinhubl SR, Berger PB, et al. Analysis of risk of bleeding complications after different doses of aspirin in 192,036 patients enrolled in 31 randomized controlled trials. Am J Cardiol 2005; 95(10):1218–22.

22. Topol EJ, Easton D, Harrington RA, et al. Randomized, double-blind, placebo-controlled, international trial of the oral IIb/IIIa antagonist lotrafiban

in coronary and cerebrovascular disease. Circulation 2003;108(4):399–406.

23. Storey RF, Sanderson HM, White AE, et al. The central role of the P(2T) receptor in amplification of human platelet activation, aggregation, secretion and procoagulant activity. Br J Haematol 2000;110(4): 925–34.

24. Rollini F, Franchi F, Angiolillo DJ. Switching P2Y12-receptor inhibitors in patients with coronary artery disease. Nat Rev Cardiol 2016;13(1):11–27.

25. Ferri N, Corsini A, Bellosta S. Pharmacology of the new P2Y12 receptor inhibitors: insights on pharmacokinetic and pharmacodynamic properties. Drugs 2013;73(15):1681–709.

26. Savi P, Nurden P, Nurden AT, et al. Clopidogrel: a review of its mechanism of action. Platelets 1998; 9(3–4):251–5.

27. Jiang XL, Samant S, Lesko LJ, et al. Clinical pharmacokinetics and pharmacodynamics of clopidogrel. Clin Pharmacokinet 2015;54(2):147–66.

28. CAPRIE Steering Committee. A randomised, blinded, trial of clopidogrel versus aspirin in patients at risk of ischaemic events (CAPRIE). CAPRIE Steering Committee. Lancet 1996;348(9038):1329–39.

29. O'Gara PT, Kushner FG, Ascheim DD, et al. 2013 ACCF/AHA guideline for the management of ST-elevation myocardial infarction: a report of the American College of Cardiology Foundation/American Heart Association Task Force on Practice Guidelines. Circulation 2013;127(4):e362–425.

30. Huber K. Prasugrel in clopidogrel nonresponders: a way to improve secondary prevention in patients after percutaneous coronary intervention? JACC Cardiovasc Interv 2015;8(12):1571–3.

31. Siller-Matula JM, Trenk D, Schror K, et al. Response variability to P2Y12 receptor inhibitors: expectations and reality. JACC Cardiovasc Interv 2013; 6(11):1111–28.

32. Bonello L, Tantry US, Marcucci R, et al. Consensus and future directions on the definition of high on-treatment platelet reactivity to adenosine diphosphate. J Am Coll Cardiol 2010;56(12):919–33.

33. Matetzky S, Shenkman B, Guetta V, et al. Clopidogrel resistance is associated with increased risk of recurrent atherothrombotic events in patients with acute myocardial infarction. Circulation 2004; 109(25):3171–5.

34. Price MJ, Berger PB, Teirstein PS, et al. Standard- vs high-dose clopidogrel based on platelet function testing after percutaneous coronary intervention: the GRAVITAS randomized trial. JAMA 2011; 305(11):1097–105.

35. Collet JP, Cuisset T, Range G, et al. Bedside monitoring to adjust antiplatelet therapy for coronary stenting. N Engl J Med 2012;367(22):2100–9.

36. Levine GN, Bates ER, Blankenship JC, et al. 2011 ACCF/AHA/SCAI guideline for percutaneous

coronary intervention: executive summary: a report of the American College of Cardiology Foundation/American Heart Association Task Force on Practice Guidelines and the Society for Cardiovascular Angiography and Interventions. Circulation 2011;124(23):2574–609.

37. Mousa SA, Jeske WP, Fareed J. Prasugrel: a novel platelet ADP P2Y(12) receptor antagonist. Methods Mol Biol 2010;663:221–8.

38. Angiolillo DJ, Bates ER, Bass TA. Clinical profile of prasugrel, a novel thienopyridine. Am Heart J 2008; 156(Suppl 2):S16–22.

39. Wiviott SD, Braunwald E, McCabe CH, et al. Prasugrel versus clopidogrel in patients with acute coronary syndromes. N Engl J Med 2007; 357(20):2001–15.

40. Udell JA, Braunwald E, Antman EM, et al. Prasugrel versus clopidogrel in patients with ST-segment elevation myocardial infarction according to timing of percutaneous coronary intervention: a TRITON-TIMI 38 subgroup analysis (Trial to Assess Improvement in Therapeutic Outcomes by Optimizing Platelet Inhibition with Prasugrel-Thrombolysis In Myocardial Infarction 38). JACC Cardiovasc Interv 2014;7(6):604–12.

41. Wiviott SD, Desai N, Murphy SA, et al. Efficacy and safety of intensive antiplatelet therapy with prasugrel from TRITON-TIMI 38 in a core clinical cohort defined by worldwide regulatory agencies. Am J Cardiol 2011;108(7):905–11.

42. Dhillon S. Ticagrelor: a review of its use in adults with acute coronary syndromes. Am J Cardiovasc Drugs 2015;15(1):51–68.

43. Dobesh PP, Oestreich JH. Ticagrelor: pharmacokinetics, pharmacodynamics, clinical efficacy, and safety. Pharmacotherapy 2014;34(10):1077–90.

44. Wallentin L, Becker RC, Budaj A, et al. Ticagrelor versus clopidogrel in patients with acute coronary syndromes. N Engl J Med 2009;361(11):1045–57.

45. Roe MT, Armstrong PW, Fox KA, et al. Prasugrel versus clopidogrel for acute coronary syndromes without revascularization. N Engl J Med 2012; 367(14):1297–309.

46. Steg PG, James S, Harrington RA, et al. Ticagrelor versus clopidogrel in patients with ST-elevation acute coronary syndromes intended for reperfusion with primary percutaneous coronary intervention: a platelet inhibition and patient outcomes (PLATO) trial subgroup analysis. Circulation 2010;122(21): 2131–41.

47. Franchi F, Rollini F, Muniz-Lozano A, et al. Cangrelor: a review on pharmacology and clinical trial development. Expert Rev Cardiovasc Ther 2013; 11(10):1279–91.

48. Akers WS, Oh JJ, Oestreich JH, et al. Pharmacokinetics and pharmacodynamics of a bolus and infusion of cangrelor: a direct, parenteral P2Y12

receptor antagonist. J Clin Pharmacol 2010;50(1): 27–35.

49. Harrington RA, Stone GW, McNulty S, et al. Platelet inhibition with cangrelor in patients undergoing PCI. N Engl J Med 2009;361(24):2318–29.

50. Bhatt DL, Stone GW, Mahaffey KW, et al. Effect of platelet inhibition with cangrelor during PCI on ischemic events. N Engl J Med 2013;368(14): 1303–13.

51. Berkowitz SD. Current knowledge of the platelet glycoprotein IIb/IIIa receptor antagonists for the treatment of coronary artery disease. Haemostasis 2000;30(Suppl 3):27–43.

52. Phillips DR, Charo IF, Parise LV, et al. The platelet membrane glycoprotein IIb-IIIa complex. Blood 1988;71(4):831–43.

53. Use of a monoclonal antibody directed against the platelet glycoprotein IIb/IIIa receptor in high-risk coronary angioplasty. The EPIC Investigation. N Engl J Med 1994;330(14):956–61.

54. Topol EJ, Ferguson JJ, Weisman HF, et al. Long-term protection from myocardial ischemic events in a randomized trial of brief integrin beta3 blockade with percutaneous coronary intervention. EPIC Investigator Group. Evaluation of Platelet IIb/IIIa Inhibition for Prevention of Ischemic Complication. JAMA 1997;278(6):479–84.

55. Brener SJ, Barr LA, Burchenal JE, et al. Randomized, placebo-controlled trial of platelet glycoprotein IIb/IIIa blockade with primary angioplasty for acute myocardial infarction. ReoPro and Primary PTCA Organization and Randomized Trial (RAPPORT) Investigators. Circulation 1998;98(8): 734–41.

56. Montalescot G, Barragan P, Wittenberg O, et al. Platelet glycoprotein IIb/IIIa inhibition with coronary stenting for acute myocardial infarction. N Engl J Med 2001;344(25):1895–903.

57. Stone GW, Grines CL, Cox DA, et al. Comparison of angioplasty with stenting, with or without abciximab, in acute myocardial infarction. N Engl J Med 2002;346(13):957–66.

58. Randomised placebo-controlled trial of effect of eptifibatide on complications of percutaneous coronary intervention: IMPACT-II. Integrilin to minimise platelet aggregation and coronary thrombosis-II. Lancet 1997;349(9063):1422–8.

59. ESPRIT Investigators. Enhanced Suppression of the Platelet IIb/IIIa Receptor with Integrilin Therapy. Novel dosing regimen of eptifibatide in planned coronary stent implantation (ESPRIT): a randomised, placebo-controlled trial. Lancet 2000; 356(9247):2037–44.

60. Inhibition of platelet glycoprotein IIb/IIIa with eptifibatide in patients with acute coronary syndromes. The PURSUIT Trial Investigators. Platelet glycoprotein IIb/IIIa in unstable angina: Receptor

suppression using integrilin therapy. N Engl J Med 1998;339(7):436–43.

61. O'Shea JC, Hafley GE, Greenberg S, et al. Platelet glycoprotein IIb/IIIa integrin blockade with eptifibatide in coronary stent intervention: the ESPRIT trial: a randomized controlled trial. JAMA 2001; 285(19):2468–73.

62. Ohman EM, Kleiman NS, Gacioch G, et al. Combined accelerated tissue-plasminogen activator and platelet glycoprotein IIb/IIIa integrin receptor blockade with Integrilin in acute myocardial infarction. Results of a randomized, placebo-controlled, dose-ranging trial. IMPACT-AMI Investigators. Circulation 1997;95(4):846–54.

63. Zeymer U, Zahn R, Schiele R, et al. Early eptifibatide improves TIMI 3 patency before primary percutaneous coronary intervention for acute ST elevation myocardial infarction: results of the randomized integrilin in acute myocardial infarction (INTAMI) pilot trial. Eur Heart J 2005;26(19):1971–7.

64. Gibson CM, Kirtane AJ, Murphy SA, et al. Early initiation of eptifibatide in the emergency department before primary percutaneous coronary intervention for ST-segment elevation myocardial infarction: results of the Time to Integrilin Therapy in Acute Myocardial Infarction (TITAN)-TIMI 34 trial. Am Heart J 2006;152(4):668–75.

65. Akerblom A, James SK, Koutouzis M, et al. Eptifibatide is noninferior to abciximab in primary percutaneous coronary intervention: results from the SCAAR (Swedish Coronary Angiography and Angioplasty Registry). J Am Coll Cardiol 2010;56(6): 470–5.

66. Effects of platelet glycoprotein IIb/IIIa blockade with tirofiban on adverse cardiac events in patients with unstable angina or acute myocardial infarction undergoing coronary angioplasty. The RESTORE Investigators. Randomized Efficacy Study of Tirofiban for Outcomes and REstenosis. Circulation 1997;96(5):1445–53.

67. Gibson CM, Goel M, Cohen DJ, et al. Six-month angiographic and clinical follow-up of patients prospectively randomized to receive either tirofiban or placebo during angioplasty in the RESTORE trial. Randomized Efficacy Study of Tirofiban for Outcomes and Restenosis. J Am Coll Cardiol 1998; 32(1):28–34.

68. Van't Hof AW, Ten Berg J, Heestermans T, et al. Prehospital initiation of tirofiban in patients with ST-elevation myocardial infarction undergoing primary angioplasty (On-TIME 2): a multicentre, double-blind, randomised controlled trial. Lancet 2008;372(9638):537–46.

69. Fan W, Plent S, Prats J, et al. Trends in P2Y Inhibitor Use in Patients Referred for Invasive Evaluation of Coronary Artery Disease in Contemporary US Practice. Am J Cardiol 2016;117(9):1439–43.

70. Sherwood MW, Wiviott SD, Peng SA, et al. Early clopidogrel versus prasugrel use among contemporary STEMI and NSTEMI patients in the US: insights from the National Cardiovascular Data Registry. J Am Heart Assoc 2014;3(2):e000849.

71. Sahlén A. Contemporary use of ticagrelor in patient with acute coronary syndrome: insight from Swedish Web System for Enhancement and Development of Evidence-Based Care in Heart Disease Evaluated According to Recommended Therapies (SWEDEHEART). Eur Heart J Cardiovasc Pharmacother 2015;5–12.

72. Larmore C, Effron MB, Molife C, et al. "Real-World" comparison of prasugrel with ticagrelor in patients with acute coronary syndrome treated with percutaneous coronary intervention in the United States. Catheter Cardiovasc Interv 2015. [Epub ahead of print].

73. Mahoney EM, Wang K, Arnold SV, et al. Cost-effectiveness of prasugrel versus clopidogrel in patients with acute coronary syndromes and planned percutaneous coronary intervention: results from the trial to assess improvement in therapeutic outcomes by optimizing platelet inhibition with Prasugrel-Thrombolysis in Myocardial Infarction TRITON-TIMI 38. Circulation 2010;121(1):71–9.

74. Nikolic E, Janzon M, Hauch O, et al, PLATO Health Economic Substudy Group. Cost-effectiveness of treating acute coronary syndrome patients with ticagrelor for 12 months: results from the PLATO study. Eur Heart J 2013;34(3):220–8.

75. Fanari Z, Weiss S, Weintraub WS. Cost effectiveness of antiplatelet and antithrombotic therapy in the setting of acute coronary syndrome: current perspective and literature review. Am J Cardiovasc Drugs 2015;15(6):415–27.

76. Rao RV, Goodman SG, Yan RT, et al. Temporal trends and patterns of early clopidogrel use across the spectrum of acute coronary syndromes. Am Heart J 2009;157(4):642–50.e1.

77. Biondi-Zoccai G, Lotrionte M, Agostoni P, et al. Adjusted indirect comparison meta-analysis of prasugrel versus ticagrelor for patients with acute coronary syndromes. Int J Cardiol 2011;150(3):325–31.

78. Steiner S, Moertl D, Chen L, et al. Network meta-analysis of prasugrel, ticagrelor, high- and standard-dose clopidogrel in patients scheduled for percutaneous coronary interventions. Thromb Haemost 2012;108(2):318–27.

79. Rafique A, Nayyar P, Baber U, et al. Optimal P2y12 inhibitor in patients with ST segment elevation myocardial infarction undergoing primary percutaneous coronary intervention: a network meta-analysis. J Am Coll Cardiol 2016;67(13_S):212.

80. Schulz S, Angiolillo DJ, Antoniucci D, et al. Randomized comparison of ticagrelor versus prasugrel in patients with acute coronary syndrome and

planned invasive strategy—design and rationale of the intracoronary stenting and antithrombotic regimen: rapid early action for coronary treatment (ISAR-REACT) 5 trial. J Cardiovasc Transl Res 2013;7(1):91–100.

81. Parodi G, Valenti R, Bellandi B, et al. Comparison of prasugrel and ticagrelor loading doses in ST-segment elevation myocardial infarction patients: RAPID (Rapid Activity of Platelet Inhibitor Drugs) primary PCI study. J Am Coll Cardiol 2013;61(15): 1601–6.

82. Boersma E, Harrington RA, Moliterno DJ, et al. Platelet glycoprotein IIb/IIIa inhibitors in acute coronary syndromes: a meta-analysis of all major randomised clinical trials. Lancet 2002;359(9302):189–98.

83. Stone GW, Maehara A, Witzenbichler B, et al. Intracoronary abciximab and aspiration thrombectomy in patients with large anterior myocardial infarction: the INFUSE-AMI randomized trial. JAMA 2012; 307(17):1817–26.

84. Sibbing D, Kastrati A, Berger PB. Pre-treatment with P2Y12 inhibitors in ACS patients: who, when, why, and which agent? Eur Heart J 2016;37(16): 1284–95.

85. Montalescot G, van 't Hof AW, Lapostolle F, et al. Prehospital ticagrelor in ST-segment elevation myocardial infarction. N Engl J Med 2014;371(11): 1016–27.

86. Perl L, Sasson L, Weissler-Snir A, et al. Effects of prasugrel pretreatment on angiographic myocardial perfusion parameters in patients with ST-elevation myocardial infarction undergoing primary percutaneous coronary intervention. Coron Artery Dis 2015;26(8):665–70.

Controversies in the Management of ST Elevation Myocardial Infarction
Thrombin Inhibition

Neeraj Shah, MD, MPH, David Cox, MD, FSCAI*

KEYWORDS

- ST elevation myocardial infarction (STEMI)
- Primary percutaneous coronary intervention (primary PCI) • Fibrinolysis • Bivalirudin
- Direct thrombin inhibitors • Unfractionated heparin (UFH)

KEY POINTS

- Anticoagulation is essential in patients with ST elevation myocardial infarction (STEMI) in order to prevent further thrombosis and to maintain patency of the infarct-related artery after reperfusion.
- In patients with STEMI undergoing primary percutaneous coronary intervention (PCI), bivalirudin provides a mortality benefit over unfractionated heparin (UFH), predominantly via a reduction in major bleeding with bivalirudin compared to UFH.
- In clinical situations such as radial artery access, use of newer oral antiplatelet agents or provisional (rather than routine) glycoprotein IIb/IIIa inhibitor use, the bleeding advantage of bivalirudin over UFH may not be as apparent.
- There is an increase in risk of stent thrombosis with bivalirudin compared with UFH in the first 24 hours after primary PCI, which can potentially be mitigated by preadministration of UFH or prolonging full-dose bivalirudin infusion after PCI for up to 4 hours.
- UFH is the preferred anticoagulant for patients with STEMI undergoing fibrinolysis. For those in whom a PCI is not planned, enoxaparin and fondaparinux may be reasonable alternatives.

INTRODUCTION

Acute ST elevation myocardial infarction (STEMI) occurs when there is rupture of a coronary artery atherosclerotic plaque with a superimposed fibrin-rich clot resulting in occlusion of the lumen of an epicardial coronary artery. The treatment of STEMI involves either emergent percutaneous coronary intervention (PCI), which involves balloon angioplasty and/or stenting, or fibrinolysis, which involves lysis of the clot with intravenous (IV) fibrinolytic agents. The role of antithrombotic therapy in the setting of STEMI

is to prevent extension or propagation of the coronary artery thrombosis and to maintain patency of the infarct-related artery after successful reperfusion.

A brief review of the coagulation cascade reveals that the intrinsic and extrinsic pathways converge to activate Factor X to Factor Xa, which converts prothrombin to thrombin. Activated thrombin converts fibrinogen to fibrin, ultimately resulting in cross-linked clot formation.[1] Antithrombin (AT)-III, a naturally occurring regulator of the coagulation cascade, inactivates both thrombin and Factor Xa. The anticoagulants

---

Disclosures/Conflicts of Interest: Dr D. Cox is on the medical advisory board of The Medicines Company.
Department of Cardiology, Lehigh Valley Heath Network, 1250 S Cedar Crest Boulevard, Allentown, PA 18103, USA
* Corresponding author.
E-mail address: david.cox@lvhn.org

used in the setting of myocardial infarction (MI) can, therefore, be divided into the following classes:

1. Indirect thrombin inhibitors: These inhibitors include unfractionated heparin (UFH); low-molecular-weight heparin (LMWH), which includes enoxaparin; and fondaparinux, which is a synthetic heparin pentasaccharide. These medications complex with AT-III and alter its conformation to result in either rapid inactivation of thrombin (eg, UFH) or Factor Xa (eg, LMWH and fondaparinux).
2. Direct thrombin inhibitors (DTIs): These medications directly inactivate thrombin. Bivalirudin, hirudin, and lepirudin are all direct thrombin inhibitors. Bivalirudin is the only clinically used DTI.

Anticoagulation in STEMI is divided into the following sections:

1. Patients with STEMI receiving primary PCI: This topic is reviewed in the context of different clinically relevant scenarios, such as access site (radial vs femoral), antiplatelet agent use (clopidogrel vs newer oral agents, such as prasugrel or ticagrelor), and glycoprotein IIb/IIIa inhibitor (GPI) use (routine vs provisional).
2. Patients with STEMI receiving fibrinolysis: In areas with limited access to health care, fibrinolysis is a frequently used option for revascularization.
3. Patients with STEMI not eligible for fibrinolysis or PCI (no reperfusion): This scenario is uncommon, and the role of anticoagulation in this setting is discussed briefly.

Primary Percutaneous Coronary Intervention

Use of anticoagulant therapy in the setting of primary PCI is a class I indication according to all major guidelines.[2,3] The following anticoagulants have been studied in this clinical setting: UFH, bivalirudin, fondaparinux, and enoxaparin.

Unfractionated heparin versus bivalirudin

For several years, UFH was the only anticoagulant available for PCI, and it was the standard medication used for primary PCI in STEMI for a long time.[4] However, UFH has several pharmacologic limitations, including high variability in action among different individuals and in the same individual over time.[5] The efficacy of UFH needs to be monitored by activated clotting time (ACT) measurements during PCI, with repeat boluses often necessary to maintain an ACT range of 200 to 250 seconds. In the recent

years, bivalirudin has emerged as a formidable alternative to UFH. Bivalirudin is administered in a fixed weight-based dose as a bolus followed by an infusion. ACT measurements do not correlate with the level of thrombin inhibition with bivalirudin and are performed simply to assure the drug has been properly given. Routine ACT monitoring with bivalirudin is not recommended except in the presence of renal failure.[6,7] Several multicenter trials have been conducted comparing bivalirudin with UFH with conflicting results (Table 1).

RANDOMIZED CONTROLLED TRIALS

Harmonizing Outcomes with Revascularization and Stents in Acute Myocardial Infarction

The Harmonizing Outcomes with Revascularization and Stents in Acute Myocardial Infarction (HORIZONS AMI) trial published in 2008 was the first major trial comparing bivalirudin with provisional GPI to UFH with routine GP IIb/IIIa inhibition. In contrast to contemporary therapy, femoral access and clopidogrel were used in most patients and UFH was combined with a GPI in a routine rather than a provisional fashion.[8] Bivalirudin had a significant mortality benefit over UFH plus GPI with reduction in cardiac death (1.8% vs 2.9%, P = .03) and all-cause mortality at 30 days (2.1% vs 3.1%, P = .047). Similar mortality benefits with bivalirudin were maintained at the 1- and 3-year follow-up.[9] There was no difference in major adverse cardiovascular events (MACE) in the two arms; however, the primary outcome of net adverse clinical events (NACE; composite of MACE and major bleeding) was significantly lower in the bivalirudin arm (4.9% vs 8.3%, P<.001), largely driven by a reduction in major bleeding. An increase in the rate of acute (within 24 hours) stent thrombosis was observed in the bivalirudin arm (1.3% vs 0.3%, P<.001). Criticisms of this trial include high proportion (94%) of femoral arterial access and GPI use in the UFH arm (94.5%), which may have contributed to the increased bleeding rates with UFH.

European Ambulance Acute Coronary Syndrome Angiography

In the European Ambulance Acute Coronary Syndrome (ACS) Angiography (EUROMAX) trial,[10] patients were randomly assigned to receive either heparin or bivalirudin (with post-PCI infusion up to 4 hours) during emergency transport for PCI. In the heparin group, 41.5% of patients did not receive routine GPI

Table 1
Patient characteristics of randomized controlled trials comparing bivalirudin with unfractionated heparin for primary percutaneous coronary intervention in ST elevation myocardial infarction

Trial	Author, Year	Country	n	n (Bival)	n (UFH)	Age[a] (y)	Men (%)	GPI Use (Bival) (%)	GPI Use (UFH) (%)	Radial Access (%)	Clopidogrel (%)	Prasugrel/ Ticagrelor (%)
HORIZONS AMI	Stone et al,[8] 2008	United States, Italy, Poland, Israel, United Kingdom, Argentina, Norway, Netherlands, Germany, Austria, Spain	3602	1800	1802	60.2	76.6	7.2	94.5	5.9	99.8	0
EUROMAX	Steg et al,[10] 2013	France, Germany, Italy, Denmark, Netherlands, Poland, Slovenia, Austria, Czech Republic	2218	1089	1109	61.0	76.4	11.5	69.1	47.0	50.7	49.1
HEAT PPCI	Shahzad et al,[12] 2014	United Kingdom (single center)	1812	905	907	63.2	72.3	13.0	15.0	81.1	10.9	89.4
BRIGHT[b]	Han et al,[13] 2015	China (82 sites)	2194	735	1459 (729/730)[c]	57.9	82.1	4.4	5.6/100[d]	78.5	100	0
BRAVE-4	Schulz et al,[14] 2014	Germany (3 centers)	546	271	277	61.4	77.4	3.0	6.1	0.2	In UFH arm[e]	In bival arm[e]
MATRIX	Valgimigli et al,[15] 2015	Italy, Netherlands, Spain, Sweden	7213[f]	3610	3603	65.4	76.2	4.6	25.9	49.9[g]	45.9	36.5

Abbreviations: Bival, bivalirudin; n, sample size/number of patients.
[a] Age expressed as mean or median age in years in the study population.
[b] Bivalirudin compared with LFH plus provisional tirofiban (UFH-alone arm) and UFH plus routine tirofiban.
[c] A total of 729 in the UFH-alone arm and 730 in the UFH-plus-tirofiban arm.
[d] GPI use was 5.6% in UFH-alone arm and 100% in UFH-plus-tirofiban arm.
[e] Only clopidogrel used in the UFH arm, and only prasugrel used in the bivalirudin arm.
[f] Only 4010 (55.6%) had STEMI.
[g] Originally randomized to radial versus femoral access (hence 50% of each); bivalirudin versus UFH comparison was nested within the original trial.

(n = 460). The patient population was more reflective of contemporary clinical practice, with 47.0% radial access and 49.1% use of prasugrel or ticagrelor. There was no significant difference in the all-cause mortality or cardiac death with bivalirudin compared with heparin. The primary outcome of major bleeding and death was reduced with bivalirudin compared with heparin (5.1% vs 8.5%, P = .007); once again this was driven by a reduction in major bleeding (2.6% vs 6%, P<.001). Notably, 8.5% patients in the heparin group received LMWH; however, rates of primary end point were not different between UFH and LMWH.[11]

In a prespecified subanalysis of the EUROMAX trial,[11] bivalirudin was compared with heparin with routine GPI use and heparin with bailout GPI use (25.4% GPI use). Bivalirudin reduced the composite outcome of death or major bleeding compared with heparin irrespective of type of GPI use. The advantage of bivalirudin over heparin persists, regardless of planned or provisional GPI use. However, it should be kept in mind that the decision of routine versus bailout GPI use was not randomized but left at the discretion of the trial investigators.

How Effective Are Antithrombotic Therapies in Primary Percutaneous Coronary Intervention

The How Effective are Antithrombotic Therapies in Primary Percutaneous Coronary Intervention (HEAT PPCI) trial was a single-center trial comparing bivalirudin with UFH.[12] In this trial, GPI use was strictly provisional and, therefore, similar in the bivalirudin and UFH arms (13% vs 15%, see Table 1). Most patients in this trial had radial access (81%) and newer antiplatelet agent use (89%). Surprisingly, there was a significantly higher incidence of death, stroke, reinfarction, or target vessel revascularization (TVR) at 28 days with bivalirudin (8.7%) compared with the UFH (5.7%, P = .01). There was no difference in major bleeding (3.5% vs 3.1%, P = .59). Incidence of acute stent thrombosis (AST) was higher with the bivalirudin arm compared with UFH (2.9% vs 0.9%, P = .007). The beneficial effect of UFH over bivalirudin was driven by a significant increase in reinfarction rate (due to stent thrombosis) in the bivalirudin group. The higher rate of stent thrombosis in this trial was attributed to a high-risk study population and lack of UFH administration before randomization. Criticisms of the single-center HEAT PPCI trial include short duration of bivalirudin infusion and a lower ACT achieved with bivalirudin compared with prior studies.[13]

Bivalirudin in Acute Myocardial Infarction Versus Heparin and Glycoprotein IIb/IIIa Inhibitor Plus Heparin

The Bivalirudin in Acute Myocardial Infarction versus Heparin and GPI plus Heparin (BRIGHT) trial[13] was designed with 3 arms: bivalirudin with post-PCI infusion (30 minutes to 4 hours), UFH alone (100 units per kilogram), and UFH with routine GPI (tirofiban). Provisional use of GPI was allowed in the bivalirudin and UFH-alone arms; but unlike EUROMAX, routine versus provisional use of GPIs with UFH was randomized in this trial. In the bivalirudin arm, after 4 hours, reduced dose infusion at 0.2 mg/kg/h could be administered up to 20 hours at physician discretion. All patients received clopidogrel and 78% had radial access. The primary outcome of NACE (death, stroke, reinfarction, TVR, or major bleeding) was 8.8% with bivalirudin compared with 13.2% with UFH alone (P = .008) and 17% with UFH plus tirofiban (P<.001). Again, this effect was driven by a reduction in major bleeding with bivalirudin compared with UFH (4.1% vs 7.5% vs 12.3%, P<.001). Interestingly, the rate of AST was not different with bivalirudin compared with the two UFH groups. The benefit of bivalirudin over UFH persisted at 1 year. Criticisms of this trial include use of a high dose of UFH (100 U/kg) in the UFH alone arm, which may have been responsible for the higher bleeding rates seen with UFH. Notably, 12% of patients in the BRIGHT trial did not have an STEMI but had a non-STEMI (NSTEMI) requiring emergent PCI.

Bavarian Reperfusion Alternatives Evaluation 4

The Bavarian Reperfusion Alternatives Evaluation (BRAVE)-4 trial was designed to compare prasugrel plus bivalirudin with clopidogrel plus UFH.[14] Routine GPI use was not permitted; therefore, only 3% of patients in the bivalirudin arm and 6.1% of patients in the UFH arm received GPI. The access site was femoral in all but one patient. The trial was stopped prematurely, enrolling only 548 out of a target of 1240 patients, because of slow recruitment. There was no different in the primary end point of death, MI, TVR, stent thrombosis, stroke, or bleeding at 30 days in the two arms (15.6% vs 14.5%, P = .68). No differences were observed in MACE (4.8% vs 5.5%, P = .89), major bleeding (14.1% vs 12.0%, P = .54), or stent thrombosis (1.1% vs 1.5%, P = .98) at 30 days between the two arms. Given the limited sample size and premature termination of this trial, these results must be interpreted with caution.

Minimizing Adverse Hemorrhagic Events by Transradial Access Site and Systemic Implementation of Angiox

The Minimizing Adverse Hemorrhagic Events by Transradial Access Site and Systemic Implementation of Angiox (MATRIX) trial[15] was designed to compare radial with femoral access in acute coronary syndromes as well as bivalirudin versus UFH use. Initially, 8404 patients with ACS were randomized to femoral versus radial access; of those, 7213 patients were further randomized to receive either bivalirudin or UFH. Patients in the bivalirudin group were randomized to receive or not to receive post-PCI bivalirudin infusion; however, the dose and duration of post-PCI bivalirudin infusion was not randomized and was left at the discretion of the physician. Almost 50% of patients had radial access, and 36.5% of patients received either prasugrel or ticagrelor. Provisional GPI use was 4.6% with bivalirudin and 25.9% with UFH. The rates of MACE (10.3% vs 10.9%, $P = .44$) or NACE (11.5% vs 12.6%, $P = .15$) were not significantly different between bivalirudin and UFH. Post-PCI infusion of bivalirudin did not significantly decrease the rate of urgent TVR, definite AST, or NACE. Only 4010 (55.9%) of patients in the MATRIX trial had an STEMI. In the STEMI subgroup of the MATRIX trial (MATRIX-STEMI), there was a significant reduction in all-cause mortality with bivalirudin compared with UFH (2.1% vs 3.1%, $P = .05$) as well as a significant reduction in major bleeding with bivalirudin (1.6% vs 2.7%, $P = .02$).

POOLED ANALYSES

Several meta-analyses have been conducted comparing bivalirudin to UFH pooling the results from prior data. The comparisons between bivalirudin and UFH can be broken down into the following sections.

Bivalirudin and Mortality

Compared with UFH, bivalirudin is associated with a significantly reduced risk of 30-day mortality after primary PCI in pooled analyses.[16] In the HORIZONS AMI and MATRIX-STEMI trials, there was a significant reduction in the risk of all-cause mortality at 30 days with bivalirudin compared with UFH by 1% (Fig. 1). Bivalirudin was also associated with reduced risk of cardiac death at 30 days in the HORIZONS AMI trial (Fig. 2).[16] One of the reasons for the mortality benefit of bivalirudin over UFH is a reduction in major bleeding with bivalirudin. Among all patients undergoing PCI, patients with STEMI are at the highest risk of developing major bleeding[17]; occurrence of major bleeding is an independent predictor of mortality in these patients.[18] Hence, a significant reduction in major bleeding with bivalirudin translates into a mortality benefit. Of note, in the HORIZONS AMI trial, reduction in cardiac death with bivalirudin was observed even in patients who did not experience a major bleeding event, suggesting a yet-undefined pleiotropic effect of bivalirudin.[19] The mortality benefit with bivalirudin persists over time, as seen in 3-year follow-up data of the HORIZONS AMI trial.[9]

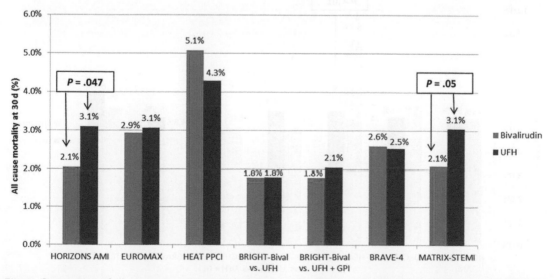

Fig. 1. Comparison of all-cause mortality at 30 days between bivalirudin and UFH arms in patients with STEMI undergoing primary PCI across major randomized controlled trials. Note: Only significant P-values (<.05) are shown. P-values for the remaining comparisons are not statistically significant. bival, bivalirudin.

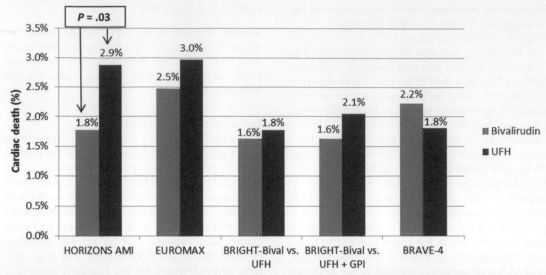

Fig. 2. Comparison of cardiac mortality at 30 days between bivalirudin and UFH arms in patients with STEMI undergoing primary PCI across major randomized controlled trials. Note: Only significant P-values (<.05) are shown in the figure. P-values for the remaining comparisons are not statistically significant. bival, bivalirudin.

Bivalirudin and Major Adverse Cardiovascular Events

Several meta-analyses have shown that compared with UFH, bivalirudin has similar rates of MACE, reinfarction, and target vessel revascularization.[16,20,21] In most of the previously discussed randomized controlled trials (RCTs), 30-day MACE rates did not differ significantly between bivalirudin and UFH (Fig. 3). Thus,

bivalirudin does not seem to have any benefit over UFH in reducing ischemic events after PCI.

Bivalirudin and Bleeding

Several studies and meta-analyses confirm that bivalirudin significantly lowers the risk of major bleeding compared with UFH ± GPI (Fig. 4).[8,10,13,15,16,20,21] Reduction in major bleeding with bivalirudin is independent of the

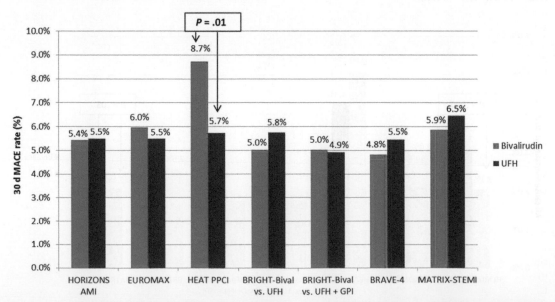

Fig. 3. Comparison of MACE at 30 days between bivalirudin and UFH arms in patients with STEMI undergoing primary PCI across major RCTs. Note: Only significant P-values (<.05) are shown. P-values for the remaining comparisons are not statistically significant. bival, bivalirudin.

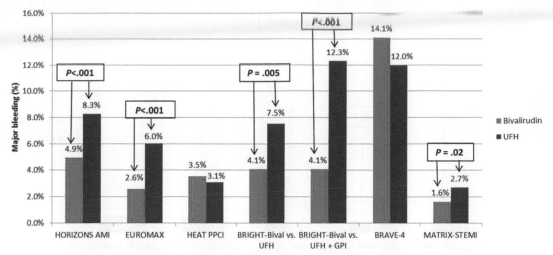

Fig. 4. Comparison of major bleeding rates at 30 days between bivalirudin and UFH arms in patients with STEMI undergoing primary PCI across major RCTs. Note: Only significant *P*-values (<.05) are shown. *P*-values for the remaining comparisons are not statistically significant. bival, bivalirudin.

baseline bleeding risk. The effect of bivalirudin on bleeding is modified by GPI use, access site, and antiplatelet agent use, with studies showing that bailout GPI use, transradial access, and newer oral P2Y12 inhibitors reduce the bleeding advantage of bivalirudin over UFH.[16,22]

The presence of bailout (rather than routine) GPI use was associated with no difference in major bleeding between bivalirudin and UFH in a few studies.[16,23] On the other hand, in the bailout GPI arm of the EUROMAX[10] and BRIGHT[13] trials, and the MATRIX-STEMI trial (whereby GPI use was not routine),[15] bivalirudin continued to exhibit a significant bleeding advantage over UFH.

Analysis of trials with predominantly radial access reveals no difference in major bleeding rates between bivalirudin and UFH.[16] Subgroup analysis of the MATRIX trial showed no bleeding advantage with bivalirudin when radial access was used[15]; however, this should be interpreted with caution because the interaction *P*-value was not significant. Of note, bivalirudin is shown to reduce both access site as well as nonaccess site bleeding[15,24] and nonaccess site bleeding is more likely to be associated with mortality.[24] Hence, the influence of the choice of access site in modifying the effect of bivalirudin on the overall bleeding risk remains controversial.

Meta-analysis of trials using predominantly prasugrel or ticagrelor showed no difference in major bleeding rates between bivalirudin and UFH[16]; however, these results were largely driven by the HEAT PPCI trial. The BRAVE-4 trial[14] also showed that using prasugrel with bivalirudin compared with clopidogrel with

UFH resulted in similar major bleeding rates in the two arms; however, these results must be interpreted with caution given the small sample size and premature termination of this study.

Bivalirudin and Acute Stent Thrombosis

Several studies have shown that the risk of AST is significantly increased with bivalirudin after primary PCI[16,20,21] (**Fig. 5**), even though the 30-day mortality is lower. The risk of AST seems to be highest in the first 4 hours following PCI and may be related to the discontinuation of bivalirudin infusion before full effect of antiplatelet medications.[8,10] Bivalirudin has a short half-life with rapid renal clearance, resulting in quick loss of drug effect once the infusion is turned off,[11] which in combination with delayed absorption, bioavailability, and onset of action of oral antiplatelet medications[25,26] in the setting of STEMI sets the stage for early stent thrombosis. Increase in AST has resulted in higher reinfarction and TVR rates in the EUROMAX[10] and HEAT PPCI[12] trials with bivalirudin.

Preadministration of UFH in the bivalirudin arm was shown to be protective for AST in the HORIZONS AMI trial.[27] Because bivalirudin has antithrombotic properties, it was theorized that prolonged (up to 4 hours) infusion of bivalirudin after PCI may provide additional protection against AST in the early risk period.[28] The lack of difference in AST between bivalirudin and UFH in the BRIGHT trial was attributed to high-dose post-PCI bivalirudin infusion for a median duration of 3 hours in the bivalirudin arm.[13] However, in the EUROMAX[10] and MATRIX[15] trials, bivalirudin infusion after PCI did not reduce the risk of

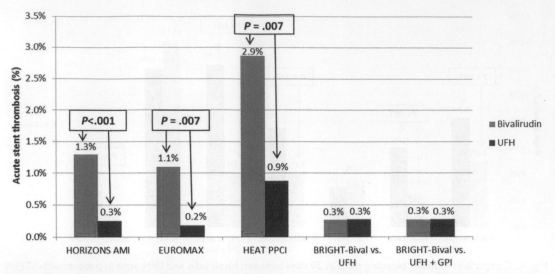

Fig. 5. Comparison of acute (within 24 hours) stent thrombosis rates between bivalirudin and UFH arms in patients with STEMI undergoing primary PCI across major RCTs. Note: Only significant P-values (<.05) are shown. P-values for the remaining comparisons are not statistically significant. bival, bivalirudin.

AST. In both trials, investigators had the option of either continuing bivalirudin infusion at the full PCI dosage of 1.75 mg/kg/h or reduced dosage of 0.25 mg/kg/h. In a subanalysis of the EURO-MAX trial, it was observed that patients who got a full dosage (1.75 mg/kg/h) post-PCI infusion of bivalirudin for a median of 4 hours had a significantly reduced risk of developing AST.[29] Similarly, explorative analysis from the MATRIX trial[15] showed that patients who received full-dose bivalirudin infusion for up to 4 hours after PCI had a significantly lower risk of AST (0.2%) compared with no post-PCI infusion (0.6%) or low-dose prolonged post-PCI infusion (0.8%), without any excess bleeding risk. However, it must be noted that in all of the aforementioned trials, the dose and duration of post-PCI bivalirudin infusion were not randomized but were at the discretion of the study investigators.

Theoretically, pretreatment with newer oral P2Y12 inhibitors (prasugrel and ticagrelor) should potentially mitigate the excess risk of AST with bivalirudin. However, subanalysis of the EUROMAX trial[29] and a recently conducted meta-analysis[22] failed to demonstrate any reduction in the risk of early stent thrombosis with bivalirudin compared with UFH with the use of newer oral P2Y12 inhibitors. Impaired gastric emptying, reduced oral absorption, and a delay in onset of antiplatelet action by 4 to 6 hours in the setting of STEMI have been proposed as possible explanations behind the lack of benefit of newer oral P2Y12 inhibitors in preventing bivalirudin-associated AST.[26,30] In this scenario, the use of an intravenous P2Y12 inhibitor with

a rapid onset of action (ie, cangrelor) becomes an attractive option. In a subgroup analysis of the CHAMPION PHOENIX trial (Clinical Trial Comparing Cangrelor to Clopidogrel Standard of Care Therapy in Subjects Who Require Percutaneous Coronary Intervention)[31] including 2059 patients who received bivalirudin, there was a trend toward less stent thrombosis at 48 hours with cangrelor compared with clopidogrel (0.7% vs 1.4%, P = .10). Hence, cangrelor infusion after PCI seems to be a promising option to reduce the excess risk of AST with bivalirudin after primary PCI.

MEDICATION DOSING

Bivalirudin is administered as an initial bolus of 0.75 mg/kg followed by an IV infusion of 1.75 mg/kg/h for at least the duration of PCI. Routine ACT monitoring with bivalirudin is not recommended, but checking an ACT value 5 minutes after bolus may have some role in confirmation of drug administration; in some trials, an additional 0.3 mg/kg bolus of bivalirudin was administered if the ACT 5 minutes after the initial bolus was less than 225 seconds.[12,13] UFH is administered as an IV bolus ranging from 60 to 100 U/kg, with higher doses (100 U/kg) used when a GPI is not coadministered. Subsequent boluses of UFH are targeted to an ACT measurement of 200 to 250 seconds.

Summary

- Bivalirudin significantly reduces the risk of major bleeding after primary PCI for

STEMI compared with UFH. It reduces both access and nonaccess site bleeding.

- Bleeding advantage of bivalirudin over UFH may be reduced with bailout (rather than routine) GPI use, radial access, or use of newer oral antiplatelet agents; however, more evidence is needed on this topic.
- Bivalirudin has no benefit over UFH for reduction in MACE or ischemic events after primary PCI.
- Bivalirudin has a significant mortality benefit over UFH after primary PCI for STEMI, which persists over time. This benefit may be explained partly by a reduction in major bleeding and a partly by a yet-undefined pleiotropic effect of bivalirudin.
- Bivalirudin significantly increases the risk of AST compared with UFH.
- The risk of AST with bivalirudin can be potentially reduced by preadministration of UFH or prolonging bivalirudin infusion at 1.75 mg/kg/h for up to 4 hours after PCI; however, more evidence is needed before a clear recommendation can be made.
- Use of newer oral P2Y12 inhibitors with bivalirudin should theoretically reduce the excess risk of AST; however, current evidence does not show any benefit with these drugs. Use of an IV P2Y12 inhibitor (cangrelor) is an attractive option to reduce the risk of AST; however, more evidence is needed to support its use.
- The choice between bivalirudin and UFH for anticoagulation in the setting of primary PCI varies among different centers. It is often dictated by availability, cost, ease of administration, and experience with a particular medication. Clinical situations, such as the use of GPI, radial versus femoral access, and the type of oral antiplatelet agent used, may influence the choice of anticoagulation.
- In summary, bivalirudin is a relatively expensive alternative to UFH for primary PCI, and it provides a significant mortality benefit at the cost of a potentially higher rate of AST.

Enoxaparin

Enoxaparin has been compared with UFH in the ATOLL trial (STEMI Treated With Primary Angioplasty and Intravenous Lovenox or Unfractionated Heparin) in 2011 involving 910 patients with STEMI undergoing primary PCI.[32] Patients were randomly assigned to receive either enoxaparin as an IV bolus of 0.5 mg/kg or UFH as an IV bolus of 70 to 100 U/kg (if no GPI) or 50 to 70 U/kg (with GPI) before primary PCI. There was a high proportion of clopidogrel use (93%), GPI use (80%), and radial access (67%) in this trial. There was no significant difference in the primary outcome of 30-day mortality, MI complication, procedure failure, or major bleeding in enoxaparin compared with UFH (28% vs 34%, $P = .06$). There was a reduction in the secondary end point of death, recurrent MI or urgent TVR with enoxaparin (7%) compared with UFH (11%, $P = .015$). The major bleeding rates did not differ between the two groups. Thus, enoxaparin significantly reduces ischemic outcomes compared with UFH, without increasing the risk of bleeding. This study is limited by the high proportion of GPI use (80%) in both arms. Two meta-analyses have revealed that LMWH significantly reduces bleeding and mortality risk on patients with STEMI undergoing primary PCI; however, these studies are limited because of significant heterogeneity in timing, dose, and route of administration of enoxaparin in different trials.[33,34]

In summary, enoxaparin can be considered over UFH at a dose of 0.5 mg/kg IV bolus before primary PCI with radial access, if no bivalirudin use is planned. The optimal dose with femoral access is not known.

Fondaparinux

Fondaparinux is not recommended for use in STEMI in patients undergoing primary PCI based on the OASIS-6 trial (Organization for the Assessment of Strategies for Ischemic Syndromes) findings[35] (discussed later).

Fibrinolysis

Fibrinolytic agents used in the setting of STEMI include streptokinase, urokinase, or fibrin-specific agents, such as the recombinant tissue plasminogen activators (t-PAs). Recombinant t-PAs approved for STEMI include alteplase, reteplase, and tenecteplase. The various anticoagulants studied in patients with STEMI undergoing fibrinolysis are discussed later.

Enoxaparin

Several RCTs have compared UFH with enoxaparin in patients with STEMI treated with fibrinolysis.[36] These trials include Baird and colleagues 2002,[37] HART II (Second Trial of Heparin and Aspirin Reperfusion Therapy),[38] ENTIRE-TIMI 23 (Enoxaparin as adjunctive antithrombin therapy for ST-elevation myocardial infarction Thrombolysis in Myocardial Infarction

Table 2
Trials comparing different classes of anticoagulants to unfractionated heparin in ST elevation myocardial infarction patients treated with fibrinolysis

Trial	Sample Size	Agent Used	Dosing Regimen of Study Drug	Duration of UFH Infusion	Outcomes
Baird et al,[37] 2002	300	Enoxaparin	40 mg IV bolus, then 40 mg SC q8h for 4 d	4 d	Significant reduction in death, reinfarction, or readmission for angina with enoxaparin at 90 d; no difference in major bleeding
HART II, 2001	400	Enoxaparin	30 mg IV bolus, then 1 mg/kg SC q12h for ≥72 h	≥77 h	Enoxaparin noninferior to UFH with regard to infarct related artery patency rates at 90 min, and reocclusion rates 5–7 d after MI; no difference in adverse events
ENTIRE-TIMI 23, 2002	483	Enoxaparin	30 mg IV bolus, then 1 mg/kg SC q12h for 8 d or discharge	≥36 h	No difference in TIMI 3 flow at 60 min; significant reduction in death/MI with enoxaparin compared with UFH; no difference in major bleeding
ASSENT-3, 2001	6095[a]	Enoxaparin	30 mg IV bolus, then 1 mg/kg SC q12h for 7 d or discharge	≥48 h	Significant reduction in death, in-hospital reinfarction, or refractory ischemia with enoxaparin compared with UFH; no difference in major bleeding
ASSENT-3 PLUS, 2003	1639	Enoxaparin	30 mg IV bolus, then 1 mg/kg SC q12h for 7 d or discharge	≥48 h	Significant reduction in 30-d mortality, in-hospital reinfarction, or refractory ischemia with enoxaparin; increase in intracranial hemorrhage with enoxaparin, especially in those aged 75 y or older
ExTRACT TIMI 25, 2006	20,475	Enoxaparin	30 mg IV bolus, then 1 mg/kg SC q12h for 8 d or discharge[b]	≥48 h	Significant reduction in 30-d mortality or reinfarction with enoxaparin; reduction in death, reinfarction, or urgent TVR with enoxaparin. Significant increase in major bleeding with enoxaparin; no increase in intracranial hemorrhage
PENTALYSE, 2001	333	Fondaparinux	4, 8, or 12 mg initial dose IV, then SC once daily for 5–7 d	48–72 h	TIMI 3 flow rates at 90 min were similar in the 4 groups; prolonged administration of fondaparinux associated with a trend toward fewer reocclusions and revascularizations; no increase in bleeding with fondaparinux

Study, Year	n	Drug	Dosing	Comparator/Duration	Findings
OASIS-6, 2006	5658	Fondaparinux	2.5 mg SC once daily for 8 d (stratum I)	Compared with placebo	Significant reduction in death or reinfarction at 30 d with fondaparinux; no difference in bleeding
OASIS-6, 2006	6434	Fondaparinux	2.5 mg IV once, then SC once daily for 8 d (stratum II)	Up to 48 h	No difference in death or reinfarction; no difference in bleeding; trend toward harm in those undergoing primary PCI
GUSTO IIb, 1998	3289	Hirudin	IV infusion to maintain aPTT 60–85 s for 3–5 d	3–5 d	Reduction in death or reinfarction at 30 d with hirudin in the streptokinase group (n = 2274), but no difference between hirudin and heparin in those receiving t-PA (n = 1015)
HIT-4, 1999	1208	Hirudin	IV bolus 0.2 mg/kg, then 0.5 mg/kg SC q12h for 5–7 d	12,500 U SC q12h for 5–7 d	All patients received streptokinase; no difference in initial TIMI 3 flow, death, reinfarction, or bleeding
HERO, 1997	412	Bivalirudin	Low dose: 0.125 mg/kg bolus followed by 0.25 mg/kg/h infusion for 12 h, then 0.125 mg/kg/h for total duration of 60 h; high dose: 0.25 mg/kg bolus followed by 0.5 mg/kg/h infusion for 12 h, then 0.25 mg/kg/h for total duration of 60 h	60 h	All patients received streptokinase; TIMI 3 flow at 90–120 min higher with bivalirudin compared with heparin; no difference in death, reocclusion, or reinfarction Lower incidence of major bleeding with both high- and low-dose bivalirudin
HERO-2, 2001	17,073	Bivalirudin	0.25 mg/kg IV bolus, then infusion at 0.5 mg/kg/h for 12 h, then 0.25 mg/kg/h for 36 h	48 h	All patients received streptokinase; no difference in mortality at 30 d; significantly fewer reinfarctions within 96 h in the bivalirudin group; higher rates of mild to moderate bleeding with bivalirudin compared with heparin; however, no difference in rates of severe bleeding and intracerebral bleeding

Abbreviations: aPTT, activated partial thromboplastin time; q12h, every 12 hours; q8h, every 8 hours; SC, subcutaneous.

[a] n = 2040 in enoxaparin and n = 2038 in UFH group; there were additional comparisons of full-dose tenecteplase with half-dose tenecteplase and abciximab.

[b] Reduced dose (0.75 mg/kg) in patients older than 75 years and reduced frequency (once a day) in patients with impaired renal function.

(TIMI) - Study 23),[39] ASSENT-3 (The Assessment of the Safety and Efficacy of a New Thrombolytic Regimen-3),[40] ASSENT-3 PLUS (The Assessment of the Safety and Efficacy of a New Thrombolytic Regimen-3 PLUS),[41] and ExTRACT-TIMI 25 (Enoxaparin and Thrombolysis Reperfusion for Acute Myocardial Infarction Treatment Thrombolysis in Myocardial Infarction - Study 25)[42] (Table 2). All trials used UFH bolus followed by infusion to adjust to an activated partial thromboplastin time (aPTT) of 2.0 to 2.5 times normal. The duration of UFH varied in among the trials, as did the dose and duration of enoxaparin. Some of the trials (ENTIRE-TIMI 23,[39] ASSENT-3[40]) involved additional comparisons of full-dose fibrinolytics with half-dose fibrinolytics combined with GPI (eg, abciximab). The newer, larger trials comparing enoxaparin with UFH in the setting of full-dose fibrinolysis (ASSENT-3 PLUS,[41] ExTRACT-TIMI 25[42]) show a benefit of week-long enoxaparin therapy compared with 48 hour UFH infusion in reducing ischemic events, but an increase in major bleeding, especially intracranial hemorrhage in patients 75 years or older.[41]

In summary, there is benefit of enoxaparin over UFH in reduction of ischemic events in patients with STEMI receiving fibrinolysis, with an increase in the risk of major bleeding. Enoxaparin can be considered as a reasonable alternative to UFH in patients with STEMI receiving fibrinolysis without a planned PCI.

Fondaparinux

The efficacy of fondaparinux in STEMI was evaluated in the PENTALYSE (Synthetic Pentasaccharide as an Adjunct to Fibrinolysis in Acute Myocardial Infarction)[43] and OASIS-6 trials[35] (see Table 2). The OASIS-6 trial enrolled 12,092 patients with STEMI who could be treated with fibrinolytic therapy, primary PCI, or no reperfusion. Patients were stratified based on whether or not there was an indication for heparin. Stratum 1 consisted of 5658 patients without planned PCI in whom heparin was not indicated. Most of these patients (78%) received fibrinolytic therapy with streptokinase. They were randomly assigned to receive fondaparinux 2.5 mg/d subcutaneously (SC) for up to 8 days versus placebo. In stratum 2, there were 6434 patients with an indication for heparin, such as fibrinolytic therapy with t-PA, primary PCI, or no reperfusion (eligible for heparin). These patients were either randomly assigned to receive fondaparinux (as discussed earlier) or UFH for 24 to 48 hours. The following outcomes were observed:

- For the entire population, there was a reduction in the primary end point of death or reinfarction at 30 days (9.7% vs 11.2%, P = .008). There was no difference in major bleeding rates.
- In stratum 1, compared with placebo, there was significant reduction in death or reinfarction at 30 days with fondaparinux (11.2% vs 14.0%, P = .002), which persisted in a subgroup analysis of patients receiving streptokinase.
- In stratum 2, there was no benefit with fondaparinux over UFH (primary end point 8.3% vs 8.7%, P = .58). There was a trend toward worse outcomes in patients undergoing primary PCI with fondaparinux (incidence of death or MI at 30 days was 6.1% with fondaparinux vs 5.1% with UFH). There was an increased incidence of guide-catheter–related thrombosis in those who received fondaparinux and underwent primary PCI.
- In a prespecified subgroup analysis, benefits of fondaparinux over UFH/placebo were confined to those receiving either fibrinolytic therapy or no reperfusion. There was a trend towards harm in those undergoing primary PCI.

Based on these findings, fondaparinux may be used in patients with STEMI undergoing fibrinolysis when a PCI is not planned or in those in whom no reperfusion therapies are planned. Of note, the US Food and Drug Administration has not approved it for use in STEMI.

Direct Thrombin Inhibitors

Studies comparing direct thrombin inhibitors with UFH in patients with STEMI undergoing fibrinolysis include GUSTO IIb (Global Use of Strategies to Open Occluded Coronary Arteries in Acute Coronary Syndromes IIb),[44] HIT-4 (Hirudin for the Improvement of Thrombolysis (HIT)-4),[45] HERO (Hirulog Early Reperfusion/Occlusion Study),[46] and HERO-2 (Hirulog Early Reperfusion/Occlusion Study (HERO)-2)[47] (see Table 2). There is some evidence of benefit of hirudin over UFH in patients with STEMI receiving streptokinase.[44] In the HERO-2 trial,[47] whereby streptokinase was used for fibrinolysis, there was a reduction in reinfarction rates at 96 hours with bivalirudin compared with UFH (1.6% vs 2.3%, P = .001). There was a trend of higher severe bleeding (0.7% vs 0.5%, P = .07) and intracerebral bleeding (0.6% vs 0.4%, P = .09) as well as significantly increased mild to moderate bleeding with bivalirudin compared with UFH. Because streptokinase is rarely used for fibrinolysis in the United States in the current era, there is no good evidence supporting the use of direct thrombin inhibitors over UFH for anticoagulation in patients with STEMI receiving fibrinolysis with fibrin-specific agents.

No reperfusion

There is a lack of randomized trials comparing UFH with placebo in patients with STEMI who are not reperfused. It is reasonable to use systemic anticoagulation with UFH in the presence of severe left ventricular (LV) dysfunction, large anterior MI, LV thrombus, atrial fibrillation, or a high risk for systemic or pulmonary embolism. Reviparin, an LMWH, administered SC twice daily for 7 days, was shown to significantly reduce the primary outcome of death, reinfarction, or stroke when compared with placebo (15.0% vs 18.3%) in a subset of 3225 patients not undergoing reperfusion in the CREATE trial (Clinical Trial of Reviparin and Metabolic Modulation in Acute Myocardial Infarction Treatment Evaluation).[48] Compared with UFH, enoxaparin showed similar incidence of death, reinfarction, or recurrent angina in a trial of 1225 patients with STEMI not receiving reperfusion.[49] The OASIS-6 trial provides evidence of benefit with fondaparinux 2.5 mg SC once daily compared with placebo in patients with STEMI undergoing no reperfusion[35] (see earlier discussion). Direct thrombin inhibitors have not been evaluated in this setting.

SUMMARY

Anticoagulation is essential in all patients with STEMI. In patients undergoing primary PCI, bivalirudin compared with UFH provides a mortality benefit, predominantly via reduction in major bleeding. Bailout (rather than routine) GPI use, transradial access, and use of newer oral P2Y12 inhibitors can potentially lessen the bleeding advantage of bivalirudin over UFH. There is an increase in the risk of acute (within 24 hours) stent thrombosis with bivalirudin compared with UFH, which can potentially be reduced by prolonging full-dose bivalirudin infusion after PCI for 4 hours. With the advent of newer oral (prasugrel and ticagrelor) and IV (cangrelor) P2Y12 inhibitors, several potential combinations can arise, which makes the choices challenging. For instance, IV cangrelor is a potentially attractive option to reduce the risk of AST with bivalirudin; however, more studies need to be undertaken to explore its role in this setting. In patients with STEMI

undergoing fibrinolysis, UFH is the preferred anticoagulant, with enoxaparin and fondaparinux being reasonable alternatives for those in whom a PCI is not planned. In patients with STEMI not undergoing reperfusion, UFH, enoxaparin or fondaparinux can be used for anticoagulation.

For the clinician, the choices of antithrombin therapy for primary PCI can be daunting. In most of the clinical trials, the choice was dichotomous; but in real-world practice, it becomes a complex calculus after factoring in decisions about radial versus femoral access, provisional versus routine GPI use, which oral antiplatelet agent to use, timing of the oral antiplatelet agent, and whether an IV P2Y12 inhibitor should be used. It is, therefore, little wonder that an individual interventional cardiologist struggles to determine if a given clinical trial fits into an algorithm to choose the optimal antithrombin strategy for a particular patient in the cardiac catheterization laboratory. There is no doubt that continued hearty debate will surround this controversy.

REFERENCES

1. Davie EW, Fujikawa K, Kisiel W. The coagulation cascade: initiation, maintenance, and regulation. Biochemistry 1991;30(43):10363–70.
2. O'Gara PT, Kushner FG, Ascheim DD, et al. ACCF/AHA guideline for the management of ST-elevation myocardial infarction: a report of the American College of Cardiology Foundation/American Heart Association Task Force on Practice Guidelines. Circulation 2013;127(4):e362–425.
3. Task Force on the management of ST-segment elevation acute myocardial infarction of the European Society of Cardiology (ESC), Steg PG, James SK, et al. ESC guidelines for the management of acute myocardial infarction in patients presenting with ST-segment elevation. Eur Heart J 2012;33(20):2569–619.
4. Rao SV, Ohman EM. Anticoagulant therapy for percutaneous coronary intervention. Circulation 2010;3(1):80–8.
5. Hirsh J, Warkentin TE, Shaughnessy SG, et al. Heparin and low-molecular-weight heparin: mechanisms of action, pharmacokinetics, dosing considerations, monitoring, efficacy, and safety. Chest 2001;119(1S):64S–94S.
6. Cho L, Kottke-Marchant K, Lincoff AM, et al. Correlation of point-of-care ecarin clotting time versus activated clotting time with bivalirudin concentrations. Am J Cardiol 2003;91(9):1110–3.
7. Koster A, Chew D, Grundel M, et al. Bivalirudin monitored with the ecarin clotting time for

anticoagulation during cardiopulmonary bypass. Anesth Analg 2003;96(2):383–6. table of contents.

8. Stone GW, Witzenbichler B, Guagliumi G, et al. Bivalirudin during primary PCI in acute myocardial infarction. N Engl J Med 2008;358(21):2218–30.

9. Stone GW, Witzenbichler B, Guagliumi G, et al. Heparin plus a glycoprotein IIb/IIIa inhibitor versus bivalirudin monotherapy and paclitaxel-eluting stents versus bare-metal stents in acute myocardial infarction (HORIZONS-AMI): final 3-year results from a multicentre, randomised controlled trial. Lancet 2011;377(9784):2193–204.

10. Steg PG, van 't Hof A, Hamm CW, et al. Bivalirudin started during emergency transport for primary PCI. N Engl J Med 2013;369(23):2207–17.

11. Zeymer U, van 't Hof A, Adgey J, et al. Bivalirudin is superior to heparins alone with bailout GP IIb/IIIa inhibitors in patients with ST-segment elevation myocardial infarction transported emergently for primary percutaneous coronary intervention: a pre-specified analysis from the EUROMAX trial. Eur Heart J 2014;35(36):2460–7.

12. Shahzad A, Kemp I, Mars C, et al. Unfractionated heparin versus bivalirudin in primary percutaneous coronary intervention (HEAT-PPCI): an open-label, single centre, randomised controlled trial. Lancet 2014;384(9957):1849–58.

13. Han Y, Guo J, Zheng Y, et al. Bivalirudin vs heparin with or without tirofiban during primary percutaneous coronary intervention in acute myocardial infarction: the BRIGHT randomized clinical trial. JAMA 2015;313(13):1336–46.

14. Schulz S, Richardt G, Laugwitz KL, et al. Prasugrel plus bivalirudin vs. clopidogrel plus heparin in patients with ST-segment elevation myocardial infarction. Eur Heart J 2014;35(34):2285–94.

15. Valgimigli M, Frigoli E, Leonardi S, et al. Bivalirudin or unfractionated heparin in acute coronary syndromes. N Engl J Med 2015;373(11):997–1009.

16. Shah R, Rogers KC, Matin K, et al. An updated comprehensive meta-analysis of bivalirudin vs heparin use in primary percutaneous coronary intervention. Am Heart J 2016;171(1):14–24.

17. Peterson ED, Dai D, DeLong ER, et al. Contemporary mortality risk prediction for percutaneous coronary intervention: results from 588,398 procedures in the National Cardiovascular Data Registry. J Am Coll Cardiol 2010;55(18):1923–32.

18. Mehran R, Rao SV, Bhatt DL, et al. Standardized bleeding definitions for cardiovascular clinical trials: a consensus report from the Bleeding Academic Research Consortium. Circulation 2011;123(23): 2736–47.

19. Stone GW, Clayton T, Deliargyris EN, et al. Reduction in cardiac mortality with bivalirudin in patients with and without major bleeding: the HORIZONS-AMI trial (Harmonizing Outcomes with Revascularization and Stents in Acute Myocardial Infarction). J Am Coll Cardiol 2014;63(1):15–20.

20. Barria Perez AE, Rao SV, Jolly SJ, et al. Meta-analysis of effects of bivalirudin versus heparin on myocardial ischemic and bleeding outcomes after percutaneous coronary intervention. Am J Cardiol 2016;117(8):1256–66.

21. Zhang S, Gao W, Li H, et al. Efficacy and safety of bivalirudin versus heparin in patients undergoing percutaneous coronary intervention: a meta-analysis of randomized controlled trials. Int J Cardiol 2016;209:87–95.

22. Bittl JA, He Y, Lang CD, et al. Factors affecting bleeding and stent thrombosis in clinical trials comparing bivalirudin with heparin during percutaneous coronary intervention. Circulation 2015;8(12): e002789.

23. Cavender MA, Sabatine MS. Bivalirudin versus heparin in patients planned for percutaneous coronary intervention: a meta-analysis of randomised controlled trials. Lancet 2014;384(9943):599–606.

24. Kilic S, Van't Hof AW, Ten Berg J, et al. Frequency and prognostic significance of access site and non-access site bleeding and impact of choice of anti-thrombin therapy in patients undergoing primary percutaneous coronary intervention. The EUROMAX trial. Int J Cardiol 2016;211:119–23.

25. Parodi G, Valenti R, Bellandi B, et al. Comparison of prasugrel and ticagrelor loading doses in ST-segment elevation myocardial infarction patients: RAPID (Rapid Activity of Platelet Inhibitor Drugs) primary PCI study. J Am Coll Cardiol 2013;61(15): 1601–6.

26. Alexopoulos D, Xanthopoulou I, Gkizas V, et al. Randomized assessment of ticagrelor versus prasugrel antiplatelet effects in patients with ST-segment-elevation myocardial infarction. Circ Cardiovasc Interv 2012;5(6):797–804.

27. Dangas GD, Caixeta A, Mehran R, et al. Frequency and predictors of stent thrombosis after percutaneous coronary intervention in acute myocardial infarction. Circulation 2011;123(16):1745–56.

28. Kimmelstiel C, Zhang P, Kapur NK, et al. Bivalirudin is a dual inhibitor of thrombin and collagen-dependent platelet activation in patients undergoing percutaneous coronary intervention. Circulation 2011;4(2):171–9.

29. Clemmensen P, Wiberg S, Van't Hof A, et al. Acute stent thrombosis after primary percutaneous coronary intervention: insights from the EUROMAX trial (European Ambulance Acute Coronary Syndrome Angiography). JACC Cardiovasc Interv 2015;8(1 Pt B):214–20.

30. Parodi G, Bellandi B, Xanthopoulou I, et al. Morphine is associated with a delayed activity of oral antiplatelet agents in patients with ST-elevation acute myocardial infarction undergoing

primary percutaneous coronary intervention. Circ Cardiovasc Interv 2015;8:e001593.

31. White HD, Bhatt DL, Gibson CM, et al. Outcomes with cangrelor versus clopidogrel on a background of bivalirudin: insights from the CHAMPION PHOENIX (A Clinical Trial Comparing Cangrelor to Clopidogrel Standard Therapy in Subjects Who Require Percutaneous Coronary Intervention [PCI]). JACC Cardiovasc Interv 2015;8(3):424–33.

32. Montalescot G, Zeymer U, Silvain J, et al. Intravenous enoxaparin or unfractionated heparin in primary percutaneous coronary intervention for ST-elevation myocardial infarction: the international randomised open-label ATOLL trial. Lancet 2011;378(9792):693–703.

33. Navarese EP, De Luca G, Castriota F, et al. Low-molecular-weight heparins vs. unfractionated heparin in the setting of percutaneous coronary intervention for ST-elevation myocardial infarction: a meta-analysis. J Thromb Haemost 2011;9(10): 1902–15.

34. Silvain J, Beygui F, Barthelemy O, et al. Efficacy and safety of enoxaparin versus unfractionated heparin during percutaneous coronary intervention: systematic review and meta-analysis. BMJ 2012;344:e553.

35. Yusuf S, Mehta SR, Chrolavicius S, et al. Effects of fondaparinux on mortality and reinfarction in patients with acute ST-segment elevation myocardial infarction: the OASIS-6 randomized trial. JAMA 2006;295(13):1519–30.

36. McCann CJ, Menown IB. New anticoagulant strategies in ST elevation myocardial infarction: trials and clinical implications. Vasc Health Risk Manag 2008; 4(2):305–13.

37. Baird SH, Menown IB, McBride SJ, et al. Randomized comparison of enoxaparin with unfractionated heparin following fibrinolytic therapy for acute myocardial infarction. Eur Heart J 2002;23(8):627–32.

38. Ross AM, Molhoek P, Lundergan C, et al. Randomized comparison of enoxaparin, a low-molecular-weight heparin, with unfractionated heparin adjunctive to recombinant tissue plasminogen activator thrombolysis and aspirin: second trial of Heparin and Aspirin Reperfusion Therapy (HART II). Circulation 2001;104(6):648–52.

39. Antman EM, Louwerenburg HW, Baars HF, et al. Enoxaparin as adjunctive antithrombin therapy for ST-elevation myocardial infarction: results of the ENTIRE-Thrombolysis in Myocardial Infarction (TIMI) 23 Trial. Circulation 2002;105(14):1642–9.

40. Assessment of the Safety and Efficacy of a New Thrombolytic Regimen (ASSENT)-3 Investigators. Efficacy and safety of tenecteplase in combination with enoxaparin, abciximab, or unfractionated heparin: the ASSENT-3 randomised trial in acute myocardial infarction. Lancet 2001;358(9282): 605–13.

41. Wallentin L, Goldstein P, Armstrong PW, et al. Efficacy and safety of tenecteplase in combination with the low-molecular-weight heparin enoxaparin or unfractionated heparin in the prehospital setting: the Assessment of the Safety and Efficacy of a New Thrombolytic Regimen (ASSENT)-3 PLUS randomized trial in acute myocardial infarction. Circulation 2003;108(2):135–42.

42. Antman EM, Morrow DA, McCabe CH, et al. Enoxaparin versus unfractionated heparin with fibrinolysis for ST-elevation myocardial infarction. N Engl J Med 2006;354(14):1477–88.

43. Coussement PK, Bassand JP, Convens C, et al. A synthetic factor-Xa inhibitor (ORG31540/ SR9017A) as an adjunct to fibrinolysis in acute myocardial infarction. The PENTALYSE study. Eur Heart J 2001;22(18):1716–24.

44. Metz BK, White HD, Granger CB, et al. Randomized comparison of direct thrombin inhibition versus heparin in conjunction with fibrinolytic therapy for acute myocardial infarction: results from the GUSTO-IIb Trial. Global Use of Strategies to Open Occluded Coronary Arteries in Acute Coronary Syndromes (GUSTO-IIb) Investigators. J Am Coll Cardiol 1998; 31(7):1493–8.

45. Neuhaus KL, Molhoek GP, Zeymer U, et al. Recombinant hirudin (lepirudin) for the improvement of thrombolysis with streptokinase in patients with acute myocardial infarction: results of the HIT-4 trial. J Am Coll Cardiol 1999;34(4):966–73.

46. White HD, Aylward PE, Frey MJ, et al. Randomized, double-blind comparison of hirulog versus heparin in patients receiving streptokinase and aspirin for acute myocardial infarction (HERO). Hirulog Early Reperfusion/Occlusion (HERO) Trial Investigators. Circulation 1997;96(7):2155–61.

47. White H. Thrombin-specific anticoagulation with bivalirudin versus heparin in patients receiving fibrinolytic therapy for acute myocardial infarction: the HERO-2 randomised trial. Lancet 2001;358(9296): 1855–63.

48. Yusuf S, Mehta SR, Xie C, et al. Effects of reviparin, a low-molecular-weight heparin, on mortality, reinfarction, and strokes in patients with acute myocardial infarction presenting with ST-segment elevation. JAMA 2005;293(4):427–35.

49. Cohen M, Gensini GF, Maritz F, et al. The safety and efficacy of subcutaneous enoxaparin versus intravenous unfractionated heparin and tirofiban versus placebo in the treatment of acute ST-segment elevation myocardial infarction patients ineligible for reperfusion (TETAMI): a randomized trial. J Am Coll Cardiol 2003;42(8):1348–56.

Controversies in the Management of ST-Segment Elevation Myocardial Infarction
Transradial Versus Transfemoral Approach

Taylor C. Bazemore, MD[a,*], Sunil V. Rao, MD[b,c]

KEYWORDS

- STEMI • Transradial approach • Transfemoral approach • PCI • Mortality • Controversy

---

KEY POINTS

- Compared with the transfemoral approach, the transradial approach for percutaneous coronary intervention (PCI) in ST-segment elevation myocardial infarction (STEMI) patients is associated improved outcomes, including a reduction in major bleeding events and decreased mortality.
- There are several controversial issues involved in the choice for catheterization access site, including the underlying mechanism of the mortality benefit and the appropriate timing for adoption of the transradial approach for primary PCI.
- Interventional cardiologists of all career stages can safely and effectively transition to the transradial approach for PCI in STEMI patients.

INTRODUCTION

Transradial access for cardiac catheterization and PCI is an effective strategy that is being adopted at an increasing rate.[1] This approach offers several advantages over transfemoral catheterization, including higher patient satisfaction and a decrease in hospital stay and associated hospital costs.[2,3] Several large trials comparing transradial and transfemoral PCI for patients with a variety of clinical presentations, including STEMI, have demonstrated superiority of transradial PCI with respect to clinical outcomes including bleeding complications and all-cause mortality.[4–6]

Despite its advantages, the systematic, center-level transition from transfemoral to transradial catheterization is often complex and requires collaboration between interventional cardiologists, cardiac catheterization laboratory staff, and hospital administration. Considering the importance of safe, effective, and expeditious PCI in patients with STEMI, the transition to a new technique for such critical procedures is controversial, because attempts by operators inexperienced with transradial catheterization

---

Financial disclosures: Dr T.C. Bazemore reports no disclosures; Dr S.V. Rao reports consulting honoraria from Terumo Interventional Systems Inc and Medtronic.

[a] Department of Internal Medicine, Duke University Medical Center, Box 3182, Durham, NC 27710, USA; [b] Division of Cardiology, Department of Internal Medicine, Duke University Medical Center, 2100 Erwin Road, Durham, NC 27705, USA; [c] Department of Cardiology, Durham VA Medical Center, 508 Fulton Street, 111A, Durham, NC 27705, USA

* Corresponding author.

E-mail address: taylor.bazemore@dm.duke.edu

Intervent Cardiol Clin 5 (2016) 513–522
http://dx.doi.org/10.1016/j.iccl.2016.06.006
2211-7458/16/$ – see front matter © 2016 Elsevier Inc. All rights reserved.

may prolong door-to-balloon times, compromise procedural outcomes, and pose unwarranted risk to patients. Nevertheless, although the systematic adoption of transradial PCI necessitates sufficient training and deliberate coordination on provider and center levels, several studies have proved that this transition can be achieved successfully and safely by interventional cardiologists at all stages of practice. This article reviews the risks and benefits of transradial catheterization in patients with STEMI and describes the established pathway for safe and effective transition to the transradial approach.

BENEFITS OF THE TRANSRADIAL APPROACH
Reduction in Procedure-Related Bleeding Events

The reduction of bleeding and major vascular complications is one of the most reproducible and clinically significant benefits of the transradial over the transfemoral approach. Bleeding events associated with cardiac catheterization in STEMI patients often occur at the site of vascular access,[7] and they are more common with transfemoral access due to the deep course of the femoral artery that does not always allow for effective external compression.[4] The risk of bleeding is particularly high in female and elderly patients and in those who undergo PCI for STEMI, which requires the use of more potent antithrombotic agents[8] and potentially because the time pressures lead to a lower likelihood of successful access into the common femoral artery.

Several large trials support the use of transradial over transfemoral approach for the reduction of bleeding complications in patients with STEMI. The Radial versus Femoral Access for Coronary Intervention (RIVAL) trial compared transradial with transfemoral access among 7021 patients with acute coronary syndrome (ACS), with or without ST-segment elevation, undergoing cardiac catheterization.[6] The primary endpoint was net adverse clinical events (NACE)—death, MI, stroke, or non–coronary artery bypass graft (CABG)-related major bleeding—at 30 days. There was no significant difference between transradial and transfemoral access with respect to the primary outcome; however, transradial access significantly reduced major vascular access-site complications and bleeding when assessed according the Acute Catheterization and Urgent Intervention Triage Strategy (ACUITY) trial definition.[6] Results in the subgroup of patients presenting with STEMI were consistent with the overall trial, showing that transradial PCI was associated with significantly fewer major vascular

complications than transfemoral PCI (1.26% vs 3.49%, $P = .002$) and a significant decrease in ACUITY major bleeding (1.99% vs 4.10%, $P = .009$).[9] The RIFLE-STEACS trial (N = 1001 STEMI patients undergoing primary PCI at 4 centers in Italy) also demonstrated a decrease in major bleeding events defined according the Bleeding Academic Research Consortium (BARC) definition in patients with STEMI undergoing transradial primary PCI (7.8% vs 12.2%, $P = .026$).[5] Finally, the STEMI-RADIAL trial (N = 707) also showed that transradial approach significantly reduced major bleeding events among STEMI patients (1.4% vs 7.2%, $P = .0001$).[10] A meta-analysis of 12 randomized controlled trials of more than 5000 patients with STEMI concluded that the odds of major bleeding with transradial PCI was approximately half that of transfemoral PCI (1.4% vs 2.9%; odds ratio [OR] 0.51; 95% CI, 0.31–0.85; $P = .01$).[11]

Registry data are consistent with the randomized trials. In the REAL registry (N = 11,068 patients from Italy), major bleeding and vascular complications in STEMI patients were significantly lower with transradial access, both at 30 days (1.1% vs 2.6%) and 2 years (4.9 vs 6.9%, $P<.001$).[4] Similarly, using the National Cardiovascular Data Registry CathPCI Registry, Baklanov and colleagues[12] examined the association between access-site and in-hospital outcomes among 294,769 patients with STEMI undergoing PCI between 2007 and 2011 and found that transradial access was associated with fewer vascular complications (0.13% vs 0.49%, $P<.001$) and lower rates of National Cardiovascular Data Registry–defined bleeding (6.88% vs 11.59%, $P<.0001$); after multivariable adjustment, the odds of bleeding were significantly lower with transradial PCI (OR 0.62; 95% CI, 0.53–0.72; $P<.0001$).

Reduction in Mortality and Other Adverse Events

An interesting finding across some clinical trials is the reduction in mortality in patients undergoing transradial versus transfemoral primary PCI. Although the primary 30-day NACE endpoint was not different between transradial and transfemoral access in the RIVAL trial among the entire study population, there was a significant reduction in this endpoint in the subgroup with STEMI (3.1% vs 5.2%, $P = .026$) (Fig. 1).[9] When analyzed individually, transradial access was also associated with a significant reduction in 30-day mortality (1.3% vs 3.2%, $P = .006$).[9] RIFLE-STEACS likewise demonstrated a reduction in 30-day NACE (composite of cardiac

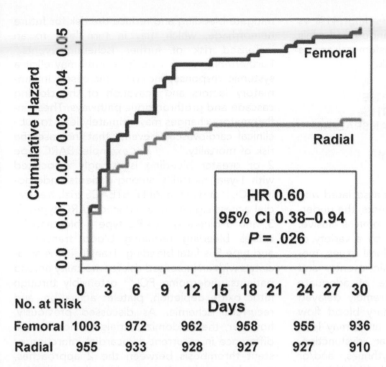

Fig. 1. Primary outcome (cardiovascular death, myocardial infarction, stroke, or non–CABG-related major bleeding) in patients with STEMI. In patients with STEMI, radial artery access reduced the primary outcome compared with femoral artery access (3.1% vs 5.2%, P = .026). HR, hazard ratio. (*Adapted from* Mehta SR, Jolly SS, Cairns J, et al. Effects of radial vs femoral artery access in patients with acute coronary syndromes with or without ST-segment elevation. J Am Coll Cardiol 2012;60(24):2494; with permission.)

death, stroke, myocardial infarction, target lesion revascularization, or bleeding) with transradial primary PCI (13.6% vs 21.0%, P = .003); a reduced risk of cardiac death was evident when this benefit was analyzed individually (5.2% vs 9.2%, P = .02).[5] Although subjects in the STEMI-RADIAL trial undergoing PCI from transradial approach did not experience a significant reduction in mortality, there was a significant decrease in net composite of adverse events, including myocardial infarction, stroke, or bleeding events.[10]

Observational data also show a consistent association between transradial access and reduced mortality among STEMI patients. For example, in the study by Baklanov using the Cath-PCI Registry, transradial access was associated with a 24% reduction in in-hospital mortality (OR 0.76; 95% CI, 0.57–0.99; P = .045).[12] With respect to longer-term outcomes, the REAL registry examined 2-year mortality and showed that transradial access was associated with a 2.6% absolute reduction in 2-year mortality (8.8% vs 11.4%, P = .025).[4] All of the available studies have been pooled into 2 meta-analyses: a 2011 study by Mamas and colleagues[13] showed that the pooled effect size of transradial approach on mortality was a approximately 47% reduction in mortality (OR 0.53; 95% CI, 0.33–0.84; P = .008), and a 2013 study by Karrowni and colleagues[11] showed similar results (2.7% vs 4.7%; OR 0.55; 95% CI, 0.40–0.76; P<.001).

Radial Approach in ST-Segment Elevation Myocardial Infarction-Associated with Cardiogenic Shock

Acute STEMI presenting with cardiogenic shock represents a high-risk scenario in which timely revascularization is essential. Although it may seem that this situation is best suited for femoral approach due to the potential need for hemodynamic support, observational data show an association between transradial access and improved outcomes. A 2015 meta-analysis by Pancholy and colleagues[14] included 8 studies with 8131 patients with cardiogenic shock undergoing PCI from transradial and transfemoral access. Adjusted risk analysis showed that transradial PCI was associated with a reduced risk of all-cause mortality (relative risk [RR] 0.55; 95% CI, 0.46–0.65; P<.001) and fewer major adverse cardiovascular events (RR 0.63; 95% CI, 0.52–0.75; P<.001) at 30 days.

The use of the radial artery for PCI preserves the femoral access site for large-bore hemodynamic support devices. One study of subjects with anterior STEMI complicated by cardiogenic shock requiring intra-aortic balloon pump showed that, compared with transfemoral approach, transradial PCI was associated with a reduction in cardiac death (25% vs 41%, P<.01), fewer access site bleeding complications (7% vs 21%, P<.01), and a reduction in a composite of adverse events, including cardiac death, myocardial infarction, stroke, target lesion revascularization, and bleeding (41% vs 67%, P<.01).[15] There are no randomized trials comparing transradial with transfemoral access specifically in patients with shock.

CONTROVERSY 1: WHAT IS THE MECHANISM UNDERLYING THE MORTALITY BENEFIT OF TRANSRADIAL APPROACH FOR PRIMARY PERCUTANEOUS CORONARY INTERVENTION?

Although transradial approach is associated with reduced mortality in STEMI patients, the underlying mechanism of this benefit remains elusive. Mortality from STEMI is driven by a variety of complications, including procedural issues, mechanical complications, ischemic events, and bleeding. For example, failure of adequate reperfusion or, potentially, extremely delayed restoration of epicardial coronary blood flow (ie, prolonged door-to-balloon time) may lead to subsequent left ventricular dysfunction, pump failure, malignant arrhythmias, and/or shock, all of which are associated with a substantially higher risk for death.[16–18] In the studies comparing the 2 approaches, there seems to be no difference in the incidence of successful PCI or stent thrombosis.[19] On the other hand, the door-to-balloon times are longer with transradial approach, with an average delay of 1.76 minutes.[20] This suggests that mortality might be higher with transradial PCI, but, as discussed previously, the opposite is true. A well-designed decision analysis showed that door-to-balloon time could potentially be significantly delayed before the mortality benefit of transradial access seen in the randomized trials was attenuated.[21] Therefore, differences in ischemic complications do not seem to explain the mortality benefit of transradial primary PCI.

The major difference between transradial and transfemoral access is in bleeding and vascular complications favoring transradial approach. Both randomized and observational studies consistently show a 30% to 50% reduction in "major" bleeding as defined by various bleeding scales and major vascular complications with transradial approach.[20] There is a strong association between bleeding and short-term and long-term mortality,[13] either through blood loss (although this degree of bleeding is rare) or cessation of secondary prevention antithrombotic therapy, which may lead to recurrent ischemic events. Any significant procedural bleeding that complicates PCI may compel clinicians to withdrawal antiplatelet agents to

mitigate bleeding and reduce the risk for future hemorrhage, which may in turn lead to an increased risk of further ischemic events.[8] Furthermore, these vascular events may elicit a systemic response, including increased inflammatory factors and activation of the clotting cascade and prothrombotic pathways. These inflammatory changes may ultimately lead to subclinical cardiovascular events that increase the risk of mortality.[8,22,23] For example, BARC type 2 or greater bleeding is strongly associated with 1-year mortality among patients undergoing PCI,[24] and in the RIFLE-STEACS trial, transradial access significantly reduced BARC types 2, 3, and 5 bleeding.[5] BARC type 3 bleeding includes bleeding requiring blood transfusion and type 5 is fatal bleeding. Transfusion is associated with an increased risk for mortality among patients undergoing PCI,[25] ostensibly through nitric oxide depletion, platelet activation, and recurrent ischemia. As discussed previously, however, the randomized trials do not show a difference in recurrent myocardial infarction or stent thrombosis between the 2 approaches, so it is not clear how the bleeding reduction with transradial access results in reduced mortality. Moreover, bleeding events in the trial were analyzed according to whether they were access-site related or non–access-site related, and transradial approach only reduced access-site bleeding. Whether access-site bleeding is associated with mortality is controversial, and an analysis of the ACUITY trial of patients with non–ST-segment elevation ACS demonstrated no association between large access-site hematomas and subsequent adverse outcomes.[26] Therefore, although it is possible that reduction in bleeding complications explains the mortality benefit of transradial approach, the data currently do not support a direct, causal relationship.

Another possibility is that the difference in mortality might be influenced by systematic, center-level differences in addition to procedural variables in themselves. Center-level factors within the health systems that perform transradial primary PCI, such as protocols for STEMI treatment that use secondary prevention strategies or other management approaches affecting outcomes, could influence mortality. In other words, transradial primary PCI may be a marker of quality rather than a mediator of survival. These variables would be expected to affect the findings of observational studies (ie, unmeasured confounding), but treatments in a randomized trial should be balanced between the randomized groups. In the trials comparing transradial and transfemoral access for STEMI, pharmacotherapy is similar between the groups. Other management, like duration of manual compression of the femoral access site, has not been reported, but is expected to be balanced across patients and sites given the large sample sizes of the trials. Thus, center-level differences may also not explain the mortality benefit of transradial access.

CONTROVERSY 2: TIMING AND STRATEGY TO ADOPT RADIAL APPROACH FOR PRIMARY PERCUTANEOUS CORONARY INTERVENTION

Although the mechanisms underlying the mortality reduction with transradial primary PCI remain elusive, the benefit is consistent across both trials and observational studies, as summarized previously. Professional society guidelines have given a strong recommendation for transradial access as the default approach for patients with ACS.[27] For centers and operators that do not have experience with transradial primary PCI, the transition from transfemoral to transradial catheterization within clinical practice can be complex. Considering the importance of timely and effective revascularization during STEMI that requires operator proficiency and confidence, interventional cardiologists trained in transfemoral PCI may be reluctant to transition to an alternate approach that, in the early stages, may prolong door-to-balloon time. Nevertheless, single-center studies have shown that the transition from transfemoral to transradial approach is highly feasible in a variety of practice models and among providers at all career stages.[28]

Although studies have shown a slight increase in fluoroscopy time and contrast use during this transition period, the benefits of the transradial approach are preserved, such that procedures performed during this transition period are associated with a reduction in bleeding and vascular events.[29,30] Among practicing cardiologists of varying career stages trained in transfemoral catheterization, this transition period is also associated with preservation of procedural success.[31,32] Outcomes have been shown superior even for primary PCI for STEMI performed during the transition period, as a recent retrospective review demonstrated that transradial PCI was associated with a significant decrease in 30-day bleeding and access-site complications as well as a decrease in mortality and MACE at both 30 days and 1 year.[33]

The Learning Curve Associated with Transradial Catheterization

The development of proficiency in transradial PCI can be likened to the learning curve for other skill sets; however, the pathway to mastery of transradial intervention is nonetheless multifaceted and dependent on multiple variables, including the quality and availability of mentorship and the complexity of cases attempted during the learning period. Furthermore, this learning curve may be nonuniform among different operators, who approach transradial catheterization from a variety of backgrounds in clinical experience. In addition to operator proficiency, transition from transfemoral to transradial approach is contingent on many institutional variables that require coordination among hospital administration and cardiac catheterization support staff to develop a successful transradial program.[28]

For providers who are first learning or transitioning to transradial catheterization, the establishment of outcome measures to characterize technical proficiency can be challenging. The infrequency of death or other major adverse events during catheterization make these outcomes inadequate in appropriately measuring proficiency, and prior studies have demonstrated that other endpoints, including radiation exposure and procedural length, are limited in characterizing operator skill due to the multiple patient, operator, and practice variables that contribute to these measures.[28,34,35] Moreover, given the rapid evolution of this clinical field with continued technological advances and the development of new practice benchmarks, the determination of a specific endpoint to describe proficiency in the transition to transradial approach is unlikely to remain up to date or clinically relevant.[28]

Despite the limited effectiveness of specific endpoints to mark an operator's place on the learning curve, continued practice with transradial catheterization reliably allows for improvement in clinical skill. Unsurprisingly, operator proficiency and confidence with transradial catheterization is positively correlated to breadth of experience, and clinical centers with high transradial case volume have proved to have better clinical outcomes. The RIVAL trial divided participating clinical centers into tertiles based on the volume of transradial procedures performed annually (low volume, ≤60 transradial PCIs per year per operator; intermediate volume, 61–146 transradial PCIs per year per operator; high volume, >146 transradial PCIs per year per operator). It was shown that within the highest-volume tertile, transradial PCI was associated with a significantly lower rate of composite adverse events than transfemoral PCI (1.6% vs 3.2%, P = .015), whereas there was no significant difference in composite adverse events between these approaches among centers with intermediate and low volumes of transradial PCI.[36] RIVAL and other studies have demonstrated that higher transradial case volume at

both the operator and center levels is associated with improved outcomes,[36–38] and a study by Hess and colleagues[37] shows that transradial access is associated with decreased fluoroscopy time and contrast use (Fig. 2).

Another factor to be considered when transitioning to transradial approach is the potential for crossover to transfemoral approach that could prolong door-to-balloon times in the setting of primary PCI. Several procedural variables are

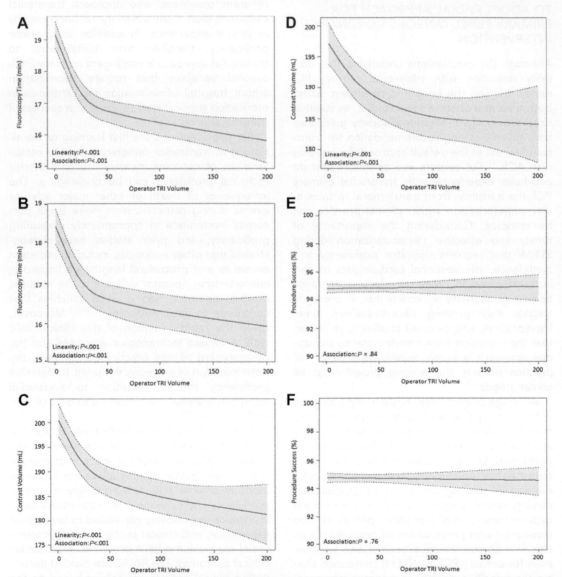

Fig. 2. Relationship between operator transradial percutaneous coronary intervention (TRI) volume and procedural outcomes. Shown are curves depicting the unadjusted and adjusted relationships between TRI volume and fluoroscopy times ([A] and [B], respectively), unadjusted relationships between TRI volume and contrast volume ([C] and [D], respectively), and unadjusted and adjusted relationships between TRI volume and procedure success ([E] and [F], respectively). Dotted lines represent 95% CIs. (*From* Hess CN, Peterson ED, Neely ML, et al. The learning curve for transradial percutaneous coronary intervention among operators in the United States: a study from the National Cardiovascular Data Registry®. Circulation 2014;129(22):2282; with permission.)

responsible for the need for crossover to an alternate site for vascular access. The most common of these causes include inability to cannulate the radial artery, radial artery spasm, and anatomic variations that may limit catheter manipulation or engagement of the coronary artery ostia with the guiding catheter.[8] Although transfemoral access is generally used if transradial approach is unsuccessful, some operators may either attempt radial access in the contralateral arm or ipsilateral ulnar access.[39,40] Transradial procedures are associated with higher rates of crossover than transfemoral cases: among STEMI patients in the RIVAL trial, 5.3% of transradial cases required femoral crossover, compared with 1.6% of transfemoral cases requiring radial crossover (P<.0001),[6] and in the RIFLE-STEACS trial, crossover was required in 9.6% of transradial and 2.8% of transfemoral cases.[5] Increasing proficiency with transradial approach decreases the odds of femoral crossover. When the centers participating in the RIVAL trial were divided into tertiles based on transradial volume, the tertile with the highest volume had a crossover rate that was lower (4.4%) that the intermediate (9.7%) and lowest (8.0%) volume tertiles.[36] Although transradial approach is associated with higher crossover rates, it is unclear if this crossover contributes to any clinically significant difference in outcomes. For example, in the RIFLE-STEACS trial, the time delay associated with crossover did not contribute to a significantly longer door-to-balloon than transfemoral interventions.[5] Inherent in these data is the concept of using time benchmarks to convert to transfemoral access in order to maintain timely reperfusion (discussed later).

Most importantly, operators should be proficient at performing elective coronary angiography and PCI via transradial access prior to transitioning to STEMI cases. Considering the relationship between PCI volume and clinical outcomes, several studies have been performed to determine the number of transradial cases needed to attain technical proficiency. These studies have shown that at least 30 to 50 transradial PCIs are required to overcome the learning curve for transradial PCI.[28] After this initial learning period, other studies suggest that an operator should perform at least 50% of cases from a transradial approach, with a minimum of 80 transradial procedures annually to maintain technical proficiency.[8,41]

The Transradial Working Group of the Society for Cardiovascular Angiography and Intervention has created a basic and advanced curriculum that can be used to ensure comprehensive training with transradial approach (Box 1), and it has provided recommendations for when it is appropriate for operators to transition to transradial primary PCI. It is recommended that operators perform 100 elective PCI cases from transradial approach with femoral crossover rate of less than or equal to 4% before performing transradial primary PCI. Bailout to contralateral radial or femoral access should be implemented if there is a delay of greater than 3 minutes in

---

Box 1
Proposed curriculum content of structured basic and advanced transradial training courses

Basic training course

Basic anatomy related to the upper extremity vasculature

Patient evaluation and selection

Patient preparation and room set-up, minimizing radiation

Obtaining radial artery access

Pharmacologic considerations (minimizing spasm and radial artery occlusion)

Catheter manipulation through the upper extremity

Catheters and guides for transradial procedures

Basic trouble-shooting during transradial approach

Recognizing and managing complications related to transradial approach

Right heart catheterization from the arm

Sheath removal and access-site management

Advanced (master's) training course

Reiteration/refinement of basic techniques

Transradial procedures in high-risk subsets (LM, CTO, etc.)

Maneuvering through the most difficult anatomy

When and how to establish a transradial STEMI program

Performing sheathless procedures

Same-day PCI

Recent advances in the field

Abbreviations: CTO, chronic total occlusion; LM, left main.

From Rao SV, Tremmel JA, Gilchrist IC, et al. Best practices for transradial angiography and intervention: a consensus statement from the society for cardiovascular angiography and intervention's transradial working group. Catheter Cardiovasc Interv 2014;83(2):234; with permission.

obtaining radial access, if there is a delay of greater than 10 minutes from introducer sheath placement to engagement of the infarct-related artery, or if there is a delay of greater than 20 minutes from placement of introducer sheath to dilation of infarct lesion. For operators new to the transradial approach, it is recommended that femoral access sites are prepared in STEMI patients in case there is need for crossover. With close monitoring of door-to-balloon times, centers can monitor progress in proficiency with transradial PCI and review whether the transradial approach may be responsible for any delays in intervention.[42]

SUMMARY

Transradial primary PCI is associated with superior clinical outcomes compared with transfemoral primary PCI, including a reduction in mortality. These findings have been replicated in both randomized and observational studies; however, there are 2 main controversial issues surrounding the use of transradial access in STEMI patients. The first is the underlying mechanism of the mortality benefit, and the second is the appropriate timing for operators to transition to using transradial approach for primary PCI. Future studies should attempt to elucidate how transradial access reduces mortality in STEMI and whether professional society recommendations for transitioning to transradial primary PCI are too conservative or aggressive.

REFERENCES

1. Feldman DN, Swaminathan RV, Kaltenbach LA, et al. Adoption of radial access and comparison of outcomes to femoral access in percutaneous coronary intervention an updated report from the National Cardiovascular Data Registry (2007–2012). Circulation 2013;127(23):2295–306.

2. Cooper CJ, El-Shiekh RA, Cohen DJ, et al. Effect of transradial access on quality of life and cost of cardiac catheterization: a randomized comparison. Am Heart J 1999;138(3):430–6.

3. Cruden NL, Teh CH, Starkey IR, et al. Reduced vascular complications and length of stay with transradial rescue angioplasty for acute myocardial infarction. Catheter Cardiovasc Interv 2007;70(5):670–5.

4. Valgimigli M, Saia F, Guastaroba P, et al. Transradial versus transfemoral intervention for acute myocardial infarction: a propensity score-adjusted and-matched analysis from the REAL (REgistro regionale AngiopLastiche dell'Emilia-Romagna) multicenter registry. JACC Cardiovasc Interv 2012; 5(1):23–35.

5. Romagnoli E, Biondi-Zoccai G, Sciahbasi A, et al. Radial versus femoral randomized investigation in ST-segment elevation acute coronary syndrome: the RIFLE-STEACS (Radial Versus Femoral Randomized Investigation in ST-Elevation Acute Coronary Syndrome) study. J Am Coll Cardiol 2012; 60(24):2481–9.

6. Jolly SS, Yusuf S, Cairns J, et al. Radial versus femoral access for coronary angiography and intervention in patients with acute coronary syndromes (RIVAL): a randomised, parallel group, multicentre trial. Lancet 2011;377(9775):1409–20.

7. Rao SV, Cohen MG, Kandzari DE, et al. The transradial approach to percutaneous coronary intervention: historical perspective, current concepts, and future directions. J Am Coll Cardiol 2010;55(20): 2187–95.

8. Kedev S. Transradial primary percutaneous coronary intervention. Interv Cardiol Clin 2015;4(2): 167–77.

9. Mehta SR, Jolly SS, Cairns J, et al. Effects of radial versus femoral artery access in patients with acute coronary syndromes with or without ST-segment elevation. J Am Coll Cardiol 2012;60(24):2490–9.

10. Bernat I, Horak D, Stasek J, et al. ST-segment elevation myocardial infarction treated by radial or femoral approach in a multicenter randomized clinical TrialThe STEMI-RADIAL Trial. J Am Coll Cardiol 2014;63(10):964–72.

11. Karrowni W, Vyas A, Giacomino B, et al. Radial versus femoral access for primary percutaneous interventions in ST-segment elevation myocardial infarction patients: a meta-analysis of randomized controlled trials. JACC Cardiovasc Interv 2013; 6(8):814–23.

12. Baklanov DV, Kaltenbach LA, Marso SP, et al. The prevalence and outcomes of transradial percutaneous coronary intervention for ST-segment elevation myocardial infarction: analysis from the National Cardiovascular Data Registry (2007 to 2011). J Am Coll Cardiol 2013;61(4):420–6.

13. Mamas MA, Ratib K, Routledge H, et al. Influence of access site selection on PCI-related adverse events in patients with STEMI: meta-analysis of randomised controlled trials. Heart. 2012;98(4): 303–11.

14. Pancholy SB, Shantha GPS, Romagnoli E, et al. Impact of access site choice on outcomes of patients with cardiogenic shock undergoing percutaneous coronary intervention: a systematic review and meta-analysis. Am Heart J 2015;170(2): 353–61.e6.

15. Romagnoli E, De Vita M, Burzotta F, et al. TCT-31 Clinical benefit of radial versus femoral approach in percutaneous coronary intervention with intra-aortic balloon pump support. J Am Coll Cardiol 2012;60(17_S):B9–10.

16. Antoniucci D, Valenti R, Migliorini A, et al. Relation of time to treatment and mortality in patients with acute myocardial infarction undergoing primary coronary angioplasty. Am J Cardiol 2002;89(11): 1248–52.

17. De Luca G, Suryapranata H, Ottervanger JP, et al. Time delay to treatment and mortality in primary angioplasty for acute myocardial infarction every minute of delay counts. Circulation 2004;109(10): 1223–5.

18. Nallamothu BK, Bradley EH, Krumholz HM. Time to treatment in primary percutaneous coronary intervention. N Engl J Med 2007;357(16):1631–8.

19. Valgimigli M, Gagnor A, Calabró P, et al. Radial versus femoral access in patients with acute coronary syndromes undergoing invasive management: a randomised multicentre trial. Lancet 2015; 385(9986):2465–76.

20. Joyal D, Bertrand OF, Rinfret S, et al. Meta-analysis of ten trials on the effectiveness of the radial versus the femoral approach in primary percutaneous coronary intervention. Am J Cardiol 2012;109(6):813–8.

21. Wimmer NJ, Cohen DJ, Wasfy JH, et al. Delay in reperfusion with transradial percutaneous coronary intervention for ST-elevation myocardial infarction: Might some delays be acceptable? Am Heart J 2014;168(1):103–9.

22. Doyle BJ, Rihal CS, Gastineau DA, et al. Bleeding, blood transfusion, and increased mortality after percutaneous coronary intervention: implications for contemporary practice. J Am Coll Cardiol 2009;53(22):2019–27.

23. Allen C, Glasziou P, Del Mar C. Bed rest: a potentially harmful treatment needing more careful evaluation. The Lancet. 1999;354(9186):1229–33.

24. Ndrepepa G, Schuster T, Hadamitzky M, et al. Validation of the Bleeding Academic Research Consortium definition of bleeding in patients with coronary artery disease undergoing percutaneous coronary intervention. Circulation 2012;125(11): 1424–31.

25. Sherwood MW, Wang Y, Curtis JP, et al. Patterns and outcomes of red blood cell transfusion in patients undergoing percutaneous coronary intervention. JAMA 2014;311(8):836–43.

26. Mehran R, Pocock SJ, Nikolsky E, et al. A risk score to predict bleeding in patients with acute coronary syndromes. J Am Coll Cardiol 2010; 55(23):2556–66.

27. Roffi M, Patrono C, Collet J-P, et al. 2015 ESC Guidelines for the management of acute coronary syndromes in patients presenting without persistent ST-segment elevation. Eur Heart J 2015;37(3): 267–315.

28. Gilchrist IC. The transradial learning curve and volume-outcome relationship. Interv Cardiol Clin 2015;4(2):203–11.

29. Leonardi RA, Townsend JC, Bonnema DD, et al. Comparison of percutaneous coronary intervention safety before and during the establishment of a transradial program at a teaching hospital. Am J Cardiol 2012;109(8):1154–9.

30. Balwanz CR, Javed U, Singh GD, et al. Transradial and transfemoral coronary angiography and interventions: 1-year outcomes after initiating the transradial approach in a cardiology training program. Am Heart J 2013;165(3):310–6.

31. Barbash IM, Gallino R, Lager R, et al. Operator learning curve for transradial percutaneous coronary interventions: implications for the initiation of a transradial access program in contemporary US practice. Cardiovasc Revasc Med 2014;15(4):195–9.

32. Nadarasa K, Robertson MC, Wong CK, et al. Rapid cycle change to predominantly radial access coronary angiography and percutaneous coronary intervention. Catheter Cardiovasc Interv 2012; 79(4):589–94.

33. Kedev S, Kalpak O, Dharma S, et al. Complete transitioning to the radial approach for primary percutaneous coronary intervention: a real-world single-center registry of 1808 consecutive patients with acute ST-elevation myocardial infarction. J Invasive Cardiol 2014;26(9):475–82.

34. Mercuri M, Mehta S, Xie C, et al. Radial artery access as a predictor of increased radiation exposure during a diagnostic cardiac catheterization procedure. JACC Cardiovasc Interv 2011;4(3):347–52.

35. Shah B, Bangalore S, Feit F, et al. Radiation exposure during coronary angiography via transradial or transfemoral approaches when performed by experienced operators. Am Heart J 2013;165(3): 286–92.

36. Jolly SS, Cairns J, Yusuf S, et al. Procedural volume and outcomes with radial or femoral access for coronary angiography and intervention. J Am Coll Cardiol 2014;63(10):954–63.

37. Hess CN, Peterson ED, Neely ML, et al. The learning curve for transradial percutaneous coronary intervention among operators in the United States: a study from the National Cardiovascular Data Registry®. Circulation 2014;129(22):2277–86.

38. Gutierrez A, Tsai TT, Stanislawski MA, et al. Adoption of transradial percutaneous coronary intervention and outcomes according to center radial volume in the veterans affairs healthcare system insights from the veterans affairs clinical assessment, reporting, and tracking (CART) Program. Circ Cardiovasc Interv 2013;6(4):336–46.

39. Kedev S, Zafirovska B, Dharma S, et al. Safety and feasibility of transulnar catheterization when ipsilateral radial access is not available. Catheter Cardiovasc Interv 2014;83(1):E51–60.

40. de Andrade PB, Tebet MA, Nogueira EF, et al. Transulnar approach as an alternative access site

for coronary invasive procedures after transradial approach failure. Am Heart J 2012;164(4):462–7.

41. Hamon M, Pristipino C, Di Mario C, et al. Consensus document on the radial approach in percutaneous cardiovascular interventions. EuroIntervention 2013;8(11):1242–51.

42. Rao SV, Tremmel JA, Gilchrist IC, et al. Best practices for transradial angiography and intervention: a consensus statement from the society for cardiovascular angiography and intervention's transradial working group. Catheter Cardiovasc Interv 2014; 83(2):228–36.

Controversies in the Treatment of Women with ST-Segment Elevation Myocardial Infarction

CrossMark

Vivian G. Ng, MD[a], Alexandra J. Lansky, MD[b],*

KEYWORDS

- ST-segment elevation myocardial infarction • Women • Gender • Outcomes

KEY POINTS

- Cardiovascular disease is the leading cause of death in women.
- Cardiovascular disease is underrecognized and undertreated in women.
- Women, especially young women, with ST-segment elevation myocardial infarctions have worse clinical outcomes than men.
- Although thrombolytic therapy improved outcomes in women, women have high rates of hemorrhagic complications.
- Primary angioplasty with stenting improves outcomes in women compared with thrombolytic therapy.

The treatment of coronary artery disease (CAD) and ST-segment elevation myocardial infarctions (STEMI) has drastically shifted from supportive care to thrombolytic therapy and now primary percutaneous coronary interventions (PCI). CAD remains the leading cause of death in women. However, the presentation and outcomes of women with STEMI are different than that in men. This article reviews the key differences in the presentation of and treatment options for women with STEMI.

EPIDEMIOLOGY AND CLINICAL PRESENTATION

Cardiovascular disease continues to be the leading cause of mortality among women in developed countries.[1,2] Although mortality rates from cardiovascular disease have decreased and the mortality gap is finally starting to narrow between men and women,[3] the rate of decline in women is slower than that in men.[1] Furthermore, compared with men, women lose more years of expected life after an acute myocardial infarction (AMI) compared with men.[4] Despite these concerning findings, CAD continues to be an underrecognized disease in women.[3,5]

Women with CAD present nearly a decade later in life than men.[6,7] The average age of a first myocardial infarction (MI) in men is 65 years, whereas the average age of a first MI in women is 70 years.[7] Furthermore, when women seek medical attention for CAD, they present with unstable angina/non–STEMI more frequently than men and manifest different symptoms of cardiac ischemia than men.[6,8–11] Among AMI patients, women are less likely to present with substernal chest pain and are more likely to complain of atypical chest pain with or without shortness of breath, abdominal pain, nausea, or fatigue.[12–20] In addition, ischemia is more often silent,[21,22] and MI is frequently unrecognized in women

Disclosures: The authors have nothing to disclose.
[a] Yale University School of Medicine, New Haven, CT, USA; [b] Heart and Vascular Clinical Research Program, Yale University School of Medicine, PO Box 208017, New Haven, CT 06520-8017, USA
* Corresponding author.
E-mail address: alexandra.lansky@yale.edu

compared with men.[23,24] Because of these differences in symptoms, women may not recognize that their complaints are cardiac in origin and are more likely to present later after symptom onset than men.[18,25–34] Thus, physicians must be attuned to these differences in symptoms to expedite care once women do present to a medical care setting.

PATHOPHYSIOLOGY OF CORONARY ARTERY DISEASE IN WOMEN

It is thought that women with CAD present a decade later in life than men as a result of the protective effects of estrogen.[6,7,35] As a result of presenting at an older age, women have higher rates of traditional risk factors such as diabetes, hypertension, and hyperlipidemia at the time of their MI.[9–11,17,28,31,34,36,37] Paradoxically, women have less extensive CAD,[38–40] a higher incidence of nonsignificant CAD,[10,15] and less plaque development compared with men.[41,42]

AMI generally is caused by rupture of a coronary plaque that has a lipid-rich core covered by a thin fibrous cap (Fig. 1). Approximately 75% of fatal MIs are caused by so-called thin cap fibroatheromas, and the remaining 25% are caused by plaque erosion rather than rupture. Plaque erosions are more common in women, particularly young smokers, whereas plaque rupture is

more common in men and older patients of both sexes,[43] a finding that may, in part, be hormonally modulated.[44–47] In the PROSPECT trial gender subanalysis, evidence of plaque rupture was significantly less common in women versus men (6.6% vs 16.3%; $P = .002$) even after adjusting for comorbidities ($P = .004$).[40] The frequency of other plaque vulnerability phenotypes was similar for men and women. Patients with plaque erosions are more likely to have a longer indolent period of angina as opposed to patients with plaque ruptures.[48,49] This difference could explain why women presenting with STEMIs are more likely to present later after symptom onset than men, who are more likely to present with sudden severe chest pain.[28,50]

GENDER AND AGE INTERACTION

Young women with STEMIs have higher early mortality rates than their male counterparts of the same age when treated medically or with angioplasty.[11,22,51–58] Furthermore, although there have been improvements in mortality rates in women overall, the improvement has been minimal among young women in the last decade.[59] A retrospective study of 1025 patients found that women who were younger than 75 years were 49% more likely to die during their hospitalization than men.[52] This difference is

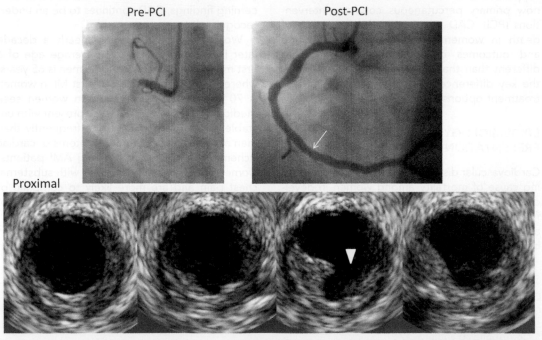

Fig. 1. Angiogram shows occluded right coronary artery. After the culprit lesion was stented, intravascular ultrasound scan showed plaque rupture in the distal vessel (*white arrow* in angiography and *white arrowhead* in intravascular ultrasound scan).

accentuated in younger age groups; women who were younger than 50 years had twice the likelihood of dying in hospital compared with age-matched men. These differences are not limited to in-hospital and short-term outcomes. Young women suffer from higher long-term mortality rates, with one study reporting a 15.6% relative increase in 2-year mortality risk for every 10-year decrease in age.[53] In addition, in the Variation in Recovery: Role of Gender on Outcomes of Young AMI Patients (VIRGO) trial, 3501 young AMI patients (less than 55 years), women had lower health status scores (symptoms, functioning, quality of life) after an AMI compared with men at 30 days and 1 year.[60] It is unknown why young premenopausal women, who are generally considered to be low-risk patients and who are thought to be protected by estrogen, have worse outcomes compared with age-matched men. Young women with STEMI may not be treated as aggressively as young men. Among 1465 young STEMI patients (younger than 55 years) enrolled in the VIRGO trial, women were more likely to be treated without reperfusion therapies (9% vs 4%; P = .002) and were more likely to have delays in care.[61] The degree to which these factors contribute to the worse outcomes seen in young women with AMI compared with men is unknown.

CORONARY REVASCULARIZATION IN WOMEN

Guidelines recommend that women receive the same medical and interventional management as men for STEMI[1,62]; however, women are less likely to have optimized medical regimens[37,63–66] or undergo revascularization procedures.[28,33,37,58,65–72] Despite the significant rates of STEMIs in both men and women (4.3% prevalence in men, 2.2% prevalence in women),[7] women comprise only the minority of patients in large clinical trials.[73,74] Most reports compare outcomes between the genders instead of among women by treatment subgroups. Nonetheless, the data provide useful information on how to best treat women with STEMI.

THROMBOLYTIC THERAPY IN WOMEN

Early reperfusion with thrombolytic therapy for STEMI improves survival and reduces infarct size and heart failure risk.[75–78] For example, in the ISIS-2 trial, 17,070 AMI patients (13,125 [76.9%] men and 3945 [23.1%] women) were randomly assigned in a 2 × 2 factorial scheme

to intravenous streptokinase, oral aspirin, both therapies, or neither,[75] and women who received streptokinase and aspirin had a 31% reduction in mortality (P value not reported for comparison). However, in all large thrombolytic trials, women had worse mortality rates than men. The ISIS-3 study, which contained 36,080 patients (9600 [26.6%] women) who underwent thrombolytic therapy for AMI, found that women were at increased risk of death at 35-day follow-up even after adjustment for age and other baseline characteristics (odds ratio [OR], 1.20 [95% confidence interval [CI], 1.11, 1.29]).[79] It is unclear why women had higher mortality rates in these studies. Women presented later in the disease time course potentially decreasing the extent of salvageable myocardium from thrombolytic administration, which likely translates into higher rates of subsequent cardiac events. There is no current evidence in angiographic studies that reperfusion rates are different between men and women.[38,80,81] Most likely, women have decreased survival after MI as a result of bleeding complications and hemorrhagic strokes. Studies have identified female sex as an independent predictor of intracranial hemorrhage after thrombolytic therapy for AMI.[82–84] It is important to emphasize that despite the higher mortality and bleeding rates in women compared with men, women clearly benefit from thrombolytic therapy when other reperfusion modalities are not available. Thus, when pharmacologic reperfusion is necessary, thrombolytics should not be withheld in women.

PRIMARY ANGIOPLASTY IN WOMEN

Despite the benefit and widespread application of fibrinolytic therapy in the treatment of STEMI, bleeding complications, including devastating hemorrhagic strokes, present a major limitation of this therapy, beyond the substantial proportion (approximately 20%–30%) of patients with failed reperfusion[85–89] and recurrent ischemia.[75,90–92] Although thrombolytics can restore epicardial coronary artery flow, it does not address the underlying unstable plaque and the exposed thrombogenic material thought to cause recurrent ischemic events.

Mechanical reperfusion with primary balloon angioplasty improved reperfusion, recurrent ischemia, and bleeding complication rates.[93–98] The benefit of primary angioplasty compared with thrombolytics is generalizable to women.[99] The Primary Angioplasty in Acute Myocardial Infarction (PAMI) trial included

395 patients (27% women) randomly assigned to either thrombolysis using tissue plasminogen activator or to angioplasty. Women treated with primary angioplasty had a 4% rate of in-hospital mortality compared with 14% for thrombolytic therapy (P = .07). Primary angioplasty compared with thrombolytic therapy independently predicted in-hospital survival in women. Although women had worse outcomes compared with men, sex was not an independent predictor of mortality after adjustment for differences in baseline characteristics. Women also had more intracranial hemorrhage events than men after thrombolysis (5.3% vs 0.7%, P = .04); however, intracranial bleeding was completely eliminated in the angioplasty groups.[99] Thus, angioplasty seemed to be a safer treatment modality narrowing the outcomes gap between men and women based on improved reperfusion rates, targeted intervention to the lesion site, and decreased bleeding complications.

PRIMARY STENTING IN WOMEN

Although primary angioplasty improves mortality rates compared with thrombolysis, it is associated with higher rates of restenosis.[90,100,101] Although initial studies evaluating primary stenting raised concerns that women may not benefit from stent implantation, subsequent analyses have found that women do have improved clinical and angiographic outcomes when treated with stents.

The CADILLAC (Controlled Abciximab and Device Investigation to Lower Late Angioplasty Complications) trial included 2082 patients (27% women) with AMI and found that patients who underwent primary stent placement with or without a glycoprotein IIb/IIIa inhibitors had improved survival rates compared with patients who received balloon angioplasty alone.[100] Among women, major adverse cardiac event (19.1% vs 28.1%; P = .013) and ischemic target revascularization (10.8% vs 20.4%; P = .002) rates were lower at 1 year with primary stenting compared with balloon angioplasty. Furthermore, female sex was an independent predictor of 1-year major adverse cardiac events in a multivariate analysis (OR, 1.64 [95% CI, 1.24, 2.17]; P = .04). Procedure-related moderate-to-severe bleeding rates were 2.5 times higher in women, with female sex being an independent predictor of moderate-to-severe bleeding complications. Importantly, female sex was not a predictor of 1-year death.[102]

Although the use of drug-eluting stents (DES) in the setting of primary PCI appears to offer a benefit in terms of prevention of target lesion revascularization, the sex-related differences in long-term benefit remain to be seen. In a subset analysis of AMI patients in the combined RESEARCH (Rapamycin-Eluting Stent Evaluated at Rotterdam Cardiology Hospital) and T-SEARCH (Taxus-Stent Evaluated at Rotterdam Cardiology Hospital) registries, women continued to have worse outcomes compared with men and had higher rates of major adverse cardiac events despite the routine use of DES (adjusted hazard ratio [HR], 1.7 [95% CI, 1.02, 1.85]).[103] A post-hoc analysis of the MULTISTRATEGY (Multicentre Evaluation of Single High-Dose Bolus Tirofiban vs Abciximab with Sirolimus-Eluting Stent or Bare Metal Stent in Acute Myocardial Infarction Study) study (N = 745; 24% women), which randomly assigned patients to sirolimus-eluting stents versus bare-metal stents, found at 3-year follow-up that sirolimus-eluting stents use was associated with a significantly lower risk of major adverse cardiac events (adjusted HR, 0.62 [95% CI, 0.41–0.94]; P = .026) and target vessel revascularization (adjusted HR, 0.35 [95% CI, 0.19–0.63]; P<.001) in men but not in women.[104] Additional studies are needed to further clarify the impact of female sex on STEMI outcomes in the era of DES.

In the first interventional study dedicated to women, the SPIRIT Women prospective, open-label multicenter study enrolled 1573 women receiving the XIENCE V everolimus-eluting stent. Compared with men in the SPIRIT V study, women in this study were older, had more clinical risk factors, and were more likely to present with atypical angina or silent ischemia. The study found that the rate of 1-year composite of all death, MI, and target vessel revascularization was 12% and 1-year stent thrombosis was 0.59%.[105] These rates are low and similar to rates seen in other XIENCE V studies. Thus, these data in an all-comer female population suggest that women benefit from advancing DES technology.

Primary stenting in women improves outcomes including mortality compared with primary angioplasty and should be considered the preferred strategy of reperfusion in treating women with STEMI. Although the gap in sex outcomes has narrowed more recently, women who undergo stenting continue to have worse short-term outcomes compared with men. Additional research is needed to further characterize the cause for this difference and ways to optimize outcomes for women with STEMI.

BLEEDING AND VASCULAR COMPLICATIONS

In studies from the 1990s, vascular complications were 3 to 4 times more frequent in women than in men. Rates of vascular complications in women have subsequently decreased with the development of less-aggressive anticoagulation regimens, weight-adjusted heparin dosing, and the availability of smaller sheath sizes made possible by the smaller profile of newer third- and fourth-generation devices.[62]

Despite improvements, women undergoing PCI (primarily through the femoral artery) continue to have a 2-fold increased risk of bleeding and vascular complications compared with men, even after adjusting for differences in baseline and procedural characteristics.[10,106] This sex difference may be even more pronounced in younger women compared with younger men.[107] Women with bleeding complications have an approximately 3-fold increased incidence of stroke, MI, and all-cause death compared with women without bleeding complications, and, even after controlling for both clinical and procedural differences, women with bleeding have a 75% increased risk of death, MI, or stroke during their index hospitalization (OR, 1.75 [95% CI, 1.23, 2.51]).[106]

The use of the direct thrombin inhibitor bivalirudin during elective PCI lowers the risk of periprocedural ischemic complications and major bleeding in both women and men; however, women have higher 1-year mortality rates (3.7% vs 2.7%; $P = .002$) than men, and 30-day major bleeding was the strongest independent predictor of 1-year mortality in women in a pooled analysis of the REPLACE-2, ACUITY, and HORIZONS-AMI studies. Women receiving bivalirudin had lower rates of 30-day non–coronary artery bypass grafting–related major bleeding (5.6% vs 9.7%; $P<.001$) and 1-year mortality (2.9% vs 4.4%; $P = .02$) compared with conventional therapy (**Fig. 2**).[108] Thus, therapies that reduce bleeding complications after PCI may be particularly beneficial to female patients and may help narrow the mortality gap between men and women.

Observational data suggest that using a radial access leads to significantly reduced bleeding and vascular complications in both sexes, and women experience an even greater benefit because of their increased baseline risk.[109,110] This finding was investigated in the multicenter randomized Study of Access Site for Enhancement of PCI for Women (SAFE PCI for Women) trial, which randomly assigned 1785 women to either radial or femoral arterial access. This study was terminated early because of lower-than-expected event rates. There was no difference in bleeding or vascular complication rates among the enrolled women receiving PCI in this study.[111]

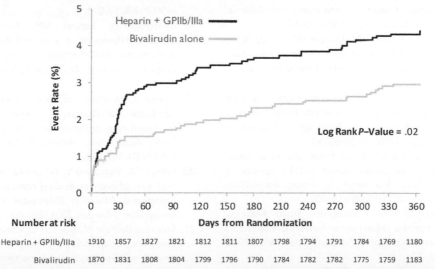

Fig. 2. Kaplan-Meier time-to-event curves of 1-year death in women according to heparin plus glycoprotein IIb/IIIa inhibitors or bivalirudin treatment in a patient level pooled analysis of the REPLACE-2, ACUITY, and HORIZONS-AMI trials.

SUMMARY

CAD remains the leading cause of death in women; however, symptoms of cardiac ischemia in women presenting with STEMI are often atypical. There have been great advances in the treatment of STEMI starting from the development of thrombolytic therapy and most recently with percutaneous coronary interventions. Although most research to date has focused on outcome disparities between men and women, despite the high-risk status of women, women clearly benefit from these therapeutic interventions. Thus, women with STEMIs should be treated aggressively and undergo the same treatment algorithms as men with particular precautions to minimize bleeding and vascular complications.

REFERENCES

1. Stramba-Badiale M, Fox KM, Priori SG, et al. Cardiovascular diseases in women: a statement from the policy conference of the European Society of Cardiology. Eur Heart J 2006;27(8): 994–1005.
2. Heron M. Deaths: leading causes for 2004. Natl Vital Stat Rep 2007;56(5):1–95.
3. Rogers WJ, Frederick PD, Stoehr E, et al. Trends in presenting characteristics and hospital mortality among patients with ST elevation and non-ST elevation myocardial infarction in the National Registry of Myocardial Infarction from 1990 to 2006. Am Heart J 2008;156(6):1026–34.
4. Bucholz EM, Normand SL, Wang Y, et al. Life expectancy and years of potential life lost after acute myocardial infarction by sex and race: a cohort-based study of medicare beneficiaries. J Am Coll Cardiol 2015;66(6):645–55.
5. Mehta LS, Beckie TM, DeVon HA, et al. Acute myocardial infarction in women: a scientific statement from the American Heart Association. Circulation 2016;133(9):916–47.
6. Lerner DJ, Kannel WB. Patterns of coronary heart disease morbidity and mortality in the sexes: a 26-year follow-up of the Framingham population. Am Heart J 1986;111(2):383–90.
7. Roger VL, Go AS, Lloyd-Jones DM, et al. Heart disease and stroke statistics–2011 update: a report from the American Heart Association. Circulation 2011;123(4):e18–209.
8. Kannel WB. The Framingham Study: historical insight on the impact of cardiovascular risk factors in men versus women. J Gend Specif Med 2002; 5(2):27–37.
9. Hochman JS, Tamis JE, Thompson TD, et al. Sex, clinical presentation, and outcome in patients with acute coronary syndromes. Global use of strategies to open occluded coronary arteries in acute coronary syndromes IIb investigators. N Engl J Med 1999;341(4):226–32.
10. Akhter N, Milford-Beland S, Roe MT, et al. Gender differences among patients with acute coronary syndromes undergoing percutaneous coronary intervention in the American College of Cardiology-National Cardiovascular Data Registry (ACC-NCDR). Am Heart J 2009;157(1):141–8.
11. Chang WC, Kaul P, Westerhout CM, et al. Impact of sex on long-term mortality from acute myocardial infarction vs unstable angina. Arch Intern Med 2003;163(20):2476–84.
12. Douglas PS, Ginsburg GS. The evaluation of chest pain in women. N Engl J Med 1996; 334(20):1311–5.
13. Milner KA, Funk M, Richards S, et al. Gender differences in symptom presentation associated with coronary heart disease. Am J Cardiol 1999; 84(4):396–9.
14. Chen W, Woods SL, Puntillo KA. Gender differences in symptoms associated with acute myocardial infarction: a review of the research. Heart Lung 2005;34(4):240–7.
15. Dey S, Flather MD, Devlin G, et al. Sex-related differences in the presentation, treatment and outcomes among patients with acute coronary syndromes: the Global Registry of Acute Coronary Events. Heart 2009;95(1):20–6.
16. Dittrich H, Gilpin E, Nicod P, et al. Acute myocardial infarction in women: influence of gender on mortality and prognostic variables. Am J Cardiol 1988;62(1):1–7.
17. Fiebach NH, Viscoli CM, Horwitz RI. Differences between women and men in survival after myocardial infarction. Biology or methodology? JAMA 1990;263(8):1092–6.
18. Meischke H, Larsen MP, Eisenberg MS. Gender differences in reported symptoms for acute myocardial infarction: impact on prehospital delay time interval. Am J Emerg Med 1998;16(4): 363–6.
19. Mosca L, Manson JE, Sutherland SE, et al. Cardiovascular disease in women: a statement for healthcare professionals from the American Heart Association. Writing Group. Circulation 1997;96(7):2468–82.
20. Milner KA, Vaccarino V, Arnold AL, et al. Gender and age differences in chief complaints of acute myocardial infarction (Worcester Heart Attack Study). Am J Cardiol 2004;93(5):606–8.
21. Stramba-Badiale M, Bonazzi O, Casadei G, et al. Prevalence of episodes of ST-segment depression among mild-to-moderate hypertensive patients in northern Italy: the Cardioscreening Study. J Hypertens 1998;16(5):681–8.

22. Canto JG, Rogers WJ, Goldberg RJ, et al. Association of age and sex with myocardial infarction symptom presentation and in-hospital mortality. JAMA 2012;307(8):813–22.

23. Kannel WB. Silent myocardial ischemia and infarction: insights from the Framingham Study. Cardiol Clin 1986;4(4):583–91.

24. Kannel WB, Dannenberg AL, Abbott RD. Unrecognized myocardial infarction and hypertension: the Framingham Study. Am Heart J 1985; 109(3 Pt 1):581–5.

25. Indications for fibrinolytic therapy in suspected acute myocardial infarction: collaborative overview of early mortality and major morbidity results from all randomised trials of more than 1000 patients. Fibrinolytic Therapy Trialists' (FTT) Collaborative Group. Lancet 1994;343(8893):311–22.

26. Gibler WB, Armstrong PW, Ohman EM, et al. Persistence of delays in presentation and treatment for patients with acute myocardial infarction: The GUSTO-I and GUSTO-III experience. Ann Emerg Med 2002;39(2):123–30.

27. Goldberg RJ, Gurwitz JH, Gore JM. Duration of, and temporal trends (1994-1997) in, prehospital delay in patients with acute myocardial infarction: the second National Registry of Myocardial Infarction. Arch Intern Med 1999;159(18):2141–7.

28. Heer T, Schiele R, Schneider S, et al. Gender differences in acute myocardial infarction in the era of reperfusion (the MITRA registry). Am J Cardiol 2002;89(5):511–7.

29. Leizorovicz A, Haugh MC, Mercier C, et al. Prehospital and hospital time delays in thrombolytic treatment in patients with suspected acute myocardial infarction. Analysis of data from the EMIP study. European Myocardial Infarction Project. Eur Heart J 1997;18(2):248–53.

30. Sheifer SE, Rathore SS, Gersh BJ, et al. Time to presentation with acute myocardial infarction in the elderly: associations with race, sex, and socioeconomic characteristics. Circulation 2000;102(14): 1651–6.

31. Sadowski M, Gasior M, Gierlotka M, et al. Gender-related differences in mortality after ST-segment elevation myocardial infarction: a large multicentre national registry. EuroIntervention 2011; 6(9):1068–72.

32. Bowker TJ, Turner RM, Wood DA, et al. A national Survey of Acute Myocardial Infarction and Ischaemia (SAMII) in the U.K.: characteristics, management and in-hospital outcome in women compared to men in patients under 70 years. Eur Heart J 2000;21(17):1458–63.

33. Marrugat J, Sala J, Masia R, et al. Mortality differences between men and women following first myocardial infarction. RESCATE Investigators. Recursos Empleados en el Sindrome Coronario Agudo y Tiempo de Espera. JAMA 1998;280(16): 1405–9.

34. Karlson BW, Herlitz J, Hartford M. Prognosis in myocardial infarction in relation to gender. Am Heart J 1994;128(3):477–83.

35. Williams JK, Adams MR, Klopfenstein HS. Estrogen modulates responses of atherosclerotic coronary arteries. Circulation 1990;81(5):1680–7.

36. Benamer H, Tafflet M, Bataille S, et al. Female gender is an independent predictor of in-hospital mortality after STEMI in the era of primary PCI: insights from the greater Paris area PCI Registry. EuroIntervention 2011;6(9):1073–9.

37. Jneid H, Fonarow GC, Cannon CP, et al. Sex differences in medical care and early death after acute myocardial infarction. Circulation 2008; 118(25):2803–10.

38. Lincoff AM, Califf RM, Ellis SG, et al. Thrombolytic therapy for women with myocardial infarction: is there a gender gap? Thrombolysis and angioplasty in Myocardial Infarction Study Group. J Am Coll Cardiol 1993;22(7):1780–7.

39. Lansky AJ, Mehran R, Cristea E, et al. Impact of gender and antithrombin strategy on early and late clinical outcomes in patients with non-ST-elevation acute coronary syndromes (from the ACUITY trial). Am J Cardiol 2009;103(9):1196–203.

40. Lansky AJ, Ng VG, Maehara A, et al. Gender and the extent of coronary atherosclerosis, plaque composition, and clinical outcomes in acute coronary syndromes. JACC Cardiovasc Imaging 2012; 5(3 Suppl):S62–72.

41. Kornowski R, Lansky AJ, Mintz GS, et al. Comparison of men versus women in cross-sectional area luminal narrowing, quantity of plaque, presence of calcium in plaque, and lumen location in coronary arteries by intravascular ultrasound in patients with stable angina pectoris. Am J Cardiol 1997; 79(12):1601–5.

42. Nicholls SJ, Wolski K, Sipahi I, et al. Rate of progression of coronary atherosclerotic plaque in women. J Am Coll Cardiol 2007;49(14):1546–51.

43. Qian J, Maehara A, Mintz GS, et al. Impact of gender and age on in vivo virtual histology-intravascular ultrasound imaging plaque characterization (from the global Virtual Histology Intravascular Ultrasound [VH-IVUS] registry). Am J Cardiol 2009;103(9):1210–4.

44. Cheruvu PK, Finn AV, Gardner C, et al. Frequency and distribution of thin-cap fibroatheroma and ruptured plaques in human coronary arteries: a pathologic study. J Am Coll Cardiol 2007;50(10): 940–9.

45. Farb A, Burke AP, Tang AL, et al. Coronary plaque erosion without rupture into a lipid core. A frequent cause of coronary thrombosis in sudden coronary death. Circulation 1996;93(7):1354–63.

46. Kramer MC, Rittersma SZ, de Winter RJ, et al. Relationship of thrombus healing to underlying plaque morphology in sudden coronary death. J Am Coll Cardiol 2010;55(2):122–32.

47. Gurfinkel E, Vigliano C, Janavel JV, et al. Presence of vulnerable coronary plaques in middle-aged individuals who suffered a brain death. Eur Heart J 2009;30(23):2845–53.

48. Hayashi T, Kiyoshima T, Matsuura M, et al. Plaque erosion in the culprit lesion is prone to develop a smaller myocardial infarction size compared with plaque rupture. Am Heart J 2005;149(2):284–90.

49. Kojima S, Nonogi H, Miyao Y, et al. Is preinfarction angina related to the presence or absence of coronary plaque rupture? Heart 2000;83(1):64–8.

50. Murabito JM, Evans JC, Larson MG, et al. Prognosis after the onset of coronary heart disease. An investigation of differences in outcome between the sexes according to initial coronary disease presentation. Circulation 1993;88(6):2548–55.

51. MacIntyre K, Stewart S, Capewell S, et al. Gender and survival: a population-based study of 201,114 men and women following a first acute myocardial infarction. J Am Coll Cardiol 2001;38(3):729–35.

52. Vaccarino V, Horwitz RI, Meehan TP, et al. Sex differences in mortality after myocardial infarction: evidence for a sex-age interaction. Arch Intern Med 1998;158(18):2054–62.

53. Vaccarino V, Krumholz HM, Yarzebski J, et al. Sex differences in 2-year mortality after hospital discharge for myocardial infarction. Ann Intern Med 2001;134(3):173–81.

54. Vaccarino V, Parsons L, Every NR, et al. Sex-based differences in early mortality after myocardial infarction. National Registry of Myocardial Infarction 2 Participants. N Engl J Med 1999;341(4):217–25.

55. Berger JS, Brown DL. Gender-age interaction in early mortality following primary angioplasty for acute myocardial infarction. Am J Cardiol 2006;98(9):1140–3.

56. Vaccarino V, Parsons L, Peterson ED, et al. Sex differences in mortality after acute myocardial infarction: changes from 1994 to 2006. Arch Intern Med 2009;169(19):1767–74.

57. Simon T, Mary-Krause M, Cambou JP, et al. Impact of age and gender on in-hospital and late mortality after acute myocardial infarction: increased early risk in younger women: results from the French nation-wide USIC registries. Eur Heart J 2006;27(11):1282–8.

58. Kostis JB, Wilson AC, O'Dowd K, et al. Sex differences in the management and long-term outcome of acute myocardial infarction. A statewide study. MIDAS Study Group. Myocardial Infarction Data Acquisition System. Circulation 1994;90(4):1715–30.

59. Wilmot KA, O'Flaherty M, Capewell S, et al. Coronary heart disease mortality declines in the United States from 1979 through 2011: evidence for stagnation in young adults, especially women. Circulation 2015;132(11):997–1002.

60. Dreyer RP, Wang Y, Strait KM, et al. Gender differences in the trajectory of recovery in health status among young patients with acute myocardial infarction: results from the variation in recovery: role of gender on outcomes of young AMI patients (VIRGO) study. Circulation 2015;131(22):1971–80.

61. D'Onofrio G, Safdar B, Lichtman JH, et al. Sex differences in reperfusion in young patients with ST-segment-elevation myocardial infarction: results from the VIRGO study. Circulation 2015;131(15):1324–32.

62. Lansky AJ, Hochman JS, Ward PA, et al. Percutaneous coronary intervention and adjunctive pharmacotherapy in women: a statement for healthcare professionals from the American Heart Association. Circulation 2005;111(7):940–53.

63. Rathore SS, Berger AK, Weinfurt KP, et al. Race, sex, poverty, and the medical treatment of acute myocardial infarction in the elderly. Circulation 2000;102(6):642–8.

64. Barakat K, Wilkinson P, Suliman A, et al. Acute myocardial infarction in women: contribution of treatment variables to adverse outcome. Am Heart J 2000;140(5):740–6.

65. Gan SC, Beaver SK, Houck PM, et al. Treatment of acute myocardial infarction and 30-day mortality among women and men. N Engl J Med 2000;343(1):8–15.

66. Chandra NC, Ziegelstein RC, Rogers WJ, et al. Observations of the treatment of women in the United States with myocardial infarction: a report from the National Registry of Myocardial Infarction-I. Arch Intern Med 1998;158(9):981–8.

67. Maynard C, Litwin PE, Martin JS, et al. Gender differences in the treatment and outcome of acute myocardial infarction. Results from the Myocardial Infarction Triage and Intervention Registry. Arch Intern Med 1992;152(5):972–6.

68. Maynard C, Every NR, Martin JS, et al. Association of gender and survival in patients with acute myocardial infarction. Arch Intern Med 1997;157(12):1379–84.

69. Kudenchuk PJ, Maynard C, Martin JS, et al. Comparison of presentation, treatment, and outcome of acute myocardial infarction in men versus women (the Myocardial Infarction Triage and Intervention Registry). Am J Cardiol 1996;78(1):9–14.

70. Udvarhelyi IS, Gatsonis C, Epstein AM, et al. Acute myocardial infarction in the Medicare population.

Process of care and clinical outcomes. JAMA 1992;268(18):2530–6.

71. Weitzman S, Cooper L, Chambless L, et al. Gender, racial, and geographic differences in the performance of cardiac diagnostic and therapeutic procedures for hospitalized acute myocardial infarction in four states. Am J Cardiol 1997; 79(6):722–6.

72. Fang J, Alderman MH. Gender differences of revascularization in patients with acute myocardial infarction. Am J Cardiol 2006;97(12):1722–6.

73. Gurwitz JH, Col NF, Avorn J. The exclusion of the elderly and women from clinical trials in acute myocardial infarction. JAMA 1992;268(11): 1417–22.

74. Lee PY, Alexander KP, Hammill BG, et al. Representation of elderly persons and women in published randomized trials of acute coronary syndromes. JAMA 2001;286(6):708–13.

75. Wilcox RG, von der Lippe G, Olsson CG, et al. Trial of tissue plasminogen activator for mortality reduction in acute myocardial infarction. Anglo-Scandinavian Study of Early Thrombolysis (ASSET). Lancet 1988;2(8610):525–30.

76. Long-term effects of intravenous thrombolysis in acute myocardial infarction: final report of the GISSI study. Gruppo Italiano per lo Studio della Streptochi-nasi nell'Infarto Miocardico (GISSI). Lancet 1987;2(8564):871–4.

77. Kennedy JW, Ritchie JL, Davis KB, et al. The western Washington randomized trial of intracoronary streptokinase in acute myocardial infarction. A 12-month follow-up report. N Engl J Med 1985; 312(17):1073–8.

78. Weaver WD, White HD, Wilcox RG, et al. Comparisons of characteristics and outcomes among women and men with acute myocardial infarction treated with thrombolytic therapy. GUSTO-I investigators. JAMA 1996;275(10):777–82.

79. Malacrida R, Genoni M, Maggioni AP, et al. A comparison of the early outcome of acute myocardial infarction in women and men. The Third International Study of Infarct Survival Collaborative Group. N Engl J Med 1998;338(1):8–14.

80. Woodfield SL, Lundergan CF, Reiner JS, et al. Gender and acute myocardial infarction: is there a different response to thrombolysis? J Am Coll Cardiol 1997;29(1):35–42.

81. Murphy SA, Chen C, Cannon CP, et al. Impact of gender on angiographic and clinical outcomes after fibrinolytic therapy in acute myocardial infarction. Am J Cardiol 2002;90(7):766–70.

82. White HD, Barbash GI, Modan M, et al. After correcting for worse baseline characteristics, women treated with thrombolytic therapy for acute myocardial infarction have the same mortality and morbidity as men except for a higher incidence of hemorrhagic stroke. The Investigators of the International Tissue Plasminogen Activator/Streptokinase Mortality Study. Circulation 1993;88(5 Pt 1):2097–103.

83. Brass LM, Lichtman JH, Wang Y, et al. Intracranial hemorrhage associated with thrombolytic therapy for elderly patients with acute myocardial infarction: results from the Cooperative Cardiovascular Project. Stroke 2000;31(8):1802–11.

84. Gurwitz JH, Gore JM, Goldberg RJ, et al. Risk for intracranial hemorrhage after tissue plasminogen activator treatment for acute myocardial infarction. Participants in the National Registry of Myocardial Infarction 2. Ann Intern Med 1998; 129(8):597–604.

85. Topol EJ, Califf RM, George BS, et al. A randomized trial of immediate versus delayed elective angioplasty after intravenous tissue plasminogen activator in acute myocardial infarction. N Engl J Med 1987;317(10):581–8.

86. Grines CL, Nissen SE, Booth DC, et al. A prospective, randomized trial comparing combination half-dose tissue-type plasminogen activator and streptokinase with full-dose tissue-type plasminogen activator. Kentucky Acute Myocardial Infarction Trial (KAMIT) Group. Circulation 1991;84(2):540–9.

87. Carney RJ, Murphy GA, Brandt TR, et al. Randomized angiographic trial of recombinant tissue-type plasminogen activator (alteplase) in myocardial infarction. RAAMI Study Investigators. J Am Coll Cardiol 1992;20(1):17–23.

88. Zijlstra F, de Boer MJ, Hoorntje JC, et al. A comparison of immediate coronary angioplasty with intravenous streptokinase in acute myocardial infarction. N Engl J Med 1993; 328(10):680–4.

89. The effects of tissue plasminogen activator, streptokinase, or both on coronary-artery patency, ventricular function, and survival after acute myocardial infarction. The GUSTO Angiographic Investigators. N Engl J Med 1993;329(22):1615–22.

90. Stone GW, Grines CL, Browne KF, et al. Implications of recurrent ischemia after reperfusion therapy in acute myocardial infarction: a comparison of thrombolytic therapy and primary angioplasty. J Am Coll Cardiol 1995;26(1):66–72.

91. Simoons ML, Serruys PW, van den Brand M, et al. Early thrombolysis in acute myocardial infarction: limitation of infarct size and improved survival. J Am Coll Cardiol 1986;7(4):717–28.

92. Schroder R, Neuhaus KL, Leizorovicz A, et al. A prospective placebo-controlled double-blind multicenter trial of intravenous streptokinase in acute myocardial infarction (ISAM): long-term mortality and morbidity. J Am Coll Cardiol 1987; 9(1):197–203.

93. Grines CL, Browne KF, Marco J, et al. A comparison of immediate angioplasty with thrombolytic therapy for acute myocardial infarction. The Primary Angioplasty in Myocardial Infarction Study Group. N Engl J Med 1993; 328(10):673–9.

94. Zijlstra F, Hoorntje JC, de Boer MJ, et al. Long-term benefit of primary angioplasty as compared with thrombolytic therapy for acute myocardial infarction. N Engl J Med 1999;341(19):1413–9.

95. Rogers WJ, Baim DS, Gore JM, et al. Comparison of immediate invasive, delayed invasive, and conservative strategies after tissue-type plasminogen activator. Results of the Thrombolysis in Myocardial Infarction (TIMI) Phase II-A trial. Circulation 1990;81(5):1457–76.

96. O'Neill W, Timmis GC, Bourdillon PD, et al. A prospective randomized clinical trial of intracoronary streptokinase versus coronary angioplasty for acute myocardial infarction. N Engl J Med 1986;314(13):812–8.

97. Weaver WD, Simes RJ, Betriu A, et al. Comparison of primary coronary angioplasty and intravenous thrombolytic therapy for acute myocardial infarction: a quantitative review. JAMA 1997;278(23): 2093–8.

98. Andersen HR, Nielsen TT, Rasmussen K, et al. A comparison of coronary angioplasty with fibrinolytic therapy in acute myocardial infarction. N Engl J Med 2003;349(8):733–42.

99. Stone GW, Grines CL, Browne KF, et al. Comparison of in-hospital outcome in men versus women treated by either thrombolytic therapy or primary coronary angioplasty for acute myocardial infarction. Am J Cardiol 1995;75(15):987–92.

100. Stone GW, Grines CL, Cox DA, et al. Comparison of angioplasty with stenting, with or without abciximab, in acute myocardial infarction. N Engl J Med 2002;346(13):957–66.

101. Keeley EC, Boura JA, Grines CL. Primary angioplasty versus intravenous thrombolytic therapy for acute myocardial infarction: a quantitative review of 23 randomised trials. Lancet 2003; 361(9351):13–20.

102. Lansky AJ, Pietras C, Costa RA, et al. Gender differences in outcomes after primary angioplasty versus primary stenting with and without abciximab for acute myocardial infarction: results of the Controlled Abciximab and Device Investigation to Lower Late Angioplasty Complications (CADILLAC) trial. Circulation 2005;111(13):1611–8.

103. Onuma Y, Kukreja N, Daemen J, et al. Impact of sex on 3-year outcome after percutaneous coronary intervention using bare-metal and drug-eluting stents in previously untreated coronary artery disease: insights from the RESEARCH (Rapamycin-Eluting Stent Evaluated at Rotterdam Cardiology Hospital) and T-SEARCH (Taxus-Stent Evaluated at Rotterdam Cardiology Hospital) Registries. JACC Cardiovasc Interv 2009;2(7):603–10.

104. Ferrante G, Presbitero P, Corrada E, et al. Sex-specific benefits of sirolimus-eluting stent on long-term outcomes in patients with ST-elevation myocardial infarction undergoing primary percutaneous coronary intervention: insights from the Multicenter Evaluation of Single High-Dose Bolus Tirofiban Versus Abciximab With Sirolimus-Eluting Stent or Bare-Metal Stent in Acute Myocardial Infarction Study trial. Am Heart J 2012;163(1):104–11.

105. Morice MC, Mikhail GW, Mauri i Ferre F, et al. SPIRIT Women, evaluation of the safety and efficacy of the XIENCE V everolimus-eluting stent system in female patients: referral time for coronary intervention and 2-year clinical outcomes. EuroIntervention 2012;8(3):325–35.

106. Ahmed B, Piper WD, Malenka D, et al. Significantly improved vascular complications among women undergoing percutaneous coronary intervention: a report from the Northern New England Percutaneous Coronary Intervention Registry. Circ Cardiovasc Interv 2009;2(5):423–9.

107. Argulian E, Patel AD, Abramson JL, et al. Gender differences in short-term cardiovascular outcomes after percutaneous coronary interventions. Am J Cardiol 2006;98(1):48–53.

108. Ng VG, Baumbach A, Grinfeld L, et al. Impact of Bleeding and Bivalirudin Therapy on Mortality Risk in Women Undergoing Percutaneous Coronary Intervention (from the REPLACE-2, ACUITY, and HORIZONS-AMI Trials). Am J Cardiol 2016; 117(2):186–91.

109. Pristipino C, Pelliccia F, Granatelli A, et al. Comparison of access-related bleeding complications in women versus men undergoing percutaneous coronary catheterization using the radial versus femoral artery. Am J Cardiol 2007;99(9):1216–21.

110. Rao SV, Ou FS, Wang TY, et al. Trends in the prevalence and outcomes of radial and femoral approaches to percutaneous coronary intervention: a report from the National Cardiovascular Data Registry. JACC Cardiovasc Interv 2008;1(4): 379–86.

111. Rao SV, Hess CN, Barham B, et al. A registry-based randomized trial comparing radial and femoral approaches in women undergoing percutaneous coronary intervention: the SAFE-PCI for Women (Study of Access Site for Enhancement of PCI for Women) trial. JACC Cardiovasc Interv 2014;7(8):857–67.

Management of Multivessel Disease and Cardiogenic Shock

Amerjeet S. Banning, BSc(Hons), MB BS, MRCP,
Anthony H. Gershlick, BSc, MB BS, FRCP*

KEYWORDS

- Cardiogenic shock • Myocardial infarction • Percutaneous coronary intervention

KEY POINTS

- Multivessel coronary artery disease has been reported in up to 60% to 70% of patients presenting with ST-elevation myocardial infarction (STEMI) complicated by cardiogenic shock.
- Current guideline recommendations for the management of multivessel disease in STEMI support revascularization treatment (by percutaneous coronary intervention [PCI]) of any noninfarct-related lesions in cardiogenic shock.
- Larger randomized studies are required to more robustly determine the benefit or otherwise of complete revascularization in STEMI patients presenting with cardiogenic shock.

INTRODUCTION

Cardiogenic shock represents a state of reduced cardiac output, resulting in insufficient end-organ perfusion and consequent multiorgan failure. Clinically, it can be defined by the following diagnostic criteria[1]:

- [a]Systolic blood pressure (SBP) less than 90 mm Hg for more than 30 minutes (or a requirement of vasopressor/inotrope therapy to maintain SBP greater than 90 mm Hg)
- Severe reduction in cardiac index (<1.8 L/min/m² or <2.2 L/min/m² with cardiovascular support)
- Elevated left ventricular (LV) filling pressure (left ventricular end diastolic pressure (LVEDP) >18 mm Hg or right ventricular end diastolic pressure (RVEDP) >10–15 mm Hg)

- [a]Evidence of end-organ hypoperfusion (altered mental status, oliguria with urine output <30 mL/h, cool peripheries)

Cardiogenic shock complicates 6% to 12% of cases with acute myocardial infarction depending on the population being tested and the definition of cardiogenic shock being used. For example, in an analysis of the US National Inpatient Sample database from 2003 to 2010, 7.9% of patients aged greater than 40 years with ST-elevation myocardial infarction (STEMI) had cardiogenic shock.[2]

Data from the British Cardiovascular Interventional Society - National Institute for Cardiovascular Outcomes Research (BCIS NICOR) database has shown in the United Kingdom, that the incidence of cardiogenic shock (registry data from multiple sites, so definition may vary) has progressively increased from 2005 to 2010, with the recent incidence reported to be

Disclosure Statement: The authors have nothing to disclose.
Leicester Cardiovascular Biomedical Research Unit, Department of Cardiovascular Sciences, The National Institute of Health Research (NIHR), University Hospitals of Leicester National Health Service (NHS) Trust, Glenfield Hospital, University of Leicester, Groby Road, Leicester, LE3 9QP, UK
* Corresponding author.
E-mail address: agershlick@aol.com

[a]Most commonly used in clinical practice.

11.8% in 2014 of all acute coronary syndrome patients.[3]

Cardiogenic shock is associated with a high degree of mortality. In the 1970s to 1980s, mortality was reported to be as high as 80%, but has now fallen to around 50% in more recent series, almost certainly as a result of prompt intervention in STEMI patients. However, the reasons for this fall are probably multifactorial, with prompt revascularization mortality leading to a smaller area of unrecoverable infarction but also fewer mechanical complications, better adjunctive pharmacology, and perhaps more complete revascularization. It should be noted, however, that the mortality for cardiogenic shock remains unacceptably high at 50% or so over the first 3 to 6 months. For example the BCIS NICOR data demonstrated 30-day mortality at 40% for cardiogenic shock.[3] Similarly, Shah and colleagues[4] have shown 1-year mortality to be closer to 60%.

Of patients presenting with cardiogenic shock in the context of STEMI, more than 50% have evidence of significant stenoses in at least 1 noninfarct-related artery (N-IRA). In the Should We Emergently Revascularize Occluded Coronaries for Cardiogenic Shock (SHOCK) trial, 60% of patients undergoing PCI had evidence of 3-vessel coronary artery disease.[1] Similarly, in a retrospective analysis of 4731 patients from the National Cardiovascular Data Registry (NCDR) CathPCI Registry undergoing primary PCI for STEMI complicated by cardiogenic shock, 63.4% of patients had greater than 50% stenosis in a noninfarct-related artery.[5] It has also been shown that the presence of multi-vessel disease (MVD) in STEMI patients with cardiogenic shock is associated with worse outcomes,[6–8] with presence of MVD being an independent predictor of in-hospital mortality. However, this does not necessarily mean that treatment of N-IRA lesions translates into improved clinical outcomes, as there may be other factors influencing the mortality in such patients.

Recently, a series of randomized controlled trials, namely PRAMI (Preventive Angioplasty in Acute Myocardial Infarction Trial),[9] CvLPRIT (Complete Versus Lesion-only Primary PCI Trial),[10] and DANAMI-3-PRIMULTI (Primary PCI in patients with ST-elevation Myocardial Infarction and Multivessel disease Trial)[11] have shown benefit in multivessel PCI (MV-PCI) in hemodynamically stable patients with STEMI presenting with MVD, leading to a change in the ACC/AHA/SCAI guidelines for the management of such patients, with PCI of N-IRA lesions being changed from a class III to a Class IIb recommendation.[12]

This article will explore the rationale and current data on the management of MVD in patients presenting with STEMI and cardiogenic shock.

PRESENCE OF MULTIVESSEL CORONARY DISEASE IN ST-ELEVATION MYOCARDIAL INFARCTION WITH CARDIOGENIC SHOCK
Impact and Pathophysiological Considerations

The presence of MVD is associated with worse outcomes. Data from the Brazilian InCor registry showed that MVD is an independent predictor of in-hospital mortality in cardiogenic shock (odds ratio [OR] 2.62; 95% confidence interval [95% CI] 1.16–5.90).[6] Similarly, the presence of 3-vessel disease was also an independent predictor of in-hospital mortality in a large European registry of cardiogenic shock patients (OR = 1.8, 95% CI = 1.4–2.4).[13]

In the Manitoba cardiogenic SHOCK registry, 210 consecutive patients presenting with cardiogenic shock were analyzed for independent predictors of in-hospital mortality. Following multivariate logistic regression of the STEMI subset with MVD (n = 101), achieving complete revascularization either with PCI or coronary artery bypass grafting (CABG) was an independent predictor of survival to discharge (OR = 2.5, 95% CI = 1.1–6.2, P = .025).[8]

Myocardial ischemia impacts the entire coronary circulation, and involves not only the culprit artery but may also exacerbate ischemia in noninfarct-related artery lesions. This may occur through a pan-myocardial inflammatory process as well as systemic hypotension maintained by the systemic inflammatory response syndrome, leading to further coronary hypoperfusion in the N-IRAs[14] and a spiral of further myocardial ischemia and further impaired function. Usually, both systolic and diastolic myocardial dysfunction are present in patients with cardiogenic shock. Metabolic derangements that impair myocardial contractility further compromise systolic ventricular function.[15]

Hence, revascularizing only the infarct-related artery may not resolve the continuing ischemia in the context of hypoperfusion that can occur within any concomitant N-IRA lesions. Thus, the rationale behind complete revascularization in this context is to improve perfusion to N-IRA territories and thus attempt to improve myocardial function and cardiac output and reverse the spiral of decline that can occur with persistent hypotension from poor cardiac output. Although this is good theory, it requires data to show that total revascularization in the context of a very sick patient does not actually worsen outcomes.

Evidence Base for Revascularization Strategy in Patients Presenting with Cardiogenic Shock

In the landmark Should we Emergently Revascularise Occluded arteries for Cardiogenic Shock (SHOCK) trial, 352 patients with acute myocardial infarction complicated with cardiogenic shock were randomized to receive either emergency revascularization with either PCI or CABG (n = 152) or initial medical stabilization (n = 150). The intra-aortic balloon counter-pulsation pump was used in 86% of cases in both groups; therefore, this study cannot be regarded as a test of cardiovascular support. Although there were no differences in 30-day mortality between the 2 groups (46.7% vs 56.0%, P = 11), the 6-month mortality rates were lower in the revascularization group (50.3% vs 63.1%, P = .027).[1] This study showed continued benefit for survival in favor of the early revascularization group in all patients and in-hospital survivors out to 6 years after randomization.[16]

Although this pivotal cardiogenic shock study indicated that early revascularization was important, with benefits seen after 6 months, it did not indicate whether revascularization to the N-IRA should also be undertaken in patients with MVD. In cardiogenic shock patients, multivessel coronary disease MVD is present in more than 50% of cases.[1,17]

The pathophysiological processes that lead to progressive spiral of reduction in cardiac output and further ischemia leading to worsening cardiac output mean that halting this spiral of decline early would intuitively result in better outcomes.

From the SHOCK trial, the timing of PCI in cardiogenic shock did not appear to influence mortality rates regardless of whether PCI was performed within 6 hours or later than 24 hours.[18] However, it is possible that even earlier intervention may be required to improve outcomes. In patients presenting with cardiogenic shock on admission in the SHOCK trial and registry, immediate revascularization was associated with reduction in mortality.[19]

This has also been shown recently in the Japanese Circulation Society (JCS) shock registry, where 30-day mortality from cardiogenic shock was significantly lower with a door-to-balloon time of less than 2 hours compared with greater than 2 hours (20.0% vs 33.6%, log-rank P = .0364).[20]

Although some evidence suggests that in the hemodynamically stable patients, a staged revascularization procedure for N-IRA lesions may be as efficacious if not better than an index procedure,[21,22] currently no studies have examined staged N-IRA PCI in cardiogenic shock patients initially treated with culprit-only PCI.

Cavender and colleagues[23] looked retrospectively at patients presenting with STEMI from the NCDR registry, and demonstrated not only that most of patients undergoing MV-PCI during the index procedure were in the context of cardiogenic shock, but also potentially poorer outcomes in these patients compared with culprit-only PCI, even after adjustment for potential confounders (adjusted HR = 1.54 [95% CI = .22 = 1.95], P<.01). A multivariate analysis revealed that presence of cardiogenic shock increased the propensity for MV-PCI in this unselected cohort of patients.

The presence of an N-IRA chronic total occlusion (CTO) confers a worse prognosis that MVD without CTO in cardiogenic shock.[24] This may present an issue with regards to the ability to achieve complete revascularization, as CTO PCI requires an operator with sufficient skills in this technically challenging subset of coronary lesions. In addition, assessment of viability may not be possible in the acute STEMI/cardiogenic shock setting, leading deferral of CTO PCI while treating any other N-IRA lesions.

The ALKK (Arbeitsgemeinschaft Leitende Kardiologische Krankenhausärzte)-PCI registry has been analyzed with regards to patients with MVD presenting with cardiogenic shock. Cardiogenic shock was presented in 6.4% of patients presenting with STEMI and 1.1% of patients with non-st-elevation myocardial infarction (NSTEMI) cardiogenic shock, and of these 71.5% had MVD without significant left main stem stenosis.[7] Only one-quarter of cardiogenic shock patients with MVD underwent MV-PCI. The registry analysis showed higher mortality in the MV-PCI group compared with culprit-only PCI, as well as higher rate of dialysis in the MV-PCI group in keeping with higher contrast volume use in this group. However, it should be noted that in this registry, there was a significantly higher impaired renal function in the MV-PCI cohort at baseline, emphasizing the problem with registry data.

Further conflicting evidence of the role of multivessel revascularization during cardiogenic shock comes from the Euro-Heart Survey-PCI registry. Although this study showed increased tendency towards in-hospital mortality with MV-PCI (48.8% vs 37.4% for culprit-only PCI, P = .07), it was noted that sicker patients on requiring ventilation were more likely to undergo MV-PCI (30% vs 19%, P = .05). Correcting for confounders using multivariate logistic regression analysis attenuated this difference in in-hospital mortality between the 2 groups (OR = 1.28, 95%CI = 0.72–2.28).[25]

Hence, much of the current evidence looking at management of MVD in the context of cardiogenic shock has been obtained from retrospective analysis of registry data and has produced heterogeneous and conflicting data (Table 1).

Two recent studies add some support to the current guideline recommendation of MV-PCI in STEMI presenting with cardiogenic shock:

1. An analysis of 31,149 patients with acute myocardial infarction (AMI) enrolled in the Korean Acute Myocardial Infarction Registry (KAMIR) demonstrated 1105 patients with STEMI and cardiogenic shock. Of these patients, 510 had evidence of MVD on angiography. Retrospective analysis of patients who underwent culprit vessel revascularization (n = 386) compared with multivessel revascularization (n = 124) revealed lower adjusted risk of in-hospital mortality (9.3% vs 2.4% for culprit-only revascularization, HR = 0.263, 95% CI = 0.149–0.462, P<.001).[28] There was also reduction in all-cause death with multivessel revascularization (13.1% vs 4.8%, HR = 0.400, 95% CI = 0.264–0.606, P<.001) and cardiac death (9.7% vs 4.8%, HR = 0.510, 95% CI = 0.329–0.790, P = .002). There was early separation of the Kaplan-Meier curves, indicating most of the benefit occurred with reduction of early death rates with complete revascularization. In-hospital death rates observed in this registry are lower than seen in other national registries.[3] The mean left ventricular ejection fraction (LVEF) in both groups was greater than 50%, higher than would be expected in patients with MVD and cardiogenic shock, and a high proportion of RCA culprit artery in both groups (66% in the culprit-only revascularization, 49% in the multivessel group); low rates of LAD-related infarction may have impacted on the in-hospital mortality rates in both groups.

2. Mylotte and colleagues[27] conducted a prospective observational study of 266 patients with STEMI and resuscitated cardiac arrest with cardiogenic shock. They demonstrated improved 6-month survival in patients with MVD undergoing multivessel PCI compared with culprit artery-only PCI (43.9% vs 20.4%, P = .0017), mediated by a reduction in recurrent cardiac arrest/shock-related death in the MV-PCI group (50.0% vs

68.0%, P = .024). Multivariate analysis demonstrated MV primary PCI in patients with MVD to be an independent predictor of 6-month survival in this cohort (HR = 0.57, 95% CI = 0.38–0.84, P = .005). It should be noted, however, in this observational study that culprit-only group was older; had longer no-reflow, arrest–defibrillation, and return of spontaneous circulation (ROSC) intervals; and were more likely to have TIMI-0 flow grade on presentation. Hence, this may have influenced the outcome rates in the culprit-only group.

Hence, the current evidence base provides no clear answer in terms of whether improved outcomes result from MV-PCI in patients with cardiogenic shock.

When evaluating the data from these studies, several points are evident:

- PCI to the N-IRA in patients with MVD was only performed in one-fourth to one-third of patients presenting with cardiogenic shock.
- Because of the retrospective and observational nature of these studies, it is difficult to ascertain the reasons why some of these patients underwent MV-PCI while others did not. This is especially so since in most cases the baseline characteristics appear similar. Thus it is likely selection bias is being seen in favor of those patients receiving multivessel revascularization, which may not be accounted for by statistical methods of adjustment for potential confounders.
- In most of these studies, a large proportion of patients with MVD had culprit PCI only. Consequentially, treatment effects may have been influenced by relatively low numbers in the respective MV-PCI groups of these studies.
- Although contrast load was increased with a strategy of multi-vessel PCI,[7] data from these registries and nonrandomized observational studies do not determine whether this resulted in worse outcomes in terms of contrast-induced nephropathy or need for renal support compared with culprit-only PCI.

Current Guideline Recommendations on Revascularization in Cardiogenic Shock

The current recommendation from the European Society of Cardiology is that in the context of cardiogenic shock, patients should undergo

Table 1
Summary of studies comparing culprit-only and multivessel PCI in cardiogenic shock

Study	Description	Outcomes
Studies demonstrating no benefit of MV-PCI		
Bauer et al,[25] 2012	Retrospective analysis of 336 patients presenting with ACS and cardiogenic shock at time of index PCI with evidence of MVD. 82 patients (24.4%) underwent MV-PCI; coronary artery disease burden similar between both groups, LMS and previous CABG excluded	No significant difference in in-hospital mortality between the 2 groups, although numerically higher mortality in the MV-PCI group (48.8% MV-PCI vs 37.4% for culprit-only PCI, $P = .07$); following adjustment for confounding variables there was no difference in in-hospital mortality between the 2 groups (OR = 1.28, 95% CI = .72–2.28)
Van Der Schaff et al,[24] 2010	Retrospective analysis of 292 patients presenting with STEMI complicated by cardiogenic shock; 161 patients had MVD, of whom 92 had MVD without a CTO, and 69 had MVD with an N-IRA CTO; MV-PCI was performed in 21 patients (23%) of patients with MVD without CTO, and 16 patients (23%) of patients with MVD and CTO	No difference in 1-y mortality between patients with MVD (+/− N-IRA CTO) who underwent culprit lesion-only PCI or MV-PCI (53% vs 60%, $P = .50$)
Yang et al,[26] 2014	Prospective multicenter observational study of *338* patients presenting with STEMI, cardiogenic shock, MVD and at least successful PCI of the Culprit vessel; MV-PCI performed in 60 (17.8%) patients; median follow-up of 224 d (Inter-quartile range = 46–383 d).	In-hospital mortality similar between MV-PCI (31.7%) and culprit-only PCI (24.5%), $P = .247$; No difference in all-cause mortality at follow-up (35.0% MV-PCI vs 30.6% culprit-only PCI, adjusted HR = 1.06, 95% CI = 0.61–1.86, $P = .831$); no difference in major adverse cardiovascular events (all-cause death, recurrent MI and any revascularization with PCI or CABG) at follow up (41.7% MV-PCI vs 37.1% culprit-only, adjusted HR = 1.03, 95% CI = 0.62–1.71, $P = .908$)
Studies demonstrating worse outcomes with MV-PCI		
Cavender et al,[23] 2009	Retrospective analysis of 3134 patients presenting with STEMI and MVD undergoing MV-PCI from the NCDR registry, subgroup of patients with STEMI and cardiogenic shock (n = 3087), of whom 433 underwent MV-PCI (14%)	Significantly higher in-hospital mortality in patients with MV-PCI (36.49% vs 27.77% in those treated with single-vessel PCI alone, $P<.01$); adjusted HR = 1.54 (95% CI = .22 = 1.95), $P<.01$
Zeymer et al,[7] 2015	Prospective multicenter German PCI registry, *735* patients presenting with cardiogenic shock, AMI and MVD; 173 patients (23.5%) within this cohort underwent MV-PCI at time of index procedure	Higher in-hospital death in MV-PCI group (46.8% vs 35.8%, $P<.01$); No difference in in-hospital MI, stroke, or bleeding between the 2 groups; MV-PCI was an independent predictor of in-hospital mortality (adjusted OR = 1.50, 95% CI = 1.15–1.84).

(continued on next page)

Study	Description	Outcomes
Studies demonstrating improved clinical outcomes with MV-PCI		
Mylotte et al,[27] 2013	Multicenter prospective observational study of STEMI patients presenting with cardiogenic shock and resuscitated cardiac arrest; 266 patients, 97 patients (36.5%) with single vessel disease and 169 patients with MV disease. In MVD cohort, 66 (39.0%) of patients underwent MV-PCI.	6-mo survival significantly greater in MV-PCI group compared with culprit-only PCI in MVD (43.9% vs 20.4%, P = .0017). MV-PCI at time of PPCI was an independent predictor of 6-mo survival (HR = 0.57, 95% CI = 0.38–0.84, P = .005)
Hussein et al,[8] 2011	210 cardiogenic shock patients, of whom 101 patients underwent MV-PCI; 17% of the PCI cohort underwent MV-PCI	Survival to discharge higher in MV-PCI group (76% vs 44% in culprit-only group, P<.001). Complete revascularization was an independent predictor of survival to discharge (OR = 6.2, 95% CI = 1.85–24.6, P = .005)
Park et al,[28] 2015	Retrospective analysis of 1105 patients with STEMI and cardiogenic shock; 510 patients had MVD; culprit-only revascularization in 386 patients, MV-PCI at time of index PCI in 124 patients	In-hospital mortality lower in MV-PCI group (2.4% vs 9.3% for culprit-only PCI)

immediate invasive evaluation and emergency PCI if coronary anatomy is amenable, or emergency CABG if not amenable to PCI (Class I, Level of evidence B).[29] The guideline also recommends MV-PCI during STEMI should be considered in patients with cardiogenic shock in the presence of multiple, critical stenosis or highly unstable lesions. Based on the authors' review, in terms of the variable quality of the data as a Class IIa, Level of evidence B recommendation, this appears more intuitive rather than evidence led.

The ACC/AHA/SCAI guidelines recommend that in patients presenting with STEMI complicated by cardiogenic shock, emergency revascularization with either PCI or CABG irrespective of the time delay from myocardial infarction onset (Class I, Level of evidence B).[30] In the presence of hemodynamic instability and cardiogenic shock, the guideline suggests that PCI of a severe stenosis in a large noninfarct-related artery "might improve haemodynamic stability and should be considered during the primary procedure," which is more in keeping with the data currently out there.

In spite of the guideline recommendations generally supporting use of multivessel revascularization in cardiogenic shock, and maybe in the absence of robust data, the EHS-PCI registry has shown that only 25% of patients with cardiogenic shock and evidence of MVD actually underwent MV-PCI.[25] Similarly low rates of MV-PCI have been shown in other studies.[23,24,28]

Future Perspective in the Management of Multivessel Disease and Cardiogenic Shock in ST-elevation myocardial infarction

The CULPRIT-SHOCK trial (Culprit Lesion Only PCI Versus Multivessel PCI in Cardiogenic Shock) is an on-going prospective multicenter, open label, trial that will randomize 706 patients presenting with cardiogenic shock with evidence of MVD at index angiography to receive either culprit vessel revascularization during the index procedure with possible staged nonculprit lesion revascularization based on ischemia later, versus multivessel revascularization at the time of primary PCI.[31] The primary outcome measure is 30-day mortality and severe renal impairment. The study permits intra-aortic balloon pump (IABP) use and mechanical support device use at the operator's discretion. This study should shed light on whether MV-PCI at the time of the index procedure results in improved clinical outcomes in patients with cardiogenic shock complicating AMI. A potential limitation of this study is advocating attempts at CTO revascularization in the acute setting, where conventionally such lesions would be treated only with evidence of ischemia and viability in the CTO territory.

The Ideal Trial and Data that are Required to Guide Management

The ideal trial should compare culprit-only PCI with complete revascularization in patients fulfilling a standard definition of cardiogenic shock, and also include analysis of the impact of adjunctive strategies to augment myocardial perfusion, including IABP (as IABP-SHOCK II had effectively a heterogeneous population with respect to not all patients undergoing complete revascularization in MVD), Impella (Abiomed, Danvers, Masachusetts), extracorporeal membrane oxygenation (ECMO), and inotropic/vasopressor support. In addition to looking at reduction in the in-hospital outcomes, the 30-day outcome reduction is another important landmark, as current data suggest there is a vulnerable period in survivors of cardiogenic shock. Long-term rates of heart failure are important metrics. Optimal timing to determine how quickly complete revascularization and use of adjunctive hemodynamic support devices should be used in cardiogenic shock may also be important to establish through future trials (eg, early use of these interventions rather than in refractory shock, since early hemodynamic support may improve LV function and rescue jeopardized myocardium).

SUMMARY

Multivessel coronary artery disease is found in up to 70% of patients presenting with cardiogenic shock. Despite guideline recommendation of undertaking complete revascularization in such patients, based on the theory that this will lead to optimal myocardial perfusion in the peri-infarct border-zones, there are limited data to robustly support this recommendation. Much of the current data is based on outcomes in studies with small numbers of patients or from retrospective, non-randomized studies. The forthcoming CULPRIT-SHOCK trial is likely to shed some insights into the optimal strategy for managing such patients in terms of revascularization strategy.

However until there are more robust data available, current best clinical practice must be to ensure prompt culprit vessel revascularization and to apply contemporary strategies to support cardiac output and maintain end organ perfusion. Decisions around undertaking complete revascularization currently need to be based on the individual patient circumstances and by individual operator considerations on benefit versus risk.

REFERENCES

1. Hochman JS, Sleeper LA, Webb JG, et al. Early revascularization in acute myocardial infarction complicated by cardiogenic shock. SHOCK Investigators. Should We Emergently Revascularize Occluded Coronaries for Cardiogenic Shock. N Engl J Med 1999;341(9):625–34.
2. Kolte D, Khera S, Aronow WS, et al. Trends in incidence, management, and outcomes of cardiogenic shock complicating ST-elevation myocardial infarction in the United States. J Am Heart Assoc 2014; 3(1):e000590.
3. Kunadian V, Qiu W, Ludman P, et al. Outcomes in patients with cardiogenic shock following percutaneous coronary intervention in the contemporary era: an analysis from the BCIS database (British Cardiovascular Intervention Society). JACC Cardiovasc Interv 2014;7(12):1374–85.
4. Shah RU, de Lemos JA, Wang TY, et al. Post-hospital outcomes of patients with acute myocardial infarction with cardiogenic shock: findings from the NCDR. J Am Coll Cardiol 2016;67(7):739–47.
5. Mehta RH, Ou F-S, Peterson ED, et al. Clinical significance of post-procedural TIMI flow in patients with cardiogenic shock undergoing primary percutaneous coronary intervention. JACC Cardiovasc Interv 2009;2(1):56–64.
6. de Castro Bienert IR, Ribeiro HB, Valim LR, et al. In-Hospital outcomes and predictors of mortality in acute myocardial infarction with cardiogenic shock treated by primary angioplasty: data from the incor registry. Rev Bras Cardiol Invasiva 2012;20(1):41–5.
7. Zeymer U, Hochadel M, Thiele H, et al. Immediate multivessel percutaneous coronary intervention versus culprit lesion intervention in patients with acute myocardial infarction complicated by cardiogenic shock: results of the ALKK-PCI registry. EuroIntervention 2015;11(3):280–5.
8. Hussain F, Philipp RK, Ducas RA, et al. The ability to achieve complete revascularization is associated with improved in-hospital survival in cardiogenic shock due to myocardial infarction: Manitoba cardiogenic SHOCK Registry investigators. Catheter Cardiovasc Interv 2011;78(4):540–8.
9. Wald DS, Morris JK, Wald NJ, et al. Randomized trial of preventive angioplasty in myocardial infarction. N Engl J Med 2013;369(12):1115–23.
10. Gershlick AH, Khan JN, Kelly DJ, et al. Randomized trial of complete versus lesion-only revascularization in patients undergoing primary percutaneous coronary intervention for STEMI and multivessel disease: the CvLPRIT trial. J Am Coll Cardiol 2015;65(10):963–72.
11. Engström T, Kelbæk H, Helqvist S, et al. Complete revascularisation versus treatment of the culprit lesion only in patients with ST-segment elevation

myocardial infarction and multivessel disease (DANAMI-3—PRIMULTI): an open-label, randomised controlled trial. Lancet 2015;386(9994):665–71.

12. Levine GN, O'Gara PT, Bates ER, et al. 2015 ACC/AHA/SCAI focused update on primary percutaneous coronary intervention for patients with ST-elevation myocardial infarction: an update of the 2011 ACCF/AHA/SCAI guideline for percutaneous coronary intervention and the 2013 ACCF/AHA guideline for the management of ST-elevation myocardial infarction. J Am Coll Cardiol 2015; 67(10):1235–50.

13. Zeymer U, Vogt A, Zahn R, et al. Predictors of in-hospital mortality in 1333 patients with acute myocardial infarction complicated by cardiogenic shock treated with primary percutaneous coronary intervention (PCI); results of the primary PCI registry of the Arbeitsgemeinschaft Leitende K. Eur Heart J 2004;25(4):322–8.

14. Kohsaka S, Menon V, Lowe AM, et al. Systemic inflammatory response syndrome after acute myocardial infarction complicated by cardiogenic shock. Arch Intern Med 2005;165(14):1643–50.

15. Reynolds HR, Hochman JS. Cardiogenic shock: current concepts and improving outcomes. Circulation 2008;117(5):686–97.

16. Hochman JS, Sleeper LA, Webb JG, et al. Early revascularization and long-term survival in cardiogenic shock complicating acute myocardial infarction. JAMA 2006;295(21):2511–5.

17. Sanborn TA, Sleeper LA, Webb JG, et al. Correlates of one-year survival inpatients with cardiogenic shock complicating acute myocardial infarction: angiographic findings from the SHOCK trial. J Am Coll Cardiol 2003;42(8):1373–9.

18. Webb JG, Sanborn TA, Sleeper LA, et al. Percutaneous coronary intervention for cardiogenic shock in the SHOCK Trial Registry. Am Heart J 2001; 141(6):964–70.

19. Jeger RV, Harkness SM, Ramanathan K, et al. Emergency revascularization in patients with cardiogenic shock on admission: a report from the SHOCK trial and registry. Eur Heart J 2006;27(6):664–70.

20. Ebina H, Tetsuya M, Masahiro M, et al. Impact of onset to balloon time and short-term mortality in patients with cardiogenic shock complicating acute coronary syndrome treated with primary percutaneous coronary intervention from JCS Shock Registry. J Am Coll Cardiol 2016;67(13):637.

21. Politi L, Sgura F, Rossi R, et al. A randomised trial of target-vessel versus multi-vessel revascularisation in ST-elevation myocardial infarction: major adverse cardiac events during long-term follow-up. Heart 2010;96(9):662–7.

22. Vlaar PJ, Mahmoud KD, Holmes DR, et al. Culprit vessel only versus multivessel and staged percutaneous coronary intervention for multivessel disease in patients presenting with ST-segment elevation myocardial infarction: a pairwise and network meta-analysis. J Am Coll Cardiol 2011; 58(7):692–703.

23. Cavender MA, Milford-Beland S, Roe MT, et al. Prevalence, predictors, and in-hospital outcomes of non-infarct artery intervention during primary percutaneous coronary intervention for ST-segment elevation myocardial infarction (from the National Cardiovascular Data Registry). Am J Cardiol 2009;104(4):507–13.

24. van der Schaaf RJ, Claessen BE, Vis MM, et al. Effect of multivessel coronary disease with or without concurrent chronic total occlusion on one-year mortality in patients treated with primary percutaneous coronary intervention for cardiogenic shock. Am J Cardiol 2010;105(7):955–9.

25. Bauer T, Zeymer U, Hochadel M, et al. Use and outcomes of multivessel percutaneous coronary intervention in patients with acute myocardial infarction complicated by cardiogenic shock (from the EHS-PCI Registry). Am J Cardiol 2012;109(7):941–6.

26. Yang JH, Hahn JY, Song PS, et al. Percutaneous coronary intervention for nonculprit vessels in cardiogenic shock complicating ST-segment elevation acute myocardial infarction. Crit Care Med 2014;42(1):17–25.

27. Mylotte D, Morice M-C, Eltchaninoff H, et al. Primary percutaneous coronary intervention in patients with acute myocardial infarction, resuscitated cardiac arrest, and cardiogenic shock: the role of primary multivessel revascularization. JACC Cardiovasc Interv 2013;6(2):115–25.

28. Park JS, Cha KS, Lee DS, et al. Culprit or multivessel revascularisation in ST-elevation myocardial infarction with cardiogenic shock. Heart 2015;101(15):1225–32.

29. Windecker S, Kolh P, Alfonso F, et al. 2014 ESC/EACTS Guidelines on myocardial revascularization: The Task Force on Myocardial Revascularization of the European Society of Cardiology (ESC) and the European Association for Cardio-Thoracic Surgery (EACTS) developed with the special contribution of the European Association of Percutaneous Cardiovascular Interventions (EAPCI). Eur Heart J 2014;35(37):2541–619.

30. O'Gara PT, Kushner FG, Ascheim DD, et al. 2013 ACCF/AHA guideline for the management of ST-elevation myocardial infarction: a report of the American College of Cardiology Foundation/American Heart Association Task Force on Practice Guidelines. J Am Coll Cardiol 2013;61(4):e78–140.

31. Thiele H, Desch S, Piek JJ, et al. Multivessel versus culprit lesion only percutaneous revascularization plus potential staged revascularization in patients with acute myocardial infarction complicated by cardiogenic shock: design and rationale of CULPRIT-SHOCK trial. Am Heart J 2016;172:160–9.

Controversies and Challenges in the Management of ST-Elevation Myocardial Infarction Complicated by Cardiogenic Shock

Byung-Soo Ko, MD, Stavros G. Drakos, MD, PhD,
Frederick G.P. Welt, MD, MS, Rashmee U. Shah, MD, MS*

KEYWORDS

- Cardiogenic shock • Acute myocardial infarction • ST-elevation myocardial infarction
- Revascularization • Mechanical circulatory support

KEY POINTS

- Despite advances in treating acute myocardial infarction, cardiogenic shock in the setting of ST-elevation myocardial infarction has a poor prognosis, with high mortality rates.
- Few randomized clinical trials focused on this patient population have been completed, a reflection of the challenges in undertaking trials in this acutely ill population.
- We have little evidence to guide treatment, particularly with respect to quality of life outcomes. As a result, controversies surrounding treatment strategies in this patient population are more common than conclusions.

INTRODUCTION

Recent data suggest that mortality improvement among ST-elevation myocardial infarction (STEMI) patients has stagnated in recent years.[1] One interpretation of these findings is that the residual mortality among STEMI patients represents the sickest patients who are beyond benefit from rapid revascularization, including patients with cardiogenic shock (CS). STEMI complicated by CS remains one of the most challenging conditions to manage. Mortality rates are high, with up to one-half of all patients dying before hospital discharge.[2,3] Timely reperfusion with primary percutaneous coronary intervention (PCI; measured by door-to-balloon time) is a class I recommendation in the American College of Cardiology Foundation/American Heart Association guidelines for the management of patients with STEMI complicated by CS.[4] Despite continued improvement in the door-to-balloon time since the implementation of the

Disclosure Statement: BSK: none; Dr Drakos currently receives research support from the NIH, AHA, Department of Veterans Affairs, Doris Duke Foundation, Intermountain Research Medical Foundation, St Jude Medical (Thoratec) and Abiomed Inc. Dr Drakos is a consultant of Novartis and Heartware Inc.; Dr Welt serves on the scientific advisory board for Medtronic; RUS: none.
Division of Cardiovascular Medicine, University of Utah School of Medicine, 30 North 1900 East, Room 4A100, Salt Lake City, UT 84132, USA
* Corresponding author.
E-mail address: Rashmee.Shah@utah.edu

Intervent Cardiol Clin 5 (2016) 541–549
http://dx.doi.org/10.1016/j.iccl.2016.06.010
2211-7458/16/$ – see front matter © 2016 Elsevier Inc. All rights reserved.

guideline[5]; however, mortality rates remain high. We discuss different management strategies and challenges that limit progress in the treatment of CS.

EPIDEMIOLOGIC TRENDS IN ST-ELEVATION MYOCARDIAL INFARCTION COMPLICATED BY CARDIOGENIC SHOCK

The incidence of CS among STEMI patients has changed little in recent decades. In 1995, the GUSTO-I (Global Utilization of Streptokinase and Tissue Plasminogen Activator for Occluded Coronary Arteries I) investigators reported a 7.2% incidence rate and a 58% 30-day mortality rate among CS patients.[6] Since then, professional guidelines have urged more aggressive use of PCI in STEMI and several registries have reported CS incidence and outcome trends. A recent publication from the ACTION Registry-GTWG reported a CS incidence of 7.4% among all patients with acute myocardial infarction (AMI), and 12.2% among STEMI patients.[2] In France, however, investigators report CS among 5.7% of all AMI patients (Fig. 1).[7]

Mortality rates are uniformly high across different studies, despite variability between populations, study methods, and definitions (see Fig. 1). Roughly one-half of patients with AMI and CS will die during hospitalization. This variation in incidence and mortality can be attributed, in part, to methodologic differences between studies. Some reports rely on chart review for case identification, whereas others rely on administrative data. Quality measurement and reporting may introduce bias toward selection of healthier patients, thus underestimating the true incidence. In addition, patients are often complex with multiple causes of shock. These issues create challenges in understanding epidemiologic trends in CS and the impact of treatment strategies on outcomes.

Regardless of the study and methodologic approach, STEMI complicated by CS is undoubtedly a highly fatal condition. These findings raise an important question: Why does the mortality from CS remain high despite timely reperfusion and what treatment strategies might alter this prognosis?

PHARMACOLOGIC THERAPY

Supportive care for STEMI patients in CS often includes vasopressors and inotropes. Milrinone and dobutamine are inotropes that can increase cardiac contractility and decrease systemic vascular resistance. Both, however, increase myocardial oxygen consumption, an undesirable feature in the setting of AMI.[8] The SOAP II (Sepsis Occurrence in Acutely Ill Patients) study compared dopamine and norepinephrine including all types of shock patients; 16.7% had

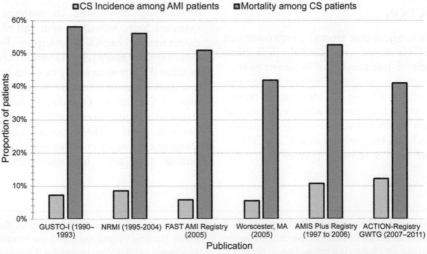

Fig. 1. Incidence and mortality rates among patients with AMI and cardiogenic shock (CS). GUSTO-I[6]: The Global Utilization of Streptokinase and Tissue Plasminogen Activator for Occluded Coronary Arteries; STEMI patients only. NRMI[3]: National Registry of Myocardial Infarction; all AMI patients. FAST AMI[7]: French Registry on Acute ST-elevation and non ST-elevation Myocardial Infarction; all AMI patients. Worcester, MA[49]: all AMI patients. AMIS Plus[50]: Acute myocardial infarction in Switzerland; STEMI patients only. ACTION Registry-GWTG[2]: Acute Coronary Treatment and Intervention Outcomes Network Registry-Get With the Guidelines; STEMI patients only. AMI, acute myocardial infarction; STEMI, ST-elevation myocardial infarction.

CS. The study was stopped early owing to lack of difference between the vasopressors, although there was a nonsignificant trend toward mortality benefit with norepinephrine in the CS subgroup.[9] To date, no other randomized controlled trials have been published that compare different inotrope/vasopressor strategies. Standard pharmacologic therapies, such as beta-blockers and angiotensin-converting enzymes inhibitors lower blood pressure and therefore are typically avoided in CS patients. The COMMIT trial (Clopidogrel and Metoprolol in Myocardial Infarction Trial), for example, showed that early, intravenous beta-blocker use is associated with an increased risk of CS, and thus should be limited to patients with demonstrated hemodynamic stability.[10]

Other pharmacologic strategies aim to decrease the infarct size by limiting reperfusion injury and addressing the inflammatory response induced by STEMI. These approaches have been used to prevent CS in STEMI patients, rather than treat CS that has already developed. Reperfusion injury is mediated by oxidative stress, intracellular calcium overload, and rapid improvement in pH that occurs when the occluded artery is opened. One hypothesis is that these factors allow a key mitochondrial membrane channel to open, which results in cell injury, death, and the development of CS.[11] Although animal and translational studies suggest that mitochondrial membrane channel inhibitors may limit infarct size, this theory has yet to be confirmed in clinical trials. The CIRCUS (Cyclosporine before PCI in Patients with Acute Myocardial Infarction) trial randomized patient with left anterior descending artery-related infarction to cyclosporine or placebo. As with most other pharmacologic trials, STEMI patients who had already developed CS were excluded, and cyclosporine did not reduce death or heart failure rates.[12]

The inflammatory response to STEMI has also been proposed as a treatment target. Myocardial ischemia triggers a systemic inflammatory response syndrome, resulting in vasoplegia despite low cardiac output, leading to multiorgan failure and death.[13] Nitric oxide is believed to play a key role in this pathologic response. Studies suggest that nitric oxide has a biphasic effects on myocardium, with a low pulsatile level providing cardioprotection and a high persistent level causing myocardial depression and vasoplegia.[14] Tilarginine, a nitric oxide synthatase inhibitor, is one of the few pharmacologic therapies that has been tested acutely among CS patients. A multicenter, randomized controlled trial (TRIUMPH [Tilarginine Acetate Injection in a Randomized International Study in Unstable MI Patients With Cardiogenic Shock]), enrolled 658 STEMI patients with CS randomized patients to tilarginine infusion or placebo. The 30-day mortality rates were similar between the tilarginine (48%) and placebo (42%) groups, and the trial was terminated early owing to futility.[15]

REVASCULARIZATION: MULTIVESSEL VERSUS CULPRIT VESSEL ONLY

Roughly one-half of patients with STEMI and CS have multivessel coronary disease and the management of nonculprit, diseased vessels is a topic of an ongoing debate. Multivessel revascularization (ie, performing PCI on culprit and nonculprit related vessels) has the theoretic benefit of restoring blood flow to ischemic territories (directly related to culprit lesion or indirectly related to hypotension or hyperdynamic noninfarct regions). These potential benefits have to be weighed against risks related to contrast, prolonged procedure times, or subacute closure. Major societal guidelines endorse multivessel revascularization as a class I indication—"Shock or severe HF is perhaps the only clinical scenario in which acute revascularization of significant stenoses in noninfarct arteries can be justified[4]"—but the risks and benefits of the 2 different strategies have yet to be tested in a randomized, controlled study. CS patients were excluded from recent randomized controlled trials comparing the 2 revascularization strategies in STEMI.[16–18]

The effect of multivessel revascularization in CS patients has been evaluated in several observational registries, and many report increased mortality with the multivessel approach.[19,20] Among STEMI patients with CS in the CathPCI Registry, for example, those treated with multivessel PCI versus culprit only PCI had higher in-hospital mortality rates (36.5% vs 27.8%).[21] One exception is an observational analysis from France, in which investigators evaluated 255 STEMI patients with CS or cardiac arrest, two-thirds had multivessel coronary disease. Death within 24 hours occurred in more than 25% of patients and rates did not differ between treatment strategies. The 6-month survival, however, was better in the multivessel group compared with the culprit only group (44% vs 21%; $P = .002$).[22] Retrospective analyses from Korea and Canada also demonstrated increased survival with a multivessel revascularization approach.[23,24] Notably, almost one-third of patients in French study had complete total occlusions and complete revascularization was achieved in only two-thirds of the multivessel PCI group. In the Korean and Canadian studies, multivessel revascularization with PCI was achieved in 17% and 24% of patients, respectively. The definitions of multivessel revascularization vary between these studies, and low success rates suggest a selection bias toward less complex coronary disease among survivors; these limitations preclude conclusions about the effect of intervention on nonculprit stenosis. A randomized trial comparing multivessel versus culprit only revascularization in all AMI patients is currently underway and should provide high-quality evidence to help inform this controversy.[25]

MECHANICAL CIRCULATORY SUPPORT

Mechanical circulatory support (MCS) devices are a potential treatment option for patients with STEMI and CS. Pharmacologic agents (inotropes and/or vasopressors) may ameliorate the noncardiac tissue hypoperfusion by increasing the cardiac output and systemic vascular resistance. However, these agents can worsen the supply–demand mismatch of the heart, especially in ischemia-induced CS. Most MCS devices, on the other hand, improve the supply–demand mismatch, and, based on several translational studies, salvage more myocardium when added to reperfusion therapy.[26–28] The intraaortic balloon pump (IABP) was the first MCS support device, initially used in the 1960s. Thiele and colleagues[29] evaluated the effect of the IABP in a randomized controlled trial of AMI patients with CS, and found that the use of IABP did not reduce 30-day mortality.

New MCS devices have emerged as the use of IABP has decreased over recent years.[30] The TandemHeart is a left atrium-to-femoral artery extracorporeal continuous flow pump that is technically challenging and time consuming to deploy. The procedure involves a transseptal puncture and is associated with ischemic complications to the lower extremity. The Impella LVAD (left ventricular assist device) system is a left ventricle-to-aorta continuous flow axial pump that is deployed through the femoral artery, a simpler approach compared with the TandemHeart. Seyfarth and colleagues[31] compared the hemodynamic effect and safety between Impella LP2.5 and IABP in a randomized study involving 26 patients with CS complicating STEMI. Hemodynamics improved to a greater degree with the Impella, without a significant

increase in complication rates. In patients with biventricular failure or concomitant respiratory failure, a venoarterial extracorporeal membrane oxygenation may be an option. Aside from observational analyses, evidence supporting the use of venoarterial extracorporeal membrane oxygenation is limited. One concern is that the device results in increased afterload, resulting in volume overload in a left ventricle with fixed contractility. The net effects are unfavorable hemodynamics, with an increase in the left ventricular end-diastolic pressure and pulmonary edema.[32]

Timing of MCS deployment, before reperfusion (upstream MCS support) versus bail out (provisional MCS support), is another source of controversy. Proponents of a provisional strategy argue that an emergent revascularization should take priority because it is the definitive therapy needed to reverse CS. One obvious advantage of this strategy is that MCS can be avoided in some patients. Proponents of the upstream strategy argue that mechanical unloading of the left ventricle by MCS prevents significant ischemic and reperfusion injury, ultimately leading to more salvaged myocardium. In support of this hypothesis, Meyns and colleagues[26] conducted a proof-of-concept study using a direct left ventricle-to-aorta continuous flow device in sheep models of myocardial infarction. The study showed that all the groups that had mechanical unloading showed a significant reduction in infarct size, and the group treated with the upstream strategy had the largest reduction. Evidence for the upstream MCS support in humans, however, is limited to observational studies. Abdel-Wahab et al[33] conducted a single-center, retrospective study of 48 CS patients complicating STEMI and showed that patients who received IABP before the PCI had significantly lower in-hospital mortality (19% vs 59%; $P = .007$) and major adverse cardiac and cerebrovascular events (23% vs 77%; $P<.001$). O'Neill and colleagues[34] identified 154 consecutive registry patients with STEMI and CS who underwent PCI and Impella 2.5 insertion and showed a similar result. These analyses are subject to selection bias, and a well-designed randomized controlled trial is needed to confirm these findings.

To date, none of the percutaneous MCS devices have been shown to improve survival in STEMI patients with CS (Table 1). A trial testing the effect of the Impella device on infarct size in STEMI patients was stopped early for unclear reasons.[35] Nevertheless, the use of these devices increased significantly over the past

Table 1
Short-term mortality of patients with cardiogenic shock treated with mechanical circulatory support

Study First Author, Publication Year	Sample Size	Type of MCS	30-d Mortality (MCS vs No MCS), %
Thiele et al,[51] 2005	41	TandemHeart vs IABP	43 vs 45; P = ns
Burkoff et al,[52] 2006	42	TandemHeart vs IABP	53 vs 64; P = ns
Seyfarth et al,[31] 2008	26	Impella 2.5 vs IABP	46 vs 46; P = ns
Combes et al,[53] 2008	81	ECMO (no comparison)	58[a,b]
Bermudez et al,[54] 2011	33	ECMO (no comparison)	36
Thiele et al,[29] 2012	600	IABP vs medical therapy	39 vs 49; P = ns
Lauten et al,[55] 2013	120	Impella 2.5 (no comparison)	64.2
O'Neill et al,[34] 2014	154	Impella 2.5 (no comparison)	50.7[a]
Kim et al,[56] 2012	27	ECMO (no comparison)	40.7[b]
Muller et al,[39] 2016	138	ECMO (no comparison)	58.7[c]

Abbreviations: ECMO, extracorporeal membrane oxygenation; IABP, intraaortic balloon pump; MCS, mechanical circulatory support.
[a] These studies reported in-hospital mortality.
[b] This study included multiple causes of cardiogenic shock, in addition to myocardial infarction.
[c] This study reported 6 month mortality.

decade[36] and providers must be aware of the risks associated with treatment. Complications include bleeding, neurologic events, and lower extremity injury, including amputation. Despite significant technological advances in modern percutaneous MCS devices, adverse events associated with the devices remain high (Table 2) and widespread MCS adoption may introduce unnecessary risk, resulting in patient harm. Lee and colleagues[37] performed a metaanalysis of 13 randomized controlled trials to evaluate the efficacy and safety of different MCS devices in patients with CS from ischemic etiology. The investigators concluded that routine use of percutaneous MCS was associated with significantly more bleeding complications without any improvement in early or late survival.

PATIENT SELECTION FOR INVASIVE AND LIFE-SUSTAINING TREATMENTS

STEMI patients with CS are extremely ill with a poor prognosis. As with any other treatment strategy, careful selection of patients who benefit the most from invasive strategies is critical. This task is especially difficult because treatment decisions related to PCI and MCS must be made immediately upon presentation, often with incomplete information regarding patient comorbidities and preferences. Various risk scores have been developed to predict in-hospital mortality among critically ill patients, but generally these scores have been used for case mix adjustment in retrospective analyses, rather than a prospective tool for patient selection. The Acute Physiology and Chronic Health

Table 2
Major adverse event rates with mechanical circulatory support devices

Event	TandemHeart[51] (%)	Impella[34] (%)	ECMO[57] (%)
Bleeding	42	18	40.8
Limb ischemia	4	21	16.9[a]
Infection	21	13	30.4
Acute renal dysfunction	21	18	55.6
Hemolysis	5	11	N/A

Abbreviations: ECMO, extracorporeal membrane oxygenation; N/A, not applicable.
[a] This study also reports lower extremity amputation in 4.7% of patients.

Evaluation score, for example, was developed to predict in-hospital mortality among a broad range of critically ill patients, included AMI patients. The model has good discrimination (area under the curve, 0.88), but is cumbersome with an extensive number of variables.[38] The electronic health record may facilitate immediate calculation of a validated risk score. An automated approach could allow for an objective measure of patient acuity before treatment decisions, if CS specific models that leverage the electronic health record are developed. Datapoints specific to CS in the setting of STEMI could include time between symptom onset and presentation, a measure of coronary disease complexity, or the presence of cardiac arrest. Muller and colleagues[39] recently published the ENCOURAGE (prEdictioN of CS OUtcome foR AMI patients salvaGed by VA-ECMO) score, a model to predict mortality in the intensive care unit, derived from 138 patients who received ECMO. The model performed better than prior AMI-specific models (area under the curve, 0.84), but requires prospective validation in a larger patient population with inclusion of patients not treated with MCS.

An automated, quantitative approach in conjunction with a multidisciplinary team may help to reduce variability in patient selection. Our institution's "Shock Team" is a multidisciplinary team comprised of advanced heart failure specialists, interventional cardiologists, cardiothoracic surgeons, and cardiac intensivists. Since April 2015, when a cardiogenic shock patient is identified in the emergency department or other areas of our hospital the team is activated through the standard hospital paging system. The on-call advanced heart failure cardiologist, interventional cardiologist, and cardiovascular intensive care unit attending evaluate the patient together, with the on-call cardiothoracic surgeon on standby. A protocol defines the sequence of diagnostic and therapeutic procedures for shock of various etiologies. It also provides specific criteria for when to consider implementing MCS. Our preliminary experience suggests that a multidisciplinary shock team approach is feasible and practical. Whether it can improve outcomes of patients with refractory cardiogenic shock requires further investigation. Proponents of a team based approach argue that having a dedicated "shock team" provides several advantages, including rapid identification of CS patients and provide immediate support to the providers. Opponents of this team-based approach argue that the strategy creates logistical challenges and will further

delay the care of critically patients with a time-sensitive condition.

PATIENT-CENTERED OUTCOMES OTHER THAN MORTALITY

Most, if not all, studies of treatment effectiveness in CS patients complicating STEMI assess mortality as a primary outcome. Still, additional outcomes such as repeat hospitalizations, functional status, and quality of life are equally important in these patients. In fact, a landmark analysis of AMI patients with CS found that 59% will die or be rehospitalized within 1 year of hospital discharge.[40] A new treatment that manages to save a patient's life only to leave the patient with disabling complications may be difficult to call a success, despite a "positive" trial. Unfortunately, there is a scarcity of data on quality of life outcomes in STEMI patients with CS.

Sleeper and colleagues[41] reported on the long-term functional status of survivors from the SHOCK trial. At 1 year, 83% of survivors had New York Heart Association functional class of I or II (57% with New York Heart Association functional class I). The authors also evaluated the Multidimensional Index of Life Quality and found that, among 1-year survivors, the mean Multidimensional Index of Life Quality score was 19 (range 4–28) and the mean score for the life satisfaction questionnaires was 7 (on a scale of 1 [worst possible life] to 10 [best possible life]). The authors concluded that patients who survived CS had good long-term functional status. Although reassuring, we must keep in mind that the sickest patients died early in both these reports, creating a survivor bias in subsequent functional outcomes. Despite our best attention, these life-saving, heroic, and invasive measures might actually prolong death in certain patient groups.

RANDOMIZED TRIALS IN ST-ELEVATION MYOCARDIAL INFARCTION PATIENTS WITH CARDIOGENIC SHOCK

All approaches to treat CS—pharmacologic, revascularization, and MCS—are difficult to test because of challenges surrounding informed consent in critically ill patients.[42] This challenge is a central barrier to improving mortality in STEMI patients with CS. The US Food and Drug Administration allows exceptions to informed consent in a narrow range of critically patients, "who are in need of emergency medical intervention but who cannot give informed consent because of their life-threatening medical condition, and who do not have a legally authorized person to represent them.[43]" STEMI patients with CS do not always fit into this exception because they are often awake and family members are present. Still, truly informed consent for CS interventions is impractical. Patients and families cannot possibly understand the nuances of clinical research within the timeframe needed to treat the patient, and providers cannot provide adequate explanation in just a few minutes. We have an imperative to improve outcomes in CS, but are faced with an ethical challenge: obtaining informed consent in the acute setting or randomizing patients under an exception of informed consent?

The issue of informed consent in AMI was recently addressed in the HEAT-PPCI (How Effective are Antithrombotic Therapies in Primary Percutaneous Coronary Intervention) trial.[44] This trial used a delayed consent process, in which patients were treated randomly with heparin or bivalirudin and consented afterward for data use; only 4 of 1820 patients declined enrollment in HEAT-PPCI.[45] Supporters of this approach argue that upfront consent would have been unethical, delayed consent was an appropriate ethical design, and the trial importantly demonstrated efficacy of a more cost-effective treatment strategy.[46] Although this approach seems feasible and acceptable to patients and regulators, an invasive intervention such as Impella or Tandem-Heart may not be as acceptable in the absence of informed consent.

SUMMARY

The prognosis of STEMI has improved dramatically since the introduction of coronary care units, revascularization, and anticoagulant strategies, but CS remains a highly fatal condition. Despite efforts to improve outcomes, the prognosis has not improved in recent decades. Controversies remain about optimal pharmacologic therapies, revascularization strategies, the role of MCS, and evidence-based patient selection—and the interaction between these parts of the care pathway. The current informed consent paradigm for clinical trials creates challenges testing treatments in CS patients, who are too ill to consent and require immediate treatment. Fortunately, several trials are underway that compare revascularization strategies[25] and MCS options.[47,48] Although the current prognosis for STEMI patients with CS is grim, careful, scientific assessment of new and existing treatments could change the course of this condition in the coming years.

REFERENCES

1. Shah RU, Henry TD, Rutten-Ramos S, et al. Increasing percutaneous coronary interventions for ST-segment elevation myocardial infarction in the United States: progress and opportunity. JACC Cardiovasc Interv 2015;8:139–46.
2. Anderson ML, Peterson ED, Peng SA, et al. Differences in the profile, treatment, and prognosis of patients with cardiogenic shock by myocardial infarction classification: a report from NCDR. Circ Cardiovasc Qual Outcomes 2013;6:708–15.
3. Babaev A, Frederick PD, Pasta DJ, et al. Trends in management and outcomes of patients with acute myocardial infarction complicated by cardiogenic shock. JAMA 2005;294:448–54.
4. O'Gara PT, Kushner FG, Ascheim DD, et al. 2013 ACCF/AHA guideline for the management of ST-elevation myocardial infarction. J Am Coll Cardiol 2013;61:e78–140.
5. Menees DS, Peterson ED, Wang Y, et al. Door-to-balloon time and mortality among patients undergoing primary PCI. N Engl J Med 2013;369:901–9.
6. Holmes DR Jr, Bates ER, Kleiman NS, et al. Contemporary reperfusion therapy for cardiogenic shock: the GUSTO-I trial experience. J Am Coll Cardiol 1995;26:668–74.
7. Aissaoui N, Puymirat E, Tabone X, et al. Improved outcome of cardiogenic shock at the acute stage of myocardial infarction: a report from the USIK 1995, USIC 2000, and FAST-MI French nationwide registries. Eur Heart J 2012;33:2535–43.
8. Nativi-Nicolau J, Selzman CH, Fang JC, et al. Pharmacologic therapies for acute cardiogenic shock. Curr Opin Cardiol 2014;29:250–7.
9. De Backer D, Biston P, Devriendt J, et al. Comparison of dopamine and norepinephrine in the treatment of shock. N Engl J Med 2010;362:779–89.
10. Chen ZM, Pan HC, Chen YP, et al, COMMIT (ClOpidogrel and Metoprolol in Myocardial Infarction Trial) collaborative group. Early intravenous then oral metoprolol in 45,852 patients with acute myocardial infarction: randomised placebo-controlled trial. Lancet 2005;366:1622–32.
11. Hausenloy DJ, Yellon DM. Myocardial ischemia-reperfusion injury: a neglected therapeutic target. J Clin Invest 2013;123:92–100.
12. Cung T-T, Morel O, Cayla G, et al. Cyclosporine before PCI in patients with acute myocardial infarction. N Engl J Med 2015;373:1021–31.
13. Drexler H. Nitric oxide synthases in the failing human heart: a doubled-edged sword? Circulation 1999;99:2972–5.

14. Feng Q, Lu X, Jones DL, et al. Increased inducible nitric oxide synthase expression contributes to myocardial dysfunction and higher mortality after myocardial infarction in mice. Circulation 2001; 104:700–4.

15. TRIUMPH Investigators The. Effect of tilarginine acetate in patients with acute myocardial infarction and cardiogenic shock: the TRIUMPH randomized controlled trial. JAMA 2007;297:1657–66.

16. Wald DS, Morris JK, Wald NJ, et al. Randomized trial of preventive angioplasty in myocardial infarction. N Engl J Med 2013;369:1115–23.

17. Gershlick AH, Khan JN, Kelly DJ, et al. Randomized trial of complete versus lesion-only revascularization in patients undergoing primary percutaneous coronary intervention for STEMI and multivessel disease: the CVULPRIT trial. J Am Coll Cardiol 2015;65:963–72.

18. Engstrom T, Kelbæk H, Helqvist S, et al. Complete revascularisation versus treatment of the culprit lesion only in patients with ST-segment elevation myocardial infarction and multivessel disease (DANAMI-3 PRIMULTI): an open-label, randomised controlled trial. Lancet 2015;386: 665–71.

19. Thiele H, Ohman EM, Desch S, et al. Management of cardiogenic shock. Eur Heart J 2015;36:1223–30.

20. Zeymer U, Hochadel M, Thiele H, et al. Immediate multivessel percutaneous coronary intervention versus culprit lesion intervention in patients with acute myocardial infarction complicated by cardiogenic shock: results of the ALKK-PCI registry. EuroIntervention 2015;11:280–5.

21. Cavender MA, Milford-Beland S, Roe MT, et al. Prevalence, predictors, and in-hospital outcomes of non-infarct artery intervention during primary percutaneous coronary intervention for ST-segment elevation myocardial infarction (from the National Cardiovascular Data Registry). Am J Cardiol 2009;104:507–13.

22. Mylotte D, Morice M-C, Eltchaninoff H, et al. Primary percutaneous coronary intervention in patients with acute myocardial infarction, resuscitated cardiac arrest, and cardiogenic shock: the role of primary multivessel revascularization. JACC Cardiovasc Interv 2013;6:115–25.

23. Park JS, Cha KS, Lee DS, et al, Korean Acute Myocardial Infarction Registry Investigators. Culprit or multivessel revascularisation in ST-elevation myocardial infarction with cardiogenic shock. Heart 2015;101:1225–32.

24. Hussain F, Philipp RK, Ducas RA, et al. The ability to achieve complete revascularization is associated with improved in-hospital survival in cardiogenic shock due to myocardial infarction: Manitoba cardiogenic shock registry investigators. Catheter Cardiovasc Interv 2011;78:540–8.

25. Thiele H, Desch S, Piek JJ, et al. Multivessel versus culprit lesion only percutaneous revascularization plus potential staged revascularization in patients with acute myocardial infarction complicated by cardiogenic shock: design and rationale of culprit-SHOCK trial. Am Heart J 2016;172:160–9.

26. Meyns B, Stolinski J, Leunens V, et al. Left ventricular support by catheter-mounted axial flow pump reduces infarct size. J Am Coll Cardiol 2003;41: 1087–95.

27. Achour H, Boccalandro F, Felli P, et al. Mechanical left ventricular unloading prior to reperfusion reduces infarct size in a canine infarction model. Catheter Cardiovasc Interv 2005;64:182–92.

28. Nanas JN, Nanas SN, Kontoyannis DA, et al. Myocardial salvage by the use of reperfusion and intraaortic balloon pump: experimental study. Ann Thorac Surg 1996;61:629–34.

29. Thiele H, Zeymer U, Neumann F-J, et al. Intra-aortic balloon support for myocardial infarction with cardiogenic shock. N Engl J Med 2012;367: 1287–96.

30. Patel H, Shivaraju A, Fonarow GC, et al. Temporal trends in the use of intraaortic balloon pump associated with percutaneous coronary intervention in the United States, 1998-2008. Am Heart J 2014; 168:363–73.e12.

31. Seyfarth M, Sibbing D, Bauer I, et al. A randomized clinical trial to evaluate the safety and efficacy of a percutaneous left ventricular assist device versus intra-aortic balloon pumping for treatment of cardiogenic shock caused by myocardial infarction. J Am Coll Cardiol 2008;52:1584–8.

32. Burkhoff D, Sayer G, Doshi D, et al. Hemodynamics of mechanical circulatory support. J Am Coll Cardiol 2015;66:2663–74.

33. Abdel-Wahab M, Saad M, Kynast J, et al. Comparison of hospital mortality with intra-aortic balloon counterpulsation insertion before versus after primary percutaneous coronary intervention for cardiogenic shock complicating acute myocardial infarction. Am J Cardiol 2010;105:967–71.

34. O'Neill WW, Schreiber T, Wohns DH, et al. The current use of Impella 2.5 in acute myocardial infarction complicated by cardiogenic shock: results from the USPella registry. J Interv Cardiol 2014;27: 1–11.

35. Clinicaltrials.Gov. Minimizing infarct size with Impella 2.5 following PCI for acute myocardial infarction. Available at: https://clinicaltrials.Gov/ct2/show/nct01319760. Accessed April 19, 2016.

36. Stretch R, Sauer CM, Yuh DD, et al. National trends in the utilization of short-term mechanical circulatory support: Incidence, outcomes, and cost analysis. J Am Coll Cardiol 2014;64:1407–15.

37. Lee JM, Park J, Kang J, et al. The efficacy and safety of mechanical hemodynamic support in patients

undergoing high-risk percutaneous coronary intervention with or without cardiogenic shock: Bayesian approach network meta-analysis of 13 randomized controlled trials. Int J Cardiol 2015;184:36–46.

38. Zimmerman J, Md F, Kramer A, et al. Acute Physiology and Chronic Health Evaluation (APACHE) IV: Hospital mortality assessment for today's critically ill patients. Crit Care Med 2006;34:1297–310.

39. Muller G, Flecher E, Lebreton G, et al. The encourage mortality risk score and analysis of long-term outcomes after VA-ECMO for acute myocardial infarction with cardiogenic shock. Intensive Care Med 2016;42:370–8.

40. Shah RU, de Lemos JA, Wang TY, et al. Post-hospital outcomes of patients with acute myocardial infarction with cardiogenic shock: findings from the NCDR. J Am Coll Cardiol 2016;67:739–47.

41. Sleeper LA, Ramanathan K, Picard MH, et al. Functional status and quality of life after emergency revascularization for cardiogenic shock complicating acute myocardial infarction. J Am Coll Cardiol 2005;46:266–73.

42. Dickert NW, Brown J, Cairns CB, et al. Confronting ethical and regulatory challenges of emergency care research with conscious patients. Ann Emerg Med 2016;67:538–45.

43. Exception from informed consent for studies conducted in emergency settings: regulatory language and excerpts from preamble- information sheet. Available at: http://www.Fda.Gov/regulatory information/guidances/ucm126482.Htm. Accessed April 11, 2016.

44. Shahzad A, Kemp I, Mars C, et al. Unfractionated heparin versus bivalirudin in primary percutaneous coronary intervention (HEAT-PPCI): an open-label, single centre, randomised controlled trial. Lancet 2014;384:1849–58.

45. Dickert NW, Miller FG. Involving patients in enrolment decisions for acute myocardial infarction trials. BMJ 2015;351:h3791.

46. Shaw D. HEAT-PPCI sheds light on consent in pragmatic trials. Lancet 2014;384:1826–7.

47. Danish cardiogenic SHOCK trial (DANSHOCK). Clinicaltrials.gov identifier: NCT01633502. Available at: https://clinicaltrials.Gov/ct2/show/nct01633502?Term=cardiogenic+shock&rank=8. Accessed April 14, 2016.

48. Clinical study of extra-corporal life support in cardiogenic shock complicating acute myocardial infarction (ECLS SHOCK). Clinicaltrials.gov identifier: Nct02544594. Available at: https://clinicaltrials.Gov/ct2/show/nct02544594?Term=cardiogenic+shock&rank=7. Accessed April 14, 2016.

49. Goldberg RJ, Spencer FA, Gore JM, et al. Thirty-year trends (1975 to 2005) in the magnitude of, management of, and hospital death rates associated with cardiogenic shock in patients with acute myocardial infarction: a population-based perspective. Circulation 2009;119:1211–9.

50. Jeger RV, Radovanovic D, Hunziker PR, et al. Ten-year trends in the incidence and treatment of cardiogenic shock. Ann Intern Med 2008;149:618–26.

51. Thiele H, Sick P, Boudriot E, et al. Randomized comparison of intra-aortic balloon support with a percutaneous left ventricular assist device in patients with revascularized acute myocardial infarction complicated by cardiogenic shock. Eur Heart J 2005;26:1276–83.

52. Burkhoff D, Cohen H, Brunckhorst C, et al. A randomized multicenter clinical study to evaluate the safety and efficacy of the TandemHeart percutaneous ventricular assist device versus conventional therapy with intraaortic balloon pumping for treatment of cardiogenic shock. Am Heart J 2006;152:469.e1-8.

53. Combes A, Leprince P, Luyt CE, et al. Outcomes and long-term quality-of-life of patients supported by extracorporeal membrane oxygenation for refractory cardiogenic shock. Crit Care Med 2008; 36:1404–11.

54. Bermudez CA, Rocha RV, Toyoda Y, et al. Extracorporeal membrane oxygenation for advanced refractory shock in acute and chronic cardiomyopathy. Ann Thorac Surg 2011;92:2125–31.

55. Lauten A, Engstrom AE, Jung C, et al. Percutaneous left-ventricular support with the Impella-2.5-assist device in acute cardiogenic shock: results of the Impella-Euroshock-registry. Circ Heart Fail 2013;6:23–30.

56. Kim H, Lim SH, Hong J, et al. Efficacy of venoarterial extracorporeal membrane oxygenation in acute myocardial infarction with cardiogenic shock. Resuscitation 2012;83:971–5.

57. Cheng R, Hachamovitch R, Kittleson M, et al. Complications of extracorporeal membrane oxygenation for treatment of cardiogenic shock and cardiac arrest: a meta-analysis of 1,866 adult patients. Ann Thorac Surg 2014;97:610–6.

Controversies in Out of Hospital Cardiac Arrest?

Rahul P. Sharma, MD[a,*], Dion Stub, MD, PhD[b]

KEYWORDS

- Cardiac arrest • Out of hospital cardiac arrest • Cardiopulmonary resuscitation • Hypothermia
- Coronary angiography

KEY POINTS

- Out-of-hospital cardiac arrest has traditionally been associated with low rates of survival.
- Long-term prognosis is poor, largely due to impaired neurocognitive function.
- Trend toward improved outcomes with implementation of key measures directed at post arrest management.

BACKGROUND

Cardiac arrest is a major cause of morbidity and mortality and is often the initial presentation of cardiovascular disease. Cardiac arrest accounts for nearly 500,000 deaths annually in the United States. In patients suffering out-of-hospital cardiac arrest (OHCA), survival is less than 15% with considerable regional variation (Fig. 1), compared with approximately 22% for in-hospital cardiac arrest (IHCA).[1–4] Although most deaths due to OHCA still occur during the initial resuscitation, an increasing proportion occur in patients hospitalized after initially successful resuscitation. In patients who initially achieve return of spontaneous circulation (ROSC) after OHCA, the significant subsequent morbidity and mortality is due to "post cardiac arrest syndrome" (Table 1), which includes anoxic brain injury, post cardiac arrest myocardial dysfunction, systemic ischemia/reperfusion response, and persistent precipitating pathology.[5,6] Until recently, most single interventions have yielded little improvement in rates of survival; however, there is growing recognition that optimal treatment strategies during the postresuscitation phase may improve outcomes.[5,7]

OHCA treatment requires a multidisciplinary approach, and the development of cardiac arrest pathways and treatment at dedicated cardiac arrest centers have been shown to improve clinical outcomes.

MANAGEMENT CONSIDERATIONS AND CONTROVERSIES

Much of the research in an effort to improving clinical outcomes has been directed to improving prehospital management[8,9] (Fig. 2). Following the most crucial initial step of ensuring ROSC, the primary objective is to maintain adequate cerebral perfusion and limit neurologic impairment.[10] Implementation of a standardized treatment protocol with a multidisciplinary approach can significantly improve clinical outcomes.[11]

Prehospital Care

The primary aim of prehospital management is minimizing time to ROSC. This in turn is dependent on whether the arrest was witnessed and the delivery of adequate cardiopulmonary resuscitation (CPR). Recent changes to resuscitation guidelines have resulted in abolition of the requirements for assisted breaths with a focus on chest compressions alone.[12] In some instances,

---

Disclosures: None of the contributing authors have financial disclosures or relationships with industry that pertain to this article.
[a] Cedars-Sinai Heart Institute, Beverly Boulevard, Los Angeles, CA 90048, USA; [b] Alfred and Western Hospital, Monash University, Baker IDI Heart and Diabetes Institute, Melbourne, Victoria, Australia
* Corresponding author.
E-mail address: rahul.sharma@cshs.org

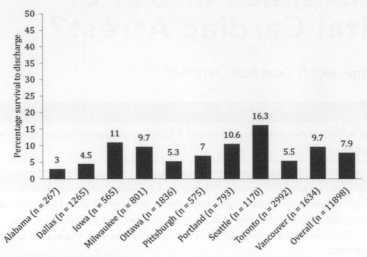

Fig. 1. Regional variation in survival of OHCA.

| Table 1 |
| Post cardiac arrest syndrome |

	Anoxic Brain Injury	Arrest-Related Myocardial Dysfunction	Systemic Ischemic/ Reperfusion Response	Persistent Precipitating Pathology
Pathophysiology	• Disrupted calcium homeostasis • Free radical formation • Cell death signaling pathways • Reperfusion injury • No-reflow Additional insults: • Pyrexia • Hyperglycemia • Hyperoxygenation	• Stunning phenomenon • Global hypokinesis • Elevated LVEDP • Preserved coronary blood flow (excluding patients with ACS)	• Intra-arrest global tissue hypotension • Reperfusion injury • Endothelial activation • Systemic inflammation • Activation of clotting cascades • Intravascular volume depletion • Disturbed vaso-regulation • Risk of infection	• ACS plaque rupture/thrombus formation • Chronic ischemic myocardial scar • Pulmonary embolism • Cardiomyopathies • Dilated • Restrictive • Hypertrophic • Genetic • Channelopathy • Congenital
Potential therapeutic approaches	• Therapeutic hypothermia • Early hemodynamic optimization • Ventilation and airway protection • Seizure control • Controlled oxygenation	• Systems of care • Revascularization • Intravenous fluid • Inotropes • IABP • ECMO • LVAD	• Goal-directed therapy • Intravenous fluids • Vasopressors • Glucose control • Hemofiltration • Antimicrobials	Address disease-specific etiology

Abbreviations: ACS, acute coronary syndrome; ECMO, extracorporeal membrane oxygenation; IABP, intra-aortic balloon pump; LVAD, left ventricular assist device; LVEDP, left ventricular end diastolic pressure.

From Stub D, Bernard S, Duffy SJ, et al. Post cardiac arrest syndrome: a review of therapeutic strategies. Circulation 2011;123:1428–35; with permission.

OHCA

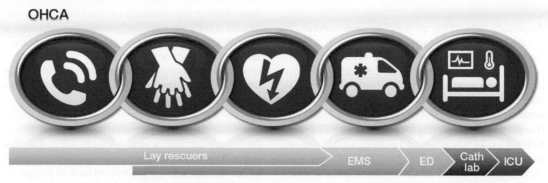

Fig. 2. American Heart Association OHCA chain of survival. Cath lab, catheterization laboratory; ED, emergency department; EMS, emergency medical services; ICU, intensive care unit. (*From* Kronick SL, Kurz MC, Lin S, et al. Part 4: Systems of Care and Continuous Quality Improvement: 2015 American Heart Association Guidelines Update for Cardiopulmonary Resuscitation and Emergency Cardiovascular Care. Circulation 2015;132(18 Suppl 2): S397–413; with permission.)

such as when CPR is given by untrained by-standers, or is required for long durations, it is difficult to maintain sustained quality CPR. However, with improved access to and ease of use of automated external defibrillators (AEDs) and new mechanical chest compression devices (eg, LUCAS [Jolife, Lund, Sweden] and AutoPulse [Zoll Circulation, Chelmsford, MA]), adequate chest compression can be established and maintained for prolonged periods. Once ROSC has been established, the aim is to stabilize the patient and transfer to a dedicated cardiac arrest center.

Cardiac Arrest Centers
The resources and experience necessary to deliver high-quality postresuscitation care may not be available uniformly across all hospitals. Based on studies reflecting marked variation in cardiac arrest survival across hospitals, expert committee recommendations advocate for regionalization of postresuscitation care in specialized centers.[13–16] Common general elements include[1] multidisciplinary collaboration (emergency medicine, cardiology, neurology, pulmonary, and critical care),[2] a designated hospital unit for admitting all post arrest patients with capability to deliver therapeutic hypothermia,[3] a standardized treatment protocol to ensure that care processes are consistent,[4] a dedicated on-call cardiac arrest consult team,[5] avoidance of early neuro-prognostication, and[6] ongoing data collection to monitor and improve quality of care.[14–17]

In-Hospital Care
Following ROSC, the aim is to maintain adequate cardio-cerebral perfusion, stable hemodynamics, and minimize ischemia-reperfusion injury.[18] Fig. 3 illustrates a stepwise approach to the management principles following OHCA.

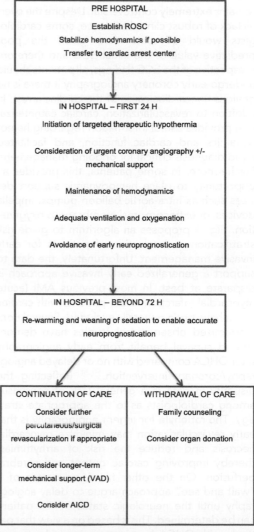

Fig. 3. Systematic approach to post-cardiac arrest care. AICD, automated implantable cardiac defibrillator; VAD, ventricular assist device.

Coronary angiography

Approximately 80% of OHCAs are cardiac in origin.[19,20] An electrocardiogram (ECG) should be recorded as soon as possible following ROSC to assess for the presence of ST elevation or new left bundle branch block.[12] These patients in particular benefit from early coronary angiography revascularization.[21–24] Current guidelines recommend early angiography for patients with ST elevation on a postresuscitation 12-lead ECG; however, the ECG has poor accuracy in this setting.[25] The absence of ST elevation does not exclude the presence of critical coronary stenosis. In one study, the negative predictive value for a critical coronary lesion was only approximately 42%, whereas 58% still had a critical lesion despite the absence of ST elevation.[19] However, the treatment of a patient with ROSC after OHCA and without ST-elevation remains extremely controversial. Despite the overall lack of robust clinical evidence, some cardiologists would advocate that, given the poor predictive value of the initial ECG and therefore irrespective of the ECG findings, all patients should undergo early coronary angiography if there is no obvious noncardiac cause of the cardiac arrest. In addition to revascularization, cardiac catheterization provides useful information regarding hemodynamics and cardiac function, and facilitated rapid diagnosis critical for ongoing management. Furthermore, in some patients, this provides an opportunity to place hemodynamic support devices such as intra-aortic balloon pumps, Impella devices, or extracorporeal membranous oxygenation. Fig. 4 proposes an algorithm to guide risk stratification and selection of patients for early invasive management. Unfortunately, the data to support a generalized early invasive approach is disparate at best. In most previous AMI (acute myocardial infarction) trials, patients with cardiac arrest have been generally excluded. Several non-randomized observational studies have demonstrated survival benefit from early angiography after OHCA compared with no or delayed angiography/coronary intervention.[19,24] Reflecting the disparity in data is a general lack of consensus among cardiologists as to the appropriate strategy. The rationale for urgent angiography is that early revascularization may minimize myocardial necrosis and reduce the risk of arrhythmias, thereby improving cardiac output and cerebral perfusion. On the other hand, advocates of a "wait and see" approach argue to delay angiography until the neurologic status of the patient can be determined. This is based on a view that patients with OHCA have a poor survival rate and often remain neurologically impaired. However, neurologic prognostication in the initial post arrest period is difficult, especially under the influence of hypothermia and sedation. Finally, in the current era of public outcomes reporting,[26] concern about the impact of poor outcomes on hospital reputation may steer clinicians toward a more conservative strategy.

Therapeutic hypothermia

Although cardiac arrest impacts all organ systems, its impact is most profound on the brain, which is exquisitely sensitive to lack of oxygen.[27] Post cardiac arrest anoxic brain injury is a major cause of morbidity and mortality and is responsible for approximately two-thirds of the deaths in the post cardiac arrest period.[28] During cardiac arrest, brain tissue becomes ischemic. After ROSC, rapid reoxygenation leads to oxygen free-radical production, which can lead to secondary cell death. Cooling slows cellular metabolism and reduces oxygen demand. Targeted therapeutic hypothermia (TTH) is a strategy of intentionally lowering body temperature with the goal of reducing ischemia-mediated and reperfusion-mediated neurologic injury.[27] TTH is the only post-ROSC intervention shown to improve survival from OHCA.[29–31]

Although prehospital cooling has not been demonstrated in randomized trials to confer a benefit in survival or neurologic recovery, there is evidence to suggest that extensive delays to institute TTH are associated with increased mortality. Indeed, one large study investigating regional systems to improve access to cooling found a 20% increase in the risk of death (95% confidence interval, 4%–39%) for every hour of delay to initiation of cooling.[32] The target temperature will depend on the clinical situation. Current guidelines suggest selecting and maintaining a temperature between 32 and 36°C.[12] Higher temperatures might be preferred in patients for whom lower temperatures convey some risk (eg, bleeding)[33,34] and lower temperatures might be preferred when patients have clinical features that are worsened at higher temperatures (eg, seizures, cerebral edema).[35–37] In clinical practice, TTH can be provided by using a number of different methods. These can be classified into surface-cooling methods (eg, use of ice packs around the body) or core-cooling methods (eg, intravenous catheters that circulate cold saline) or a combination approach. Once target temperature is achieved, it should be maintained for a period of 12 to 24 hours. Sedatives and paralytic agents are usually necessary to ensure comfort and prevent shivering.

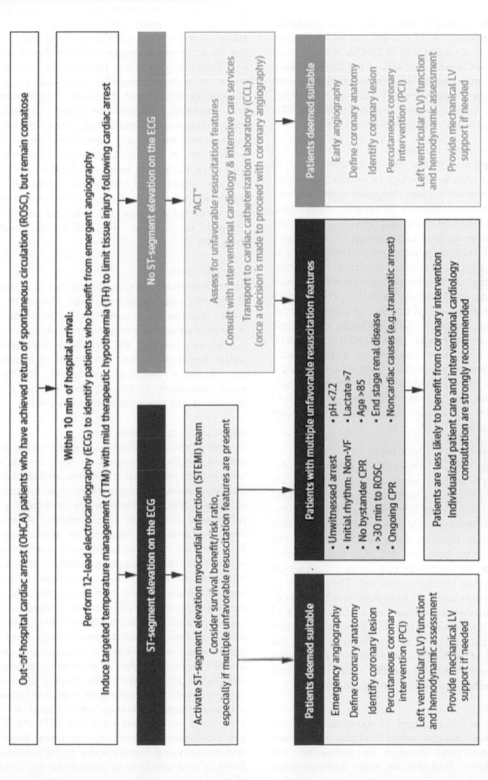

Fig. 4. Algorithm for risk stratification of cardiac arrest patients. ACT, assessment, consultation, transport; VF, ventricular fibrillation. (*From* Rab T, Kern KB, Tamis-Holland JE, et al. A Treatment algorithm for emergent invasive cardiac procedures in the resuscitated comatose patient. J Am Coll Cardiol 2015;66(1):62–73; with permission.)

Rewarming should be accomplished slowly at 0.25 to 0.5°C per hour with special care to avoid hyperthermia.[27]

Despite strong evidence and clear guideline recommendations, TTH is still not widely implemented. In a recent trial of OHCA in the United States and Canada, just 48% of the 2289 enrolled patients admitted to hospital were treated with therapeutic hypothermia.[38] Lack of resources, cost, and logistical difficulties of instituting TTH may serve as barriers to implementation.

Antiarrhythmic therapy

Antiarrhythmic drugs are used commonly in OHCA for shock-refractory ventricular fibrillation or pulseless ventricular tachycardia, but without proven survival benefit. A recent randomized, double-blind trial compared parenteral amiodarone, lidocaine, and saline placebo, along with standard care, in adults who had nontraumatic OHCA, shock-refractory ventricular fibrillation or pulseless ventricular tachycardia after at least one shock, and vascular access.[39] The primary outcome was survival to hospital discharge; the secondary outcome was favorable neurologic function at discharge. Overall, neither amiodarone nor lidocaine resulted in a significantly higher rate of survival or favorable neurologic outcome than the rate with placebo among patients with OHCA due to initial shock-refractory ventricular fibrillation or pulseless ventricular tachycardia.[39]

Hemodynamic management

Following OHCA, patients are often hemodynamically unstable, due to a combination of factors including the precipitating cause of arrest and the subsequent ischemia-reperfusion injury. Although immediately correcting and avoiding hypotension (systolic pressure <90 mm Hg and mean arterial pressure <65 mm Hg) is clearly beneficial, the optimum postresuscitation blood pressure has not been defined. The goal is to maintain cerebral perfusion despite impaired cerebral autoregulation but not at the expense of increased myocardial demand. Inotropic support (pharmacologic and/or mechanical) may be required to maintain cardiac output during the initial period of myocardial dysfunction and ensure adequate end-organ perfusion.

Oxygen

During the initial stages of reperfusion, excessive tissue oxygen concentrations may compound neuronal damage by increasing the production of free radicals, which damage mitochondria. A clinical registry study that included more than 6000 patients, based on the first documented arterial blood gas sample, postresuscitation hyperoxemia was associated with worse outcome than both normoxemia and hypoxemia.[40] However, another clinical registry study of more than 12,000 patients that used the lowest arterial oxygen pressure (PaO_2) value and controlling for more potential confounders (such as sickness severity) did not show a convincing association between hypervolemia and mortality.[41] Based on these conflicting data, unnecessary arterial hyperoxemia should be avoided, particularly during the initial post cardiac arrest period. Guidelines recommend that once ROSC has been established and the oxygen saturation of arterial blood ($SaO2$) can be monitored reliably (by pulse oximetry and/or arterial blood gas analysis), inspired oxygen is titrated to achieve an $SaO2$ of greater than 94%.[12]

Glycemic control

Attempted intensive glucose control in critically ill patients has repeatedly been shown to increase the risk for severe hypoglycemia, which is associated with worse outcomes. Accordingly, guidelines state that the benefit of any specific target range of glucose management is uncertain. From a practical standpoint, it would seem reasonable to correct severe hyperglycemia and avoid episodes of hypoglycemia.

Neuroprognostication

Despite significant advances in postresuscitative care, a significant proportion of patients will have a poor neurologic outcome. Accurate and timely neurologic prognostication is important to ensure the appropriateness and timing of withdrawal of active management. A study from the American Academy of Neurology in 2006 showed that at 72 hours, incomplete recovery of brainstem reflexes, myoclonus, extension posturing or absent motor response to pain, and bilaterally absent somatosensory cortical evoked potentials (N20) were described as being associated with a 0% false-positive rate for poor outcome (ie, lack of awakening). Furthermore, serum neuron-specific enolase and cerebral MRI were regarded as promising to help in identifying patients with little chance of neurologic recovery.[42] However, an important caveat was that these guidelines were based almost exclusively on data from the pre-TTH era. TTH can significantly impact normal body function and recovery and therefore use of the previously listed criteria can lead to premature withdrawal of care. Moreover, sedative and paralytic agents commonly used during targeted temperature management can accumulate due to a reduction in drug clearance, making neurologic assessment difficult. Therefore, the American Heart Association and the International Liaison Committee on Resuscitation strongly recommend that assessment of neurologic prognosis should be delayed for at least 72 hours after rewarming.[43] At that point, clinical examination findings that may predict a poor neurologic outcome include absence of pupillary light reflex and status myoclonus. An abnormal motor examination may identify patients who will require further prognostic testing. Electroencephalogram (absence of activity or persistent burst suppression) and evoked potentials (bilateral absence of somatosensory evoked potentials) are useful in predicting poor outcome. Computed tomography imaging with evidence of edema manifest as reduced gray-white ratio is predictive of poor neurologic outcome. Blood markers should not be used alone to predict outcomes.[12]

Organ donation

Up to 16% of patients who achieve sustained ROSC after cardiac arrest develop clinical brain death and can be considered for organ donation.[44] Transplant outcomes from the use of these organs are similar to those achieved with organs from other brain-dead donors.[45] All patients who fail to show signs of neurologic recovery after OHCA should be actively considered for organ donation.[46] Current guideline recommendations suggest that all patients who are resuscitated from cardiac arrest but who subsequently progress to death or brain death be evaluated for organ donation.[12]

SUMMARY

OHCA has traditionally been associated with extremely poor clinical outcomes, particularly low rates of survival. For those who do survive to discharge, optimism regarding long-term prognosis is guarded, largely due to impaired neurocognitive function. However, in recent years, with the implementation of a number of key advances in cardiac arrest management, there has been a trend toward improved outcomes. These advances include[1] changes to CPR guidelines to focus on compressions alone[2]; improved access to AEDs to enable sustained delivery of quality CPR[3]; development of hypothermia protocols to ensure rapid initiation and maintenance of cooling[4]; improved understanding of neuroprognostication methods to avoid inappropriate withdrawal of management[5]; and development of dedicated cardiac arrest centers with provisions for urgent coronary intervention, cooling, critical care and multidisciplinary expert clinical management. Further improvements in clinical outcomes will be possible only with improved uptake and implementation of these key elements across health care systems.

REFERENCES

1. Nichol G, Thomas E, Callaway CW, et al. Regional variation in out-of-hospital cardiac arrest incidence and outcome. JAMA 2008;300(12):1423–31.
2. Sasson C, Rogers MA, Dahl J, et al. Predictors of survival from out-of-hospital cardiac arrest: a systematic review and meta-analysis. Circ Cardiovasc Qual Outcomes 2010;3:63–81.
3. Chan PS, McNally B, Tang F, et al. Recent trends in survival from out-of-hospital cardiac arrest in the United States. Circulation 2014;130:1876–82.
4. Girotra S, Nallamothu BK, Spertus JA, et al. Trends in survival after in-hospital cardiac arrest. N Engl J Med 2012;367:1912–20.
5. Peberdy MA, Callaway CW, Neumar RW, et al. Part 9: post-cardiac arrest care: 2010 American Heart Association guidelines for cardiopulmonary resuscitation and emergency cardiovascular care. Circulation 2010;122:S768–86.
6. Neumar RW, Nolan JP, Adrie C, et al. Post-cardiac arrest syndrome: epidemiology, pathophysiology, treatment, and prognostication. A consensus statement from the International Liaison Committee on Resuscitation (American Heart Association, Australian and New Zealand Council on Resuscitation, European Resuscitation Council, Heart and Stroke Foundation of Canada, InterAmerican Heart Foundation, Resuscitation Council of Asia, and the Resuscitation Council of Southern Africa); the American Heart Association Emergency Cardiovascular Care Committee; the Council on Cardiovascular Surgery and Anesthesia; the Council on Cardiopulmonary, Perioperative, and Critical Care; the Council on Clinical Cardiology; and the Stroke Council. Circulation 2008;118:2452–83.
7. Morrison LJ, Neumar RW, Zimmerman JL, et al. Strategies for improving survival after in-hospital cardiac arrest in the United States: 2013 consensus recommendations: a consensus statement from the American Heart Association. Circulation 2013;127: 1538–63.
8. Meier P, Baker P, Jost D, et al. Chest compressions before defibrillation for out-of-hospital cardiac arrest: a meta-analysis of randomized controlled clinical trials. BMC Med 2010;8:52.
9. Perkins G, Brace S, Smyth M, et al. Out of hospital cardiac arrest: recent scientific and technological advances and their effect on outcomes. Heart 2012;98:529–35.

10. Nolan JP, Neumar RW, Adrie C, et al. Post-cardiac arrest syndrome: epidemiology, pathophysiology, treatment, and prognostication. A scientific statement from the international liaison committee on resuscitation; the American Heart Association Emergency Cardiovascular Care Committee; the council on cardiovascular surgery and anesthesia; the council on cardiopulmonary, perioperative, and critical care; the council on clinical cardiology; the council on stroke. Resuscitation 2008;79:350–79.

11. Sunde K, Pytte M, Jacobsen D, et al. Implementation of a standardised treatment protocol for post resuscitation care after out-of-hospital cardiac arrest. Resuscitation 2007;73:29–39.

12. Callaway CW, Donnino MW, Fink EL, et al. Part 8: post–cardiac arrest care: 2015 American Heart Association guidelines update for cardiopulmonary resuscitation and emergency cardiovascular care. Circulation 2015;132(Suppl 2):S465–82.

13. Herlitz J, Engdahl J, Svensson L, et al. Major differences in 1-month survival between hospitals in Sweden among initial survivors of out-of-hospital cardiac arrest. Resuscitation 2006;70:404–9.

14. Nichol G, Aufderheide TP, Eigel B, et al. Regional systems of care for out-of-hospital cardiac arrest: a policy statement from the American Heart Association. Circulation 2010;121:709–29.

15. Graham KJ, Strauss CE, Boland LL. Has the time come for a National Cardiovascular Emergency Care System? Circulation 2012;125:2035–44.

16. Donnino MW, Rittenberger JC, Gaieski D, et al. The development and implementation of cardiac arrest centers. Resuscitation 2011;82:974–8.

17. Stub D, Bernard S, Duffy SJ, et al. Post cardiac arrest syndrome: a review of therapeutic strategies. Circulation 2011;123:1428–35.

18. Gaieski DF, Band RA, Abella BS, et al. Early goal-directed hemodynamic optimization combined with therapeutic hypothermia in comatose survivors of out-of-hospital cardiac arrest. Resuscitation 2009;80:418–24.

19. Dumas F, Cariou A, Manzo-Silberman S, et al. Immediate percutaneous coronary intervention is associated with better survival after out-of-hospital cardiac arrest: insights from the PROCAT (Parisian Region Out of hospital Cardiac ArresT) registry. Circ Cardiovasc Interv 2010;3:200–7.

20. Arntz HR, Bossaert LL, Danchin N, et al. European resuscitation council guidelines for resuscitation 2010 Section 5. Initial management of acute coronary syndromes. Resuscitation 2010;81:1353–63.

21. Bendz B, Eritsland J, Nakstad AR, et al. Long-term prognosis after out-of-hospital cardiac arrest and primary percutaneous coronary intervention. Resuscitation 2004;63:49–53.

22. Gorjup V, Radsel P, Kocjancic ST, et al. Acute ST-elevation myocardial infarction after successful cardiopulmonary resuscitation. Resuscitation 2007;72:379–85.

23. Hosmane VR, Mustafa NG, Reddy VK, et al. Survival and neurologic recovery in patients with ST-segment elevation myocardial infarction resuscitated from cardiac arrest. J Am Coll Cardiol 2009;53:409–15.

24. Radsel P, Knafelj R, Kocjancic S, et al. Angiographic characteristics of coronary disease and postresuscitation electrocardiograms in patients with aborted cardiac arrest outside a hospital. Am J Cardiol 2011;108:634–8.

25. Sideris G, Voicu S, Dillinger JG, et al. Value of post-resuscitation electrocardiogram in the diagnosis of acute myocardial infarction in out-of-hospital cardiac arrest patients. Resuscitation 2011;82:1148–53.

26. Rab T, Kern KB, Tamis-Holland JE, et al. Cardiac arrest: an algorithm for emergent invasive cardiac procedures in the comatose patient. J Am Coll Cardiol 2015;66(1):62–73.

27. Girotra S, Chan PS, Bradley SM. Post-resuscitation care following out-of-hospital and in-hospital cardiac arrest. Heart 2015;101:1943–9.

28. Laver S, Farrow C, Turner D, et al. Mode of death after admission to an intensive care unit following cardiac arrest. Intensive Care Med 2004;30:2126–8.

29. Walters JH, Morley PT, Nolan JP. The role of hypothermia in post-cardiac arrest patients with return of spontaneous circulation: a systematic review. Resuscitation 2011;82:508–16.

30. Hypothermia after Cardiac Arrest Study Group. Mild therapeutic hypothermia to improve the neurologic outcome after cardiac arrest. N Engl J Med 2002;346:549–56.

31. Bernard SA, Gray TW, Buist MD, et al. Treatment of comatose survivors of out-of-hospital cardiac arrest with induced hypothermia. N Engl J Med 2002;346:557–63.

32. Mooney MR, Unger BT, Boland LL, et al. Therapeutic hypothermia after out-of-hospital cardiac arrest: evaluation of a regional system to increase access to cooling. Circulation 2011;124:206–14.

33. Watts DD, Trask A, Soeken K, et al. Hypothermic coagulopathy in trauma: effect of varying levels of hypothermia on enzyme speed, platelet function, and fibrinolytic activity. J Trauma 1998;44:846–54.

34. Lavinio A, Scudellari A, Gupta AK. Hemorrhagic shock resulting in cardiac arrest: is therapeutic hypothermia contraindicated? Minerva Anestesiol 2012;78:969–70.

35. Guilliams K, Rosen M, Buttram S, et al. Hypothermia for pediatric refractory status epilepticus. Epilepsia 2013;54:1586–94.

36. Corry JJ, Dhar R, Murphy T, et al. Hypothermia for refractory status epilepticus. Neurocrit Care 2008;9: 189–97.

37. Guluma KZ, Oh H, Yu SW, et al. Effect of endovascular hypothermia on acute ischemic edema: morphometric analysis of the ICTuS trial. Neurocrit Care 2008;8:42–7.

38. Aufderheide TP, Nichol G, Rea TD, et al. A trial of an impedance threshold device in out-of-hospital cardiac arrest. N Engl J Med 2011;365: 798–806.

39. Kudenchuk PJ, Brown SP, Daya M, et al, Resuscitation Outcomes Consortium Investigators. Amiodarone, lidocaine, or placebo in out-of-hospital cardiac arrest. N Engl J Med 2016;374:1711–22.

40. Kilgannon JH, Jones AE, Shapiro NI, et al. Association between arterial hyperoxia following resuscitation from cardiac arrest and in-hospital mortality. JAMA 2010;303:2165–71.

41. Bellomo R, Bailey M, Eastwood GM, et al. Arterial hyperoxia and in-hospital mortality after resuscitation from cardiac arrest. Crit Care 2011;15:R90.

42. Wijdicks EF, Hijdra A, Young GB, et al. Practice parameter: prediction of outcome in comatose survivors after cardiopulmonary resuscitation (an evidence-based review): report of the Quality Standards Subcommittee of the American Academy of Neurology. Neurology 2006;67:203–10.

43. Morrison LJ, Deakin CD, Morley PT, et al. Part 8: advanced life support: 2010 international consensus on cardiopulmonary resuscitation and emergency cardiovascular care science with treatment recommendations. Circulation 2010;122(16 Suppl 2):S345–421.

44. Adrie C, Haouache H, Saleh M, et al. An underrecognized source of organ donors: patients with brain death after successfully resuscitated cardiac arrest. Intensive Care Med 2008;34:132–7.

45. Sandroni C, Adrie C, Cavallaro F, et al. Are patients brain-dead after successful resuscitation from cardiac arrest suitable as organ donors? A systematic review. Resuscitation 2010;81:1609–14.

46. Collins T, Fraser J, McVeigh G, et al. Organ donation for transplantation: improving donor identification and consent rates for deceased organ donation. London: National Institute for Health and Clinical Excellence; 2011. Available at: http://www.nice.org.uk/guidance/CG135.

Public Reporting in ST Segment Elevation Myocardial Infarction

Michael C. McDaniel, MD[a], S. Tanveer Rab, MD[b],*

KEYWORDS

- STEMI • Public reporting • Cardiac arrest • Cardiogenic shock • Risk averse behavior

---

KEY POINTS

- With health care reform, there is increased use of public reporting and merit-based payment.
- Risk-adjusted mortality is contentious with some evidence of harm.
- Cardiac arrest and cardiogenic shock need to be better defined, before they are publicly reported.

INTRODUCTION

Health care in the United States is rapidly changing, moving from a volume-based "fee-for-service" reimbursement model to one focused on rewarding quality and value. These health care reforms aim to provide increasing transparency about the quality of care that patients receive. It is envisioned that the public reporting of health care outcomes and quality-based reimbursements will incentivize practice improvements and systems of care that promote quality at lower costs. Furthermore, there is a fundamental belief that patients have a right to know about the quality of care that they are likely to receive. Although these are noble goals, the challenge for hospitals and providers in this new health care era is to ensure that public reporting and quality-based reimbursements occur in fair, accurate, and meaningful ways that benefit patients and minimize the possibilities of negative unintended consequences. This is especially true for patients with acute ST segment elevation myocardial infarction (STEMI).

HISTORY OF REPORTING

Public reporting of cardiovascular health care outcomes is not new. In 1987, the Health Care Financing Administration published the risk adjusted hospital-specific mortality from coronary artery bypass graft (CABG) surgery.[1] This was later withdrawn owing to objections of using administrate claims data and concerns regarding the risk adjustment methodology. However, these efforts ultimately resulted in the creation of the Society of Thoracic Surgeons' National Cardiac Surgery Database in 1989. The New York State Department of Health started issuing public reports of CABG surgery in 1992 and percutaneous coronary intervention (PCI) outcomes in 1995, and this has since been a very divisive topic.[2] Massachusetts followed with public reporting of CABG and PCI in 2003.[3] The Centers for Medicare and Medicaid Services reestablished hospital-level public reporting for Medicare patients in 2005 with implementation of the "Hospital Compare" website for process measures of many common conditions including acute myocardial infarction and heart failure.[4] In

---

Conflict of Interest: None.

[a] Cardiac Catheterization Laboratory, Division of Cardiology, Grady Memorial Hospital, Emory University School of Medicine, 80 Jesse Hill Jr Drive, SE, Atlanta, GA 30303, USA; [b] Division of Cardiology/Interventional Cardiology, Emory University Hospital, Emory University School of Medicine, F-606, 1364 Clifton Road, Northeast, Atlanta, GA 30222, USA

* Corresponding author.
E-mail address: srab@emory.edu

2006, the Centers for Medicare and Medicaid Services attempted to collect physician specific data through the Physician Voluntary Reporting Program; however, participation in this program was limited. In 2010, the Society of Thoracic Surgeons partnered with *Consumer Reports* to report performance metrics publicly for CABG surgery using quality data from the Society of Thoracic Surgeons' Database.[3] It was the passage of the Patient Protection and Affordable Care Act in 2010 that accelerated the focus on transparency and alternative payment models based on value.[4] As part of the Patient Protection and Affordable Care Act, the National Quality Forum was selected to identify important performance measures, provide input on the reporting of these metrics, and align performance-based payments. The Medicare Access and Children's Health Insurance Program Reauthorization Act of 2015 has furthered merit-based payment systems, alternative payment models, and increased transparency.

CONTROVERSIES WITH PUBLIC REPORTING AND MERIT-BASED PAYMENTS

At the heart of all these efforts is the belief that transparency in quality data will positively impact decisions and behaviors of health care providers to improve health care delivery and outcomes. Although paved with noble intentions, the benefits of merit-based payments and public reporting of PCI outcomes have never been proven and may have unintended consequences.[5,6] As such, the PCI quality metrics used for merit-based payments and public reporting in STEMI must be carefully selected, because many outcomes often depend more on the patient selection and less on the quality of the procedure. In addition, merit-based payments and public reporting may motivate unnecessary performance reporting and potential "gaming" of the system, without addressing issues most important to patient care.[3] Patient's quality concerns tend to focus more on access to empathetic and engaged physicians that meet an acceptable standard of care.[3,7,8]

Ultimately, to compare quality outcomes between institutions, risk adjustment methods are necessary, given the wide variations in volume and case mix between institutions. However, in practice, risk adjustment is imperfect and physicians often do not trust that the risk adjustment methodology will accurately reflect the risk of procedure, especially for patients at greatest risk for adverse outcomes. For example, in New York State, where 85% of cardiologists felt that the risk adjustment methodology was inadequate to avoid penalizing physicians who perform higher risk interventions.[9] In these cases, the use of public reporting and merit-based incentives such as Quality-In-Sights Hospital Incentive Program have the potential to incentivize risk adverse behaviors through withholding of appropriate treatment to some of the highest risk sickest patients who might actually benefit most from the procedure, such as patients with cardiac arrest and cardiogenic shock.

Understanding the use of public reporting and merit-based incentives in STEMI is particularly important because studies suggest that public reporting may promote risk adverse behaviors that may actually lead to worse mortality. The 3 public reporting states (New York, Massachusetts and Pennsylvania) rank 31st, 47th, and 49th for use of PCI in acute MI with out-of-hospital cardiac arrest (OHCA) and/or cardiogenic shock, a guideline-supported indication.[10] Furthermore, the adjusted total mortality for patients presenting with STEMI was 35% higher in states with public reporting compared with those without public reporting.[10] This may be in part related to lower use of angiography and PCI in patients with STEMI (61.8% vs 68%; odds ratio [OR], 0.73; 95% CI, 0.59–0.89; $P = .002$) and shock or cardiac arrest (41.5% vs 46.7%; OR, 0.79; 95% CI, 0.64–0.98; $P = .03$) compared with states that do not publicly report mortality outcomes. Interestingly, in Massachusetts the rates of PCI were similar to other nonreporting states before public reporting, but began to diverge after public reporting was implemented, strongly implicating public reporting for a decrease in optimal care. In Massachusetts, being identified as a "negative outlier" in risk-adjusted mortality (RAM) was associated with a significant decrease in predicted mortality in the subsequent years, suggesting that public reporting led to risk averse behaviors and the exclusion of critically ill patients.[11]

The lower use of revascularization and higher mortality for patients with STEMI in states with public reporting was echoed in an analysis of 84,121 patients from the Nationwide Inpatient Sample database.[12] In this analysis, after adjustment, public reporting was again associated with significantly lower use of PCI (OR, 0.58; 95% CI, 0.47–0.70) in cardiac arrest and cardiogenic shock. Importantly, public reporting states had a higher total mortality in acute MI (OR, 1.21; 95% CI, 1.06–1.37) compared with nonreporting states. In this Nationwide Inpatient

Sample analysis, for publicly reporting states the mortality for patients who underwent PCI was actually lower (OR, 0.71; 95% CI, 0.62–0.83), but mortality was significantly higher for patients who did not undergo PCI (OR, 1.30; 95% CI, 1.13–1.50; interaction P<.001). This may suggest that there is a "risk avoidance creep" where sicker patients with cardiac arrest and cardiogenic shock are not taken for cardiac catheterization and PCI in publicly reporting states.[2]

Advocates of RAM as a quality indicator for PCI believe that that there is evidence that treating high-risk PCI cases does not adversely affect hospital RAM rates and should not promote risk adverse behaviors. In support of this belief are data from 624,286 cases from 1168 sites from the National Cardiovascular Data Registry (NCDR) Cath/PCI registry. Hospitals treating the highest overall expected risk PCI patients (the top 20% of high-risk cases) had better RAM ratings than centers treating lower risk cases (1.25% vs 1.51%).[13] In addition, combining the highest risk patients over a 2-year period into a single year did not change significantly the average RAM or the number of hospital outliers. Although the total numbers of outliers did not change significantly, this does not imply that individual hospitals were not impacted and the analysis would be more telling to compare the changes in the individual hospitals.[14] Furthermore, these data may not apply to lower volume hospitals and individual physicians. Finally, this analysis does not address the real issue of using RAM in quality reporting, which is the evidence for public harm because of procedures that were deferred. Until there are diagnosis-based registries that include all patients with cardiac arrest and cardiogenic shock who do not undergo PCI procedures, using the NCDR Cath/PCI registry will only look at "one side of the coin" and not accurately measure the true quality of care for patients with STEMI, cardiac arrest, and/or cardiogenic shock.

Based on concerns of risk adverse behaviors related to public reporting, the New York State Department of Health in 2006 excluded cardiogenic shock from RAM reporting, and there was an immediate increase in the number of PCI cases for shock performed in the subsequent years.[15] In addition, in 2006 in Massachusetts, compassionate use criteria were added for patients to improve risk prediction. These criteria included percutaneous ventricular assist device, cardiopulmonary bypass, PCI with ongoing CPR, or with coma (Glasgow Coma Scale <7).[16] The inclusion of the combination of these variable in the NCDR Cath/PCI mortality model did improve the c-statistic for the prediction of mortality (0.87–0.90; P<.001). In 2011, New York also excluded a subset of patients with anoxic encephalopathy from RAM.

The real issues with the use of RAM as a PCI quality metric is that it inappropriately implies that the mortality outcome is linked with quality of the PCI procedure. However, patients with cardiogenic shock and cardiac arrest have a 5- to 10-fold higher mortality, and most of the mortality in patients with cardiac arrest is owing to neurologic complications or multiorgan failure despite receiving appropriate care.[17] Moreover, the majority of PCI-related deaths are unrelated to complications of the interventional procedure or cardiac catheterization.[18] Using RAM as a quality outcome in merit-based payments and public reporting inadvertently places clinicians in the difficult situation of having to choose between what may be in their patient's interest and what may be best for their own quality metrics or their hospital-reported outcomes. Because no physician can always accurately choose between a futile procedure and one where there is small but meaningful chance at survival, this can shift the paradigm from, "Let's give them a shot" to "It probably won't make a difference.[6]" Moreover, public reporting is designed to empower patients to make choices about their health care, yet in emergency situations such as STEMI with cardiac arrest and/or cardiogenic shock, patients often have little chance to exercise their choice in selection of physicians and hospitals, because they are taken to the closest facility and the physician selected is the one on call.

Given these limitations, the American Heart Association (AHA) put forth a scientific statement on the topic stating

> OHCA cases should be tracked but not publicly reported or used for overall PCI performance ranking, which would allow accountability for their management but would not penalize high-volume cardiac resuscitation centers (CRCs) for following the 2010 AHA Guidelines for CPR and ECC. Until an adequate risk adjustment model is created to account for the numerous out-of-hospital and in-hospital variables that impact survival more than the performance of PCI, we believe that categorizing OHCA STEMI-PCI cases separately from other STEMI-PCI cases should occur. These patients should not be included in public reporting.[19]

Similar recommendations are seen in the 2013 American College of Cardiology (ACA)/American

Heart Association Foundation 2013 STEMI guidelines, which state "It is important for organizations that collect and publicly report STEMI and PCI data to consider resuscitated OHCA patients separately from their hospital land individual operator quality 'scorecards' because such patients, even with optimal care, have a much higher mortality rate.[20]"

The majority of interventional cardiologists in the United States agree with these recommendations. In 2015, in a national survey conducted by the Interventional Council of the ACC of 1297 interventionalists in the United States, 86% felt that public reporting of mortality rates after PCI should exclude patients with cardiac arrest patients and 76% thought the same for patients with cardiogenic shock.[21] Although the resuscitated comatose cardiac arrest patient with return of spontaneous circulation is a group that can be easily categorized,[12] for the purposes of exclusion cardiogenic shock is less easily defined and a universal standardized definition is urgently needed from the NCDR with input from the ACC and the Society of Cardiac Angiography and Interventions.[22]

DATA SOURCES FOR QUALITY METRICS

The source of data used for reporting quality metrics is extremely important, because outcomes can differ based on the database. The Centers for Medicare and Medicaid Services reports on the Medicare website using administrative billing claims data. However, there are many issues with administrative data, because these financial instruments were not designed for clinical use and there are significant issues in risk

adjustment using these data. In addition, administrative data can be 1 to 2 years behind, and thus may not represent contemporary practices. Since 1997, the ACC in partnership with the Society of Cardiac Angiography and Interventions created the NCDR Cath/PCI Registry to collect, audit, benchmark, and report clinical data and outcomes. The ACC has endorsed the use of the NCDR Cath/PCI registry for public reporting and merit-based payments.

FUTURE OF PUBLIC REPORTING

Although the specific details of the merit-based payments and public reporting are evolving, what is clear is that these reforms are not going away. Furthermore, the ACC believes that the organization has the responsibility to move the profession toward acceptance of public reporting using clinical data from the NCDR and developed a policy statement in 2008 defining 6 core principals regarding public reporting (Box 1).[1,3] Although not stated specifically, these same principals should likely be applied to all merit-based payment reforms. The ACC has also established the Public Reporting Advisory Group to guide the implementation of this program.[3] At present, hospital participation in public reporting of their NCDR data is voluntary and the metrics reported from the NCDR will only be at the hospital level.[3] The data will be available at the ACC's Cardiosmart website and all reported metrics must be endorsed by National Quality Forum and derived from the NCDR (Fig. 1).[3] The initial performance metrics from NCDR to be reported are listed in Table 1.[3] These initial metrics focus on discharge process

---

Box 1
ACC Foundation's Principles of Public Reporting

The driving force behind physician performance measurement and reporting systems should be to promote quality improvement.

Public reporting programs should be based on performance measures with scientific validity.

Public reporting programs should be developed in partnership with physicians.

Every effort should be made to use standardized data elements to assess and report performance and to make the submission process uniform across all public reporting programs.

Performance reporting should occur at the appropriate level of accountability.

Public reporting programs should include a formal process for evaluating the impact of the program on the quality and cost of health care, including an assessment of unintended consequences.

Abbreviation: ACC, American College of Cardiology.

Adapted from Drozda JP Jr, Hagan EP, Mirro MJ, et al. ACCF 2008 health policy statement on principles for public reporting of physician performance data: a report of the American College of Cardiology Foundation Writing Committee to develop principles for public reporting of physician performance data. J Am Coll Cardiol 2008;51:1995–7; with permission.

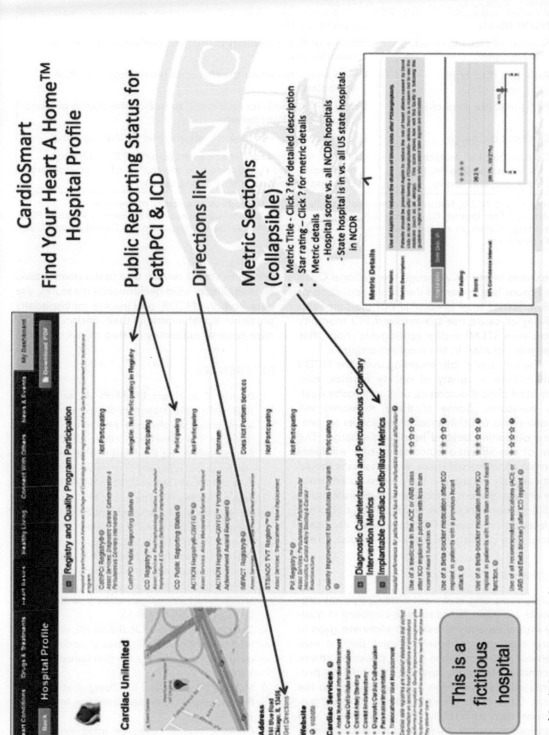

Fig. 1. Example of CardioSmart Hospital profile page. ACE, angiotensin-converting enzyme; ARB, angiotensin receptor blocker; GWTG, get with the guidelines; ICD, implantable cardiac defibrillator. (*Adapted from* Dehmer GJ, Jennings J, Madden RA, et al. The National Cardiovascular Data Registry Voluntary Public Reporting Program: an interim report from the NCDR Public Reporting Advisory Group. J Am Coll Cardiol 2016;67(2):211; with permission.)

Table 1
Initial NCDR CathPCI voluntary public reporting metrics

NCDR Metric	CardioSmart Title
Number of PCI/angioplasty procedures	Number of PCI/angioplasty procedures performed during the calendar year.
Aspirin at discharge	Use of aspirin to reduce the chance of blood clots after PCI/angioplasty.
$P2Y_{12}$ inhibitor at discharge	Use of a $P2Y_{12}$ inhibitor medication to reduce the chance of blood clots after PCI/angioplasty.
Statins at discharge	Use of a statin to decrease cholesterol after PCI/angioplasty.
Composite of all medications at discharge (aspirin, $P2Y_{12}$ inhibitor, and statin)	Use of all recommended medications (aspirin, $P2Y_{12}$ inhibitor medication, and statin) to reduce the chance of blood clots and decrease cholesterol after PCI/angioplasty.

Abbreviations: NCDR, National Cardiovascular Data Registry; PCI, percutaneous coronary intervention.

Adapted from Dehmer GJ, Jennings J, Madden RA, et al. The National Cardiovascular Data Registry Voluntary Public Reporting Program: an interim report from the NCDR Public Reporting Advisory Group. J Am Coll Cardiol 2016;67(2):209; with permission.

measures after PCI. Although the National Quality Forum has endorsed the public reporting of risk-adjusted total in-hospital PCI mortality and 30-day all-cause risk-standardized PCI mortality rates with STEMI and/or cardiogenic shock, this was not included in the initial reporting.[4]

The future of public reporting using the NCDR will include a variety of quality metrics, risk-adjusted clinical outcomes, and composite quality measures. Some of these measures will require links to other external databases to measure outcomes beyond hospital discharge. The use of risk-adjusted outcome metrics will likely remain controversial issues and physicians should stay actively engaged in this process to advocate for optimal patient outcomes through minimizing adverse behaviors. This is critical for outcomes related to emergency PCI procedures, especially those with cardiogenic shock and cardiac arrest.

SUMMARY

Public reporting and merit-based payment programs are intended to engage clinicians in quality improvement processes to eliminate gaps in care that may adversely impact patient outcomes. However, when poorly designed, these incentive programs have the potential to promote adverse behaviors that run counter to the goal. Patients at greatest risk for adverse outcomes such as STEMI with cardiac arrest and cardiogenic shock may be most vulnerable to this risk aversion. Because public reporting and merit-based payments will only increase in the coming years, it is important for physicians to remain engaged in the process by which quality metrics are developed and implemented. These programs should remain true to the goals: based on scientifically valid performance measures, use data from the NCDR, and involve multispecialty physician stakeholders in their design to minimize adverse outcomes related to risk aversion.

REFERENCES

1. Drozda JP Jr, Hagan EP, Mirro MJ, et al. ACCF 2008 health policy statement on principles for public reporting of physician performance data: a report of the American College of Cardiology Foundation Writing Committee to develop principles for public reporting of physician performance data. J Am Coll Cardiol 2008;51:1993–2001.
2. Resnic FS, Welt FG. The public health hazards of risk avoidance associated with public reporting of risk-adjusted outcomes in coronary intervention. J Am Coll Cardiol 2009;53:825–30.
3. Dehmer GJ, Jennings J, Madden RA, et al. The National Cardiovascular Data Registry Voluntary Public Reporting Program: an interim report from the NCDR Public Reporting Advisory Group. J Am Coll Cardiol 2016;67:205–15.
4. Dehmer GJ, Drozda JP Jr, Brindis RG, et al. Public reporting of clinical quality data: an update for cardiovascular specialists. J Am Coll Cardiol 2014;63:1239–45.
5. McMullan PW Jr, White CJ. Doing what's right for the resuscitated. Catheter Cardiovasc Interv 2010;76:161–3.
6. Pinto DS, Pride YB. Paved with good intentions and marred by half-truths. J Am Coll Cardiol 2013;62:416–7.
7. Metersky ML. Point: will public reporting of healthcare quality measures inform and educate patients? Yes. Chest 2011;140:1115–7.

8. Kullgren JT, Werner RM. Counterpoint: will public reporting of health-care quality measures inform and educate patients? No. Chest 2011;140:1117–20 [discussion: 1120–2].

9. Narins CR, Dozier AM, Ling FS, et al. The influence of public reporting of outcome data on medical decision making by physicians. Arch Intern Med 2005;165:83–7.

10. Joynt KE, Blumenthal DM, Orav E, et al. Association of public reporting for percutaneous coronary intervention with utilization and outcomes among Medicare beneficiaries with acute myocardial infarction. JAMA 2012;308:1460–8.

11. McCabe JM, Joynt KE, Welt FG, et al. Impact of public reporting and outlier status identification on percutaneous coronary intervention case selection in Massachusetts. JACC Cardiovasc Interv 2013;6:625–30.

12. Waldo SW, McCabe JM, O'Brien C, et al. Association between public reporting of outcomes with procedural management and mortality for patients with acute myocardial infarction. J Am Coll Cardiol 2015;65:1119–26.

13. Sherwood MW, Brennan JM, Ho KK, et al. The impact of extreme-risk cases on hospitals' risk-adjusted percutaneous coronary intervention mortality ratings. JACC Cardiovasc Interv 2015;8:10–6.

14. Miner S, Nield L. The imperfections and perils of procedure-based risk scores. JACC Cardiovasc Interv 2015;8:1003–4.

15. Hannan EL. The public reporting risk of performing high-risk procedures: perception or reality? JACC Cardiovasc Interv 2015;8:17–9.

16. Resnic FS, Normand SL, Piemonte TC, et al. Improvement in mortality risk prediction after percutaneous coronary intervention through the addition of a "compassionate use" variable to the National Cardiovascular Data Registry CathPCI dataset: a study from the Massachusetts Angioplasty Registry. J Am Coll Cardiol 2011;57:904–11.

17. Rab T, Kern KB, Tamis-Holland JE, et al. Cardiac arrest: a treatment algorithm for emergent invasive cardiac procedures in the resuscitated comatose patient. J Am Coll Cardiol 2015;66:62–73.

18. Aggarwal B, Ellis SG, Lincoff AM, et al. Cause of death within 30 days of percutaneous coronary intervention in an era of mandatory outcome reporting. J Am Coll Cardiol 2013;62:409–15.

19. Peberdy MA, Donnino MW, Callaway CW, et al. Impact of percutaneous coronary intervention performance reporting on cardiac resuscitation centers: a scientific statement from the American Heart Association. Circulation 2013;128:762–73.

20. American College of Emergency Physicians, Society for Cardiovascular Angiography and Interventions, O'Gara PT, et al. 2013 ACCF/AHA guideline for the management of ST-elevation myocardial infarction: executive summary: a report of the American College of Cardiology Foundation/American Heart Association Task Force on Practice Guidelines. J Am Coll Cardiol 2013;61: 485–510.

21. Rab T, Interventional Council, Wilson H, et al. Public reporting of mortality after PCI in cardiac arrest and cardiogenic shock: an opinion from the Interventional Council and the Board of Governors of the American College of Cardiology. JACC Cardiovasc Interv 2016;9:496–8.

22. Brennan JM, Curtis JP, Dai D, et al. Enhanced mortality risk prediction with a focus on high-risk percutaneous coronary intervention: results from 1,208,137 procedures in the NCDR (National Cardiovascular Data Registry). JACC Cardiovasc Interv 2013;6:790–9.

Global Challenges and Solutions

Role of Telemedicine in ST-Elevation Myocardial Infarction Interventions

Sameer Mehta, MD*, Roberto Botelho, MD, PhD,
Jamil Cade, MD, Marco Perin, MD, Fredy Bojanini, MD,
Juan Coral, MD, Daniela Parra, MD,
Alexandra Ferré, MD, Marco Castillo, MD,
Pablo Yépez, MD

KEYWORDS

- Telemedicine • Primary PCI • Thrombolysis • Pharmaco-invasive • Door-to-balloon time • LATIN

KEY POINTS

- Primary percutaneous coronary intervention (PCI) is the most effective technique to treat acute myocardial infarction.
- Access to primary PCI is restricted in developing countries.
- Telemedicine greatly facilitates access of primary PCI to vast populations.

INTRODUCTION

Primary percutaneous coronary intervention (PCI) has revolutionized the management of acute myocardial infarction (AMI). Although thrombolysis is still the mainstay of treatment in various parts of the world, primary PCI is vastly superior. Scientific guidelines[1,2] maintain a class I indication for treating AMI with primary PCI if performed in a timely manner by an experienced provider.[3] To mandate the urgency in performing primary PCI, parameters of door-to-balloon (D2B) times have been added.[4] Short D2B times (<90 minutes) are desirable, although this recommendation is not universal.

In developing countries, lack of infrastructure, insurance, facilities, and skilled providers greatly hamper the use of primary PCI. For example, in the entire continent of South America, less than 8% of the population has access to cardiac catheterization laboratories. In parts of Africa and some Asian countries, the situation is similarly abysmal. In these developing parts of the world, thrombolysis, often with Streptokinase, is still the predominant modality. Other developing countries predominantly use a pharmaco-invasive approach. This strategy clearly has numerous advantages: a patient with AMI receives urgent thrombolysis and is then transported for possible PCI. In sharp contrast, in various developed countries, there is a comprehensive utilization of primary PCI for an entire population.[5–8] These advanced countries use regional systems of care to optimize timeliness of reperfusion therapy.[9–11] Pre-hospital management is the norm and considerable reduction in morbidity and mortality has been achieved.[12–16]

The disparities of care between developed and developing countries for the management of AMI represent one of the largest global challenges in ST-elevation myocardial infarction (STEMI) interventions.

Conflicts of Interest: None.
Lumen Foundation, 185 Shore Drive South, Miami, FL 33133, USA
* Corresponding author. Lumen Foundation, 185 Shore Drive South, Miami, FL 33133.
E-mail address: sameer.lumenglobal@gmail.com

Intervent Cardiol Clin 5 (2016) 569–581
http://dx.doi.org/10.1016/j.iccl.2016.06.013
2211-7458/16/$ – see front matter © 2016 Elsevier Inc. All rights reserved.

Telemedicine appears an effective modality for significantly increasing access for millions of patients to appropriate STEMI care.[17,18] Remotely located experts guide accurate interpretation of the electrocardiogram (ECG) and enable teleconsultation of the patient with STEMI.[19–21] A comprehensive utilization of thrombolysis, pharmaco-invasive management, and primary PCI is possible with the use of telemedicine.[17,18] Reduction of D2B times and improvement in STEMI outcomes have been demonstrated.[20,22–24] Telemedicine may also be cost-effective, in particular, when it facilitates prehospital triage.[25–27]

In this article, we discuss the various advantages of using telemedicine and our experience of using this technology to improve populated-based STEMI care in developing countries.

We tested the hypothesis that telemedicine has 4 distinct advantages in STEMI interventions.[17,18] These included (1) increased accuracy, (2) increased access, (3) guidance of comprehensive STEMI management, and (4) increased cost-effectiveness.

AMI is unique in that its diagnosis can be instantaneously made on accurate interpretation of the presenting ECG. This accuracy can be augmented by a quick clinical evaluation. In the rapid STEMI evaluation, confirmation with cardiac biomarkers is often not required. Still, there are discrepancies in the accurate interpretation of the ECG. Fig. 1 is a graphic illustration of this disparity. The accuracy of ECG in diagnosing STEMI dramatically increases between small clinics to tertiary cardiac centers. These remarkable characteristics of ECG interpretation make the use of telemedicine an exceptional modality for treating STEMI interventions. The remote cardiologist significantly augments the accuracy of ECG interpretation and STEMI diagnosis. This particular observation makes telemedicine a pragmatic and cost-effective strategy. In our experience with the Latin America Telemedicine Infarct Network (LATIN), the accuracy of ECG interpretation increased from less than 50% in small referral clinics to greater than 95% when interpreted by a remotely located, expert cardiologist. The increased accuracy is complemented by an ability to teleconsult the STEMI process as depicted in Fig. 2. With this methodology, the expert cardiologist navigates the patient with STEMI to a more scientific and pragmatic management.

There are numerous known methods to conduct the ECG analysis. These include transtelephonic, fax, and wireless transmission. Table 1 compares these modalities with telemedicine and it illustrates the relative merits of telemedicine. Numerous telemedicine protocols[17,18,21] have been used to obtain remote consultation. We have used an integrated software platform to reliably transmit ECGs and safeguard patient privacy (Fig. 3). Often, an argument is advanced that simple and inexpensive mobile phone transmission (with applications such as WhatsApp) are comparable to using a

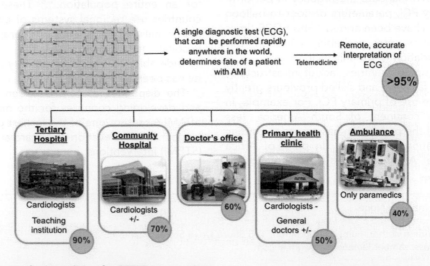

Fig. 1. Essence of telemedicine for STEMI interventions.

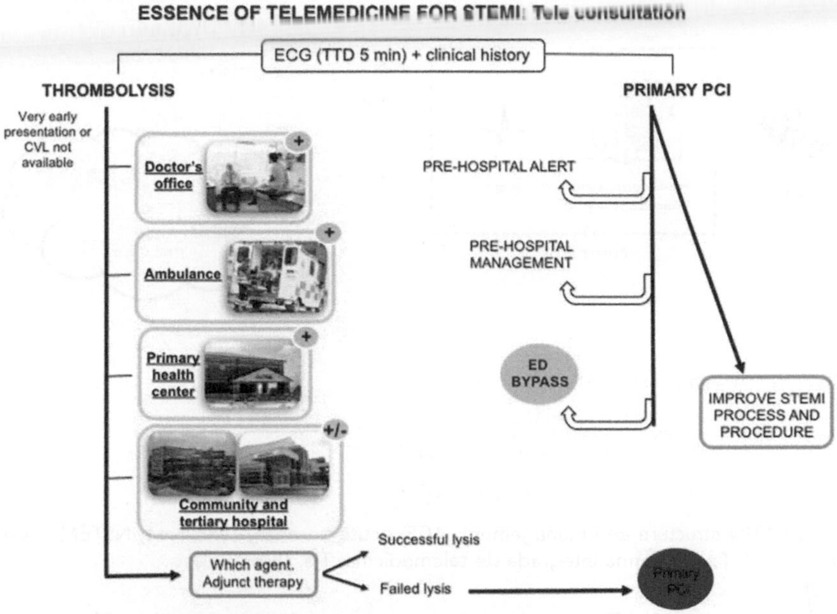

Fig. 2. Telemedicine – teleconsultation. CVL, cardiovascular laboratory.

dedicated telemedicine platform, but Table 2 demonstrates some limitations of using a mobile phone for accurate ECG interpretation.

The largest disparity in STEMI care between developed and developing countries pertains to access. Because there are tremendous structural, financial, and personnel shortages, millions of patients do not have access to contemporary STEMI treatment. Telemedicine is the novel technology that dramatically increases the access of patients to AMI care. Fig. 4 describes a telemedicine strategy that we have used in several poorer countries in South America to increase STEMI access.

METHODS

In demonstrating the effectiveness of telemedicine in STEMI interventions, we describe the creation of 2 novel, population-based STEMI programs, that used telemedicine as a foundation

pillar. These 2 programs include LATIN and Rajasthan Heart Attack Treatment (RAHAT). Both programs use a hub and spoke strategy. The hub performs primary PCI and the spoke triages the patient into 1 of the 3 STEMI management pathways: thrombolysis, pharmaco-invasive strategy, and primary PCI (see Fig. 4). The main difference between the structure used for LATIN and RAHAT was the number of hubs and spokes and the respective distance between these facilities. The distance between hub and spoke determines the extent of the geographic reach of a population-based program. It takes into consideration the geographic distance, the population density, the availability of catheterization laboratories, and the traffic patterns. The other major distinction between these diverse programs included different transmission methodologies. In LATIN, we used a sophisticated and dedicated, integrated software platform, whereas in RAHAT, the more common and less expensive mobile telephone applications were used (Figs. 5 and 6).

Latin America Telemedicine Infarct Network
This revolutionary program has populated vast areas of Brazil and Colombia with 104 LATIN telemedicine sites. The foundation of LATIN was to provide AMI management for poor patients in less developed countries. LATIN selected Brazil and Colombia for demonstrating the utility of telemedicine to improve AMI outcomes. In Brazil, the program includes 7 cities that have networked large rural areas, up

Table 1 Comparison of 4 modes of electrocardiogram transmission				
Attributes	Phone	Fax	Wireless	TM
Accuracy	+++	+++	+++	++++
Access	++++	+++	+	++++
Cost-effective	+++	++	+	+++
Timeliness	++	+++	+++	++

Abbreviation: TM, telemedicine.

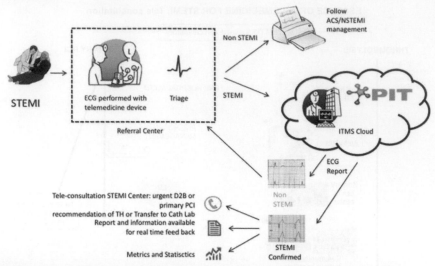

Fig. 3. Proposed LATIN structure and management. ACS, acute coronary syndrome; NSTEMI, non-ST-elevation myocardial infarction; PIT, plataforma integrada de telemedicina; TH, thrombolysis.

to 250 miles away, with LATIN spokes. In Colombia, almost 42% of the country's 48 million people are now covered by LATIN networks. In designing this program, we confronted enormous variability in ECG interpretation and in AMI care. The LATIN spokes consist primarily of small clinics, primary health centers, and community hospitals that did not have resources to

Table 2
Limitations of using mobile phone for accurate electrocardiogram interpretation

Attributes	TM	Mobile Phone
Vectorization	✓	—
ECG specific measurements	✓	—
HIPAA compliance	✓	—
Security	✓	—
Time	✓	—
Receipt of confirmation	✓	—
Codification of diagnosis	✓	—
EMR	✓	—
Accredited reviewer	✓	—
Optional teleconsultation	✓	—
Audit availability	✓	—
ICD-10 compatibility	✓	—

Abbreviations: ECG, electrocardiogram; EMR, electronic medical record; HIPPA, Health Insurance Portability and Accountability Act; ICD-10, International Classification of Diseases, 10th Revision.

treat patients with AMI. This was done in an effort to advance AMI care to patients and facilities that lacked these assets. Several of these spokes were in a very remote, hilly regions and jungles of the 2 countries. Most of these spokes had rudimentary skills in accurately diagnosing STEMI. A strategic decision was made to transmit ECG on all patients presenting with chest pain and to back up the strategy by creating efficient and inexpensive telemedicine platforms. Figs. 7 and 8 demonstrate the enormous reach of the LATIN program with its deep penetration into remote and poor regions of Brazil and Colombia. Selection of the hubs and spokes was paramount. The selection of the hubs is relatively easy because there are only a few that are available. The hubs were mandated to provide 24/7 STEMI coverage and have reliable ambulance transportation. The spokes were chosen mainly to increase coverage and access by poor patients. A single standardized STEMI management protocol was used for all LATIN hubs and spokes. Figs. 9 and 10 depict this protocol and Fig. 11 is a further illustration based on the availability of ambulances.

Spoke efficiencies were increased by mandating excellent triage of the patient presenting with chest pain. The ECG was promptly transmitted and interpreted by an expert cardiologist located at 4 sites: Bogota, Colombia; Uberlandia and Sao Paulo, Brazil; and Santiago, Chile. Primary PCI was encouraged at all hubs and spokes, and to facilitate this, ambulance arrangements were immediately made after confirmation of ECG. We simplified a 3 T's strategy for LATIN spokes: Triage, Transmit, and

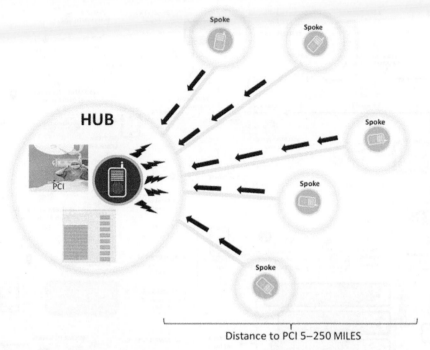

Fig. 4. Hub and spoke methodology for LATIN.

Transport. Prehospital management was routinely advocated and prehospital alert with a single phone activation was performed. In several centers, this led to emergency department (ED) bypass and reduced D2B times. The

spokes provided early pharmacologic management, medical stabilization, and patient education. Training of personnel with technology was emphasized and efficient triage was supervised. Ambulance availability was the single

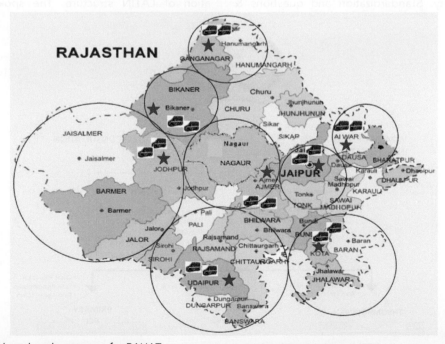

Fig. 5. Hub and spoke strategy for RAHAT.

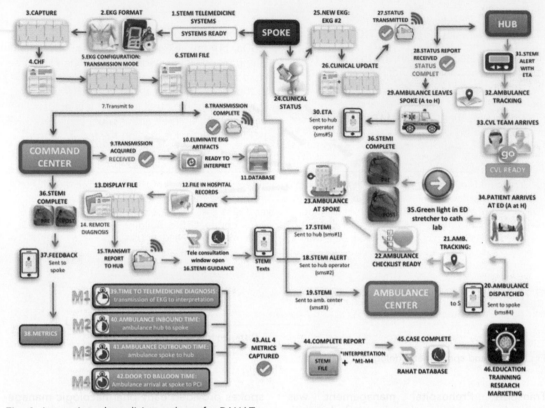

Fig. 6. Innovative telemedicine pathway for RAHAT.

biggest challenge and numerous local, community, and regional stakeholders were encouraged to provide this life-saving service for the community. Standardization and questions &

answers were mandated and a comprehensive LATIN database was created.

Brazil and Colombia differ notably in the creation of LATIN structure. The spokes were

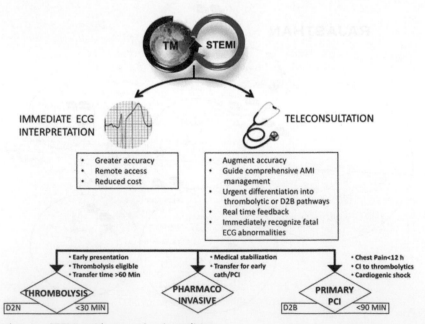

Fig. 7. Comprehensive STEMI guidance with telemedicine.

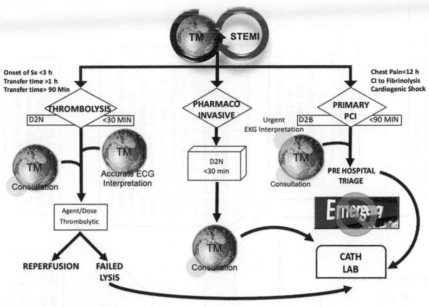

Fig. 8. LATIN protocol. Sx, syndrome.

located farther apart in Brazil but there was geographically more difficult terrain in Colombia. Both countries had infrastructure deficiencies and both had financial constraints. Brazil possessed sophisticated telemedicine knowledge, as the technology has been prevalent for decades.[22,28] Insurance approval for STEMI interventions was challenging in both countries. Lack of intensive care unit beds was another hurdle, although this deficit improved

as the program advanced. It was obvious to LATIN sites that with our rapid STEMI intervention, the need for intensive beds decreases. Public awareness was advanced in both countries.

Rajasthan Heart Attack Treatment

This telemedicine-centered, population-based STEMI program covers approximately 65 million patients of India's most populous state. It covers the size of Finland and the population of France.

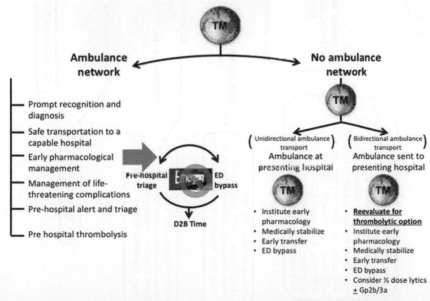

Fig. 9. Telemedicine ambulance management.

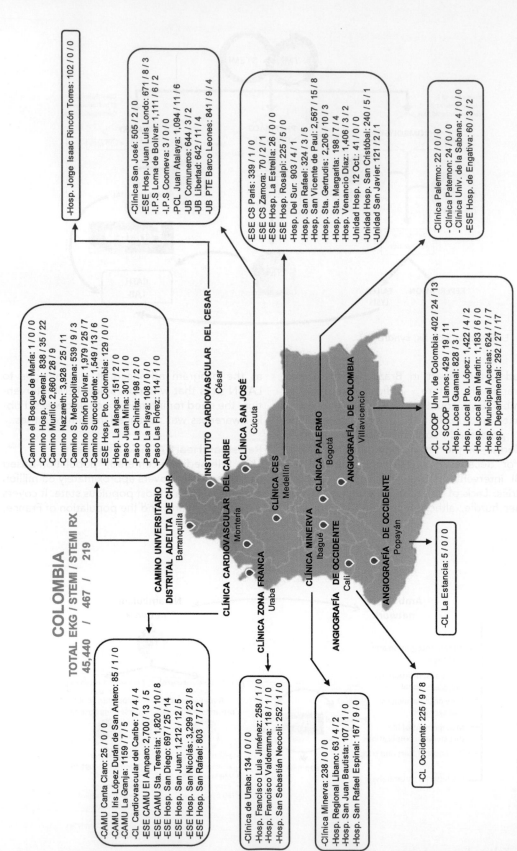

COLOMBIA

TOTAL EKG / STEMI / STEMI RX

45,440 / 467 / 219

-Hosp. Jorge Isaac Rincón Torres: 102 / 0 / 0

-Clínica San José: 505 / 2 / 0
-ESE Hosp. Juan Luis Londo: 671 / 8 / 3
-I.P.S Loma de Bolívar: 1,111 / 6 / 2
-I.P.S Coomeva: 3 / 0 / 0
-PCL Juan Atalaya: 1,094 / 11 / 6
-UB Comuneros: 644 / 3 / 2
-UB Libertad: 642 / 11 / 4
-UB PTE Barco Leones: 841 / 9 / 4

INSTITUTO CARDIOVASCULAR DEL CESAR
César

-ESE CS París: 339 / 1 / 0
-ESE CS Zamora: 70 / 2 / 1
-ESE Hosp. La Estrella: 26 / 0 / 0
-ESE Hosp. Rosalpi: 225 / 5 / 0
-Hosp. Del Sur: 903 / 4 / 1
-Hosp. San Rafael: 324 / 3 / 5
-Hosp. San Vicente de Paul: 2,567 / 15 / 8
-Hosp. Sta. Gertrudis: 2,206 / 10 / 3
-Hosp. Sta. Margarita: 198 / 7 / 4
-Hosp. Venancio Díaz: 1,406 / 3 / 2
-Unidad Hosp. 12 Oct.: 41 / 0 / 0
-Unidad Hosp. San Cristóbal: 240 / 5 / 1
-Unidad San Javier: 121 / 2 / 1

-Clínica Palermo: 22 / 0 / 0
- Clínica Patemon: 24 / 0 / 0
- Clínica Univ. de la Sabana: 4 / 0 / 0
-ESE Hosp. de Engativa: 60 / 3 / 2

-Camino el Bosque de María: 1 / 0 / 0
-Camino Hosp. General: 838 / 35 / 22
-Camino Murillo: 2,660 / 26 / 9
-Camino Nazareth: 3,928 / 25 / 11
-Camino S. Metropolitana: 539 / 9 / 3
-Camino Simón Bolívar: 1,979 / 25 / 7
-Camino Suroccidente: 1,549 / 13 / 6
-ESE Hosp. Pto. Colombia: 129 / 0 / 0
-Hosp. La Manga: 151 / 2 / 0
-Paso Juan Mina: 301 / 1 / 0
-Paso La Chinita: 198 / 2 / 0
-Paso La Playa: 108 / 0 / 0
-Paso Las Flórez: 114 / 1 / 0

CAMINO UNIVERSITARIO DISTRITAL ADELITA DE CHAR
Barranquilla

CLÍNICA CARDIOVASCULAR DEL CARIBE
Montería

CLÍNICA SAN JOSÉ
Cúcuta

CLÍNICA CES
Medellín

CLÍNICA PALERMO
Bogotá

ANGIOGRAFÍA DE COLOMBIA
Villavicencio

CLÍNICA ZONA FRANCA
Uraba

CLÍNICA MINERVA
Ibagué

ANGIOGRAFÍA DE OCCIDENTE
Cali

ANGIOGRAFÍA DE OCCIDENTE
Popayán

-CL COOP Univ. de Colombia: 402 / 24 / 13
-CL SCOOP Llanos: 429 / 19 / 11
-Hosp. Local Guamal: 828 / 3 / 1
-Hosp. Local Pto. López: 1,422 / 4 / 2
-Hosp. Local San Martin: 1,183 / 6 / 0
-Hosp. Municipal Acacias: 624 / 7 / 7
-Hosp. Departamental: 292 / 27 / 17

-CAMU Canta Claro: 25 / 0 / 0
-CAMU Iris López Durán de San Antero: 85 / 1 / 0
-CAMU La Granja: 1159 / 7 / 5
-CL Cardiovascular del Caribe: 7 / 4 / 4
-ESE CAMU El Amparo: 2,700 / 13 / 5
-ESE CAMU Sta. Teresita: 1,820 / 10 / 8
-ESE Hosp. San Diego: 697 / 25 / 14
-ESE Hosp. San Juan: 1,212 / 12 / 5
-ESE Hosp. San Nicolás: 3,299 / 23 / 8
-ESE Hosp. San Rafael: 803 / 7 / 2

-Clínica de Uraba: 134 / 0 / 0
-Hosp. Francisco Luis Jiménez: 258 / 1 / 0
-Hosp. Francisco Valderrama: 118 / 1 / 0
-Hosp. San Sebastián Necocli: 252 / 1 / 0

-Clínica Minerva: 238 / 0 / 0
-Hosp. Regional Libano: 63 / 4 / 2
-Hosp. San Juan Bautista: 107 / 1 / 0
-Hosp. San Rafael Espinal: 167 / 9 / 0

-CL La Estancia: 5 / 0 / 0

-CL Occidente: 225 / 9 / 8

Fig. 10. LATIN: Colombia telemedicine structure.

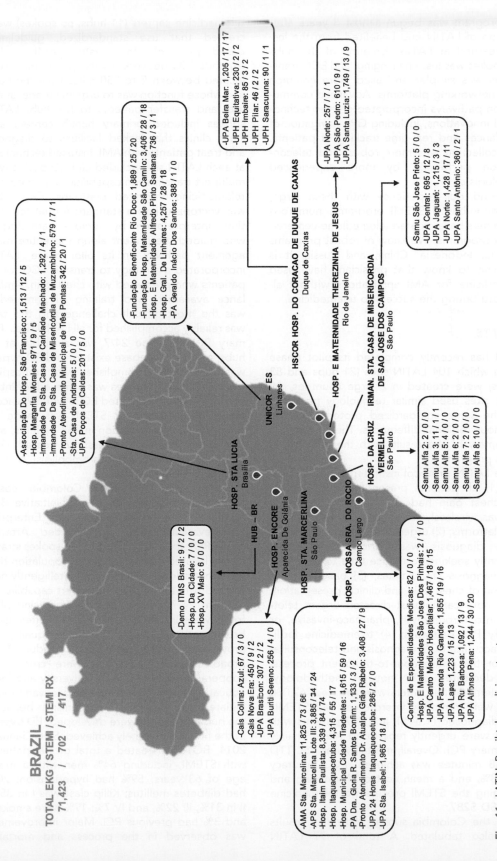

BRAZIL

TOTAL EKG / STEMI / STEMI RX

71,423 / 702 / 417

-Associação Do Hosp. São Francisco: 1,513 / 12 / 5
-Hosp. Margarita Morales: 971 / 9 / 5
-Irmandade Da Sta. Casa de Caridade Machado: 1,292 / 4 / 1
-Irmandade Da Sta. Casa de Misericórdia de Muzambinho: 579 / 7 / 1
-Pronto Atendimento Municipal de Três Pontas: 342 / 20 / 1
-Sta. Casa de Andradas: 5 / 0 / 0
-UPA Poços de Caldas: 201 / 5 / 0

-Fundação Beneficente Rio Doce: 1,889 / 25 / 20
-Fundação Hosp. Maternidade São Camilo: 3,406 / 28 / 18
-Hosp. E Maternidade Alfredo Pinto Santana: 736 / 3 / 1
-Hosp. Gral. De Linhares: 4,257 / 28 / 18
-PA Geraldo Inácio Dos Santos: 388 / 1 / 0

-UPA Beira Mar: 1,205 / 17 / 17
-UPH Equitativa: 230 / 2 / 2
-UPH Imbaíre: 85 / 3 / 2
-UPH Pilar: 46 / 2 / 2
-UPH Saracununa: 90 / 1 / 1

-UPA Norte: 257 / 7 / 1
-UPA São Pedro: 610 / 9 / 1
-UPA Santa Luzia: 1,749 / 13 / 9

-Samu São Jose Prieto: 5 / 0 / 0
-UPA Central: 695 / 12 / 8
-UPA Jaguaré: 1,215 / 3 / 3
-UPA Norte: 1,428 / 17 / 11
-UPA Santo Antônio: 360 / 2 / 1

HSCOR HOSP. DO CORAÇÃO DE DUQUE DE CAXIAS
Duque de Caxias

HOSP. E MATERNIDADE THEREZINHA DE JESUS
Rio de Janeiro

IRMAN. STA. CASA DE MISERICÓRDIA DE SAO JOSE DOS CAMPOS
São Paulo

UNICOR – ES
Linhares

HOSP. STA LUCIA
Brasília

HOSP. DA CRUZ VERMELHA
São Paulo

-Samu Alfa 2: 2 / 0 / 0
-Samu Alfa 3: 11 / 1 / 1
-Samu Alfa 5: 4 / 0 / 0
-Samu Alfa 6: 2 / 0 / 0
-Samu Alfa 7: 2 / 0 / 0
-Samu Alfa 8: 10 / 0 / 0

HUB – BR

HOSP. ENCORE
Aparecida De Goiânia

HOSP. STA. MARCELINA
São Paulo

HOSP. NOSSA SRA. DO ROCIO
Campo Largo

-Demo ITMS Brasil: 9 / 2 / 2
-Hosp. Da Cidade: 7 / 0 / 0
-Hosp. XV Maio: 6 / 0 / 0

-Cais Colíria: Azul: 67 / 3 / 0
-Cais Nova Era: 450 / 9 / 2
-UPA BrasiEcon: 307 / 2 / 2
-UPA Buriti Sereno: 256 / 4 / 0

-AMA Sta. Marcelina: 11,825 / 73 / 66
-APS Sta. Marcelina Lote III: 3,885 / 34 / 24
-Hosp. Itaim Paulista: 8,339 / 84 / 74
-Hosp. Itaquaquecetuba: 4,315 / 55 / 17
-Hosp. Municipal Cidade Tiradentes: 4,615 / 59 / 16
-PA Dra. Glória R. Santos Bonfim: 1,133 / 3 / 2
-Pronto Atendimento Dr. Atualpa Girão Rabelo: 3,408 / 27 / 9
-UPA 24 Horas Itaquaquecetuba: 286 / 2 / 0
-UPA Sta. Isabel: 1,965 / 18 / 1

-Centro de Especialidades Medicas: 82 / 0 / 0
-Hosp. E Matemidades São Jose Dos Pinhais: 2 / 1 / 0
-UPA Centro Medico Hospitalar: 1,467 / 18 / 15
-UPA Fazenda Rio Grande: 1,855 / 19 / 16
-UPA Lapa: 1,223 / 15 / 13
-UPA Ru Barbosa: 1,092 / 13 / 9
-UPA Alfonso Pena: 1,244 / 30 / 20

Fig. 11. LATIN: Brazil telemedicine structure.

This program was begun almost 3 years after initiation of LATIN and benefited from the lessons learned at LATIN. Creation of the hubs and spokes was less challenging, and ECG transmission was simpler and used more common social-networking platforms. Advanced communication pathways incorporated greater technological innovations, including GPS navigation of ambulances and real-time tracking of patients. Data collection was more robust and teleconsultation performed by more experienced cardiologists.

Beyond our experience with these large, population-based STEMI programs, numerous researchers have created telemedicine-centered STEMI programs. We know of robust programs in India, Indonesia, China, and Russia. It is intriguing to know that physicians have used telemedicine for AMI applications without always attributing the success to telemedicine.

RESULTS

LATIN has recently completed its pilot phase during which 104 LATIN sites (21 hubs and 83 spokes) were created in 2 large countries. All LATIN sites used similar technology platforms and the same standardized protocol despite enormous regional differences. The following is a summary of the results with the pilot phase of this program.

The LATIN protocol instituted a 4-part strategy: (1) all patients presenting to the spoke with chest pain had an urgent 12-lead ECG that was wirelessly transmitted using telemedicine platforms; (2) urgent, cost-effective, and accurate diagnosis was performed remotely, constantly seeking to reduce time to telemedicine diagnosis (TTD) times; (3) based on the duration of chest pain and clinical presentation, the remote cardiologist directed urgent teletriage into thrombolysis, pharmaco-invasive, or primary PCI pathways; (4) telemedicine facilitated accurate ECG diagnosis and teleconsultation for the entire door-to-treatment process. Using dedicated LATIN network methodology, 104 telemedicine centers were created, 62,000 ECGs were remotely interpreted, 642 STEMIs were diagnosed (1.04%), and 297 patients with STEMI were urgently reperfused (46%), mainly by primary PCI. Overall, mortality was 8%. TTD of 5.58 minutes was achieved. ECG accuracy was 98%, and a mean cost of diagnosing and managing the STEMI process via telemedicine was USD $287.

For the Colombia subset, individual results were also tabulated. A total of 77 LATIN telemedicine centers (11 hubs, 66 spokes) were created that use standardized, guidelines-based protocols for treating AMI. LATIN expanded its network via its spokes that were located between 5 to 250 miles from the hubs and whose function was to urgently triage, stabilize, and transfer patients to the hub. LATIN spokes included primary health centers and small clinics that lacked facilities to diagnose and treat patients with AMI. Installed technology at each LATIN site included an ECG device with multiport transmission capabilities and patented telemedicine-integrated platforms. Each ECG was vectorized into a standard format for real-time interpretation by remote cardiologists who guided the patient along the entire management pathway. In its pilot phase, LATIN incorporated a strategy to transmit ECG for all patients who presented with chest pain. Ambulance availability and training of paramedics was the most difficult challenge and this task was reliably accomplished for all LATIN sites. Primary PCI coverage 24/7 was available at all hubs, a robust database existed, and ED bypass was successfully accomplished with prehospital alert. TTD of 5.7 minutes was achieved for interpreting 47,000 transmitted ECGs with 99% accuracy. The diagnosis of STEMI was made by remote ECG interpretation in 467 patients, and 219 patients were successfully treated (215 PCI/pharmaco-invasive, 4 thrombolysis). Mortality data are being collected.

Barranquilla, the large Colombia costal town, had a regional LATIN-based initiative: Barranquilla Operational Telemedicine Enterprise for Revascularization of Occluded Arteries (BOTERO). It collected data for 11 spokes strategically located in areas of dense population that were meticulously selected and intelligently networked with a hub that had expert capability to perform 24/7 primary PCI. Telemedicine platforms were installed at all BOTERO sites using broadband technology. Continuous quality improvements were implemented to reduce TTD. Broad education initiatives were created in cooperation with Antioquia University and local educational societies. Single call activation was initiated and feedback mechanisms between the hub and spokes were developed. ED bypass at the hub was routinely achieved. Since January 2014, BOTERO treated a total of 100 patients with STEMI, including 64% men with a mean age of 63 years; 59% had hypertension; 20% had diabetes mellitus; Killip class was I in 35%, II in 31%, III 22%, and IV 7%; 19% were smokers and 3% had previous PCI. Major improvement was observed in the process and mortality parameters between 2014 and 2015. Time to first medical contact (FMC) was reduced from 247 to 207 minutes (*P*<.4) and symptom to balloon times (S2B) from 384 to 167 minutes (*P*<.0001). TTD was 5.9 minutes for the entire cohort and 98% accuracy of diagnosis was achieved. Thirty-day mortality was reduced from 11.1% to 3.2%.

Extremely encouraging results were also noted in Hospital Santa Marcelina in Sao Paulo, Brazil, which caters to the poorest population of Brazil and it demonstrated a 50% reduction in mortality after completion of the pilot phase of LATIN.

DISCUSSION

The gains of primary PCI must be provided to patients in developing countries. The disparities in STEMI care are overwhelming and inversely correlated with GDP, particularly in poorer countries of Africa, Asia, and South America. These suffocating limitations will require considerable time to resolve. Capital infusion, human resources development, and structural improvements will be necessary before primary PCI can be made available to the millions vulnerable to AMI. During this phase, thrombolytic therapy will remain the dominant modality. However, often the administration of this therapy is constrained by the same financial infrastructure limitations that prevent primary PCI. The narrow therapeutic window for thrombolysis is another challenge. A lack of patient awareness remains a major deterrent for both thrombolysis and primary PCI. With uneducated patients and a shortage of trained experts and facilities, it is unrealistic to expect patients in poorer countries to provide thrombolytic therapy in the very short 3-hour treatment opportunity. Poor countries, therefore, face a double dilemma: primary PCI is simply lacking and thrombolytic therapy is often delayed. Therefore, as noted previously, many patients with STEMI do not receive reperfusion therapy at all.

In the presence of these pervasive challenges, telemedicine provides a desirable modality. It increases access for millions of patients to STEMI management, as demonstrated in LATIN.[17,18] The advantages of telemedicine also have been observed by numerous other telemedicine networks[19,20,23–25,28] that report the feasibility of treating large populations with telemedicine. A report by Matsuda and colleagues[28] shows that the LATIN protocol can be applied for developing countries to improve access to PCI. A single hub with multiple spokes between 7.6 miles

of distance (±1.5 miles) in the east side of Sao Paulo reported that in 34 patients with STEMI, 91.1% received primary PCI and 2.8% received pharmaco-invasive treatment, with a mean spoke-to-hub time of 188 minutes and a mean D2B time of 40 minutes (±18.7 minutes). Applications of telemedicine were also demonstrated in Quebec, Canada. Between 2006 and 2012, in Chaudière-Appalaches, Tanguay and colleagues,[23] implemented a telemedicine platform to improve patient care in the prehospital setting. The 208 patients in the study were divided into 3 groups: patients on the way toward a PCI center when STEMI was diagnosed, patients initially directed to the nearest hospital and subsequently rerouted to a PCI center after STEMI diagnosis, and patients directed to a local hospital without transfer for PCI. Measure of different time intervals was done, showing a reduced time from positive ECG to hospital arrival among patients of the first group (18 minutes), compared with those of the second group (29 minutes), *P*<.001. Another prehospital ECG network in Apula, Italy, created by Brunetti and his group of investigators,[25] reported the data from the 594,140 ECGs interpreted over 9 years. Fifteen percent of patients with chest pain were abnormal, 6178 had ST elevation, and 40,106 patients had other ECG abnormalities, allowing direct access to catheterization laboratory or hospitalization for these patients.

A further demonstration of access of patients to AMI care was revealed in work done by Rasmussen and his researchers,[24] which reported 81% of the study population was able to be treated in less than 120 minutes, even to longest distance of greater than 95 km; 89% of the patients were treated before that time frame.

Another study to assess the importance of prehospital diagnosis of STEMI was conducted by Sørensen and colleagues[20] in Denmark. This group took into consideration whether the patient was from a rural or urban community. In 759 patients, the proportion of patients able to achieve less than 120 minutes D2B time was 86% with prehospital diagnosis, compared with 32% in patients without it (*P*<.001). In a median of 4.3 years' follow-up, all-cause mortality was 18% in patients with prehospital diagnosis compared with 31% in patients without it (*P* = .003).

The use of telemedicine for prehospital ECG diagnosis may reduce treatment time regardless of whether thrombolysis or primary PCI is required. Rapid ECG availability can shorten D2B time from 20 to 81 minutes.[29] Sanchez-Ross and colleagues[26] compared 92 patients with prehospital ST elevation using a wireless network versus 50 who used alternative methods and reported shorter D2B time (63 minutes in the wireless network vs 119 minutes in control, $P<.00004$), lower peak troponin (39.5 ng/mL vs 87.6 ng/mL, $P = .005$), higher left ventricular ejection fractions (50% vs 35%, $P = .004$) and shorter length of hospitalization (3.0 days vs 5.5 days, $P<.001$).

Dallan and colleagues[21] conducted a study between 2013 and 2014 comparing the number of patients treated before and after the implementation of the LATIN protocol, using telemedicine to transmit the ECG directly from remote hospital to referral centers with cardiologists available 24/7 so as to make the correct diagnosis, and allowing patients with STEMI to go straight to the catheterization laboratory, bypassing the ED. The authors reported the D2B time using the LATIN protocol was 32 minutes compared with 85 minutes using the previous protocol ($P<.05$). Furthermore, the volume of patients increased from 25 patients in 9 months to 25 patients in only 3 months with the application of LATIN protocol.

Cost-effectiveness has also been extensively researched. Yoculan and colleagues[22] determined that in a possible scenario in which the rate of performed PCI increases from 19% to 60%, the savings could be $13 million, related to the decrease in indirect cost of mortality, disabilities, and pharmacologic treatment. In Italy, Brunetti and colleagues[27] demonstrated the savings per ECG was from €8.10 to €38.41, and 69 lives per year were saved with a cost per quality-adjusted life year gained of €1927.

In our assessment, telemedicine is a promising modality that can increase access, augment accuracy, and provide a comprehensive management strategy while being cost-effective. Several of these programs are pilot studies and have incorporated first-generation telemedicine technology. These innovations will clearly improve and the economies of scale will lower the cost of telemedicine applications. Simplification of the protocols will also occur. Our LATIN protocol, although innovative in acquiring ECGs at small, remotely located clinics, is not cost-effective for routine ECGs. The newer protocols mandate presence of ECG and at least 2 risk factors before transmitting ECGs. Ambulance availability and trained paramedics remain the Achilles heel in resource-constrained, poorer countries. Improving ambulance availability and structure is critical, and barriers such as insurance denials will fall as the benefits of primary PCI become evident.

REFERENCES

1. Antman EM, Anbe DT, Armstrong PW, et al. ACC/AHA guidelines for the management of patients with ST-elevation myocardial infarction—Executive summary: a report of the American College of Cardiology/American Heart Association Task Force on Practice Guidelines (Writing Committee to Revise the 1999; Guidelines for the Management of Patients with Acute Myocardial Infarction). Circulation 2004;110:588–636.

2. Antman EM, Hand M, Armstrong PW, et al. Focused update of the ACC/AHA 2004 guidelines for the management of patients with ST-elevation myocardial infarction: a report of the American College of Cardiology/American Heart Association Task Force on Practice Guidelines. Circulation 2008;117:296–329.

3. Bhatt D. Timely PCI for STEMI—Still the treatment of choice. N Engl J Med 2013;368:1442–7.

4. Henry TD, Atkins JM, Cunningham MS, et al. ST elevation myocardial infarction: recommendations on triage of patients to cardiovascular centers of excellence. J Am Coll Cardiol 2006;47:1339–45.

5. Le May MR, Davies RF, Labinaz M. Hospitalization costs of primary stenting versus thrombolysis in acute myocardial infarction: cost analysis of the Canadian STAT Study. Circulation 2003;108:2624–30.

6. Mehta S, Kostela JC, Oliveros E, et al. Global acute myocardial infarction perspectives: beyond door-to-balloon interventions. Interv Cardiol Clin 2012;1(4):479–84.

7. Le May MR, So DY, Dionne R, et al. A citywide protocol for primary PCI in ST-segment elevation myocardial infarction. N Engl J Med 2008;358(3):231–40.

8. Schoos MM, Sejersten M, Hvelplund A, et al. Reperfusion delay in patients treated with primary percutaneous coronary intervention: insight from a real world Danish ST-segment elevation myocardial infarction population in the era of telemedicine. Eur Heart J Acute Cardiovasc Care 2012;1(3):200–9.

9. Morrison LJ, Verbeek PR, McDonald AC, et al. Mortality and pre-hospital thrombolysis for acute myocardial infarction: a meta-analysis. JAMA 2000;283:2686–92.

10. Ting HH, Rihal CS, Gersh BJ, et al. Regional systems of care to optimize timeliness of reperfusion therapy for ST-elevation myocardial infarction: The Mayo Clinic STEMI protocol. Circulation 2007;116:729–36.

11. Terkelsen CJ, Lassen JF, Nørgaard BL, et al. Reduction of treatment delay in patients with ST-elevation myocardial infarction: impact of pre-hospital diagnosis and direct referral to primary percutaneous coronary intervention. Eur Heart J 2005;26:770–7.

12. Rokos IC, Larson DM, Henry TD, et al. Rationale for establishing regional ST-elevation myocardial infarction receiving center (SRC) networks. Am Heart J 2006;152(4):661–7.

13. Brown JP, Mahmud E, Dunford JV, et al. Effect of pre hospital 12-lead electrocardiogram on activation of the cardiac catheterization laboratory and door-to-balloon time in ST-segment elevation acute myocardial infarction. Am J Cardiol 2008;101:158–61.

14. Steg PG, Cambou JP, Goldstein P, et al. Bypassing the emergency room reduces delays and mortality in ST elevation myocardial infarction: the USIC 2000 registry. Heart 2006;92:1378–83.

15. Amit G, Cafri C, Gilutz H, et al. Benefit of direct ambulance to coronary care unit admission of acute myocardial infarction patients undergoing primary percutaneous intervention. Int J Cardiol 2007;119:355–8.

16. Mumma BE, Kontos MC, Peng SA, et al. Association between pre hospital electrocardiogram use and patient home distance from the percutaneous coronary intervention center on total reperfusion time in ST-segment-elevation myocardial infarction patients: a retrospective analysis from the National Cardiovascular Data Registry. Am Heart J 2014;167(6):915–20.

17. Mehta S, Botelho R, Rodriguez D, et al. A tale of two cities: STEMI interventions in developed and developing countries and the potential of telemedicine to reduce disparities in care. J Interv Cardiol 2014;27(2):155–66.

18. Mehta S, Reynbakh O, Kostela JC, et al. Building population-based AMI management systems using telemedicine as a foundation pillar. Eur Heart J 2014;35:1172.

19. Clemmensen P, Schoos MM, Lindholm MG, et al. Pre-hospital diagnosis and transfer of patients with acute myocardial infarction—a decade long experience from one of Europe's largest STEMI networks. J Electrocardiol 2013;46(6):546–52.

20. Sørensen JT, Terkelsen CJ, Nørgaard BL, et al. Urban and rural implementation of pre-hospital diagnosis and direct referral for primary percutaneous coronary intervention in patients with acute ST-elevation myocardial infarction. Eur Heart J 2011;32(4):430–6.

21. Dallan L, Pazolini V, Matsuda C, et al. CRT-124 Telemedicine as a landmark in the reduction of the door-to-balloon time in STEMIs in distant areas in a developing country. J Am Coll Cardiol Intv 2015;8(2_S):S15.

22. Yoculan A, Kim E, Eggington S, et al. Economic value of STEMI program investment in Sao Paulo, Brazil. Value Health 2015;18(7):A861.

23. Tanguay A, Dallaire R, Hébert D, et al. Rural patient access to primary percutaneous coronary intervention centers is improved by a novel integrated telemedicine prehospital system. J Emerg Med 2015;49(5):657–64.

24. Rasmussen MB, Frost L, Stengaard C, et al. Diagnostic performance and system delay using telemedicine for prehospital diagnosis in triaging and treatment of STEMI. Heart 2014;100(9):711–5.

25. Brunetti ND, De gennaro L, Dellegrottaglie G, et al. All for one, one for all: remote telemedicine hub pre-hospital triage for public Emergency Medical Service 1-1-8 in a regional network for primary PCI in Apulia, Italy. Eur Res Telemed 2014;3(1):9–15.

26. Sanchez-Ross M, Oghlakian G, Maher J, et al. The STAT-MI (ST-Segment Analysis Using Wireless Technology in Acute Myocardial Infarction) trial improves outcomes. JACC Cardiovasc Interv 2011;4(2):222–7.

27. Brunetti ND, Dellegrottaglie G, Lopriore C. Prehospital telemedicine electrocardiogram triage for a regional public emergency medical service: is it worth it? A preliminary cost analysis. Clin Cardiol 2014;37(3):140–5.

28. Matsuda C, Cade J, Janella B, et al. Implementação do Sistema de Telemedicina no Atendimento Inicial dos Pacientes com Infarto Agudo do Miocárdio com Supradesnivelamento do Segmento ST na Zona Leste da Cidade de São Paulo. Paper presented at: 40th Congress of the Brazilian Society of Hemodynamics and Interventional Cardiology. Brasilia, Brazil, June 26, 2015.

29. Clemmensen P, Loumann-Nielsen S, Sejersten M. Telemedicine fighting acute coronary syndromes. J Electrocardiol 2010;43(6):615–8.

Moving?

Make sure your subscription moves with you!

To notify us of your new address, find your **Clinics Account Number** (located on your mailing label above your name), and contact customer service at:

Email: journalscustomerservice-usa@elsevier.com

800-654-2452 (subscribers in the U.S. & Canada)
314-447-8871 (subscribers outside of the U.S. & Canada)

Fax number: 314-447-8029

Elsevier Health Sciences Division
Subscription Customer Service
3251 Riverport Lane
Maryland Heights, MO 63043

*To ensure uninterrupted delivery of your subscription, please notify us at least 4 weeks in advance of move.

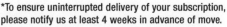